Derrik Mercer is a former managing editor of the *Sunday Times* and Editor of ITN's Channel 4 News. He co-edited the bestselling *Sunday Times Book of Body Maintenance* and *The Book of the Countryside*. Gillian Mercer is a freelance journalist who has contributed . to *Good Housekeeping* and *Mother* magazines.

They currently live in London, with their twin sons, aged 11.

DERRIK AND GILLIAN MERCER

Children
First and Always

A portrait of Great Ormond Street

Futura

Photographs by Peter Pugh-Cook

A Futura Book

Copyright © Derrik and Gillian Mercer 1986

First published in Great Britain in 1986
by Macdonald & Co (Publishers) Ltd
London & Sydney

This edition published in 1987
by Futura Publications, a Division of
Macdonald & Co (Publishers) Ltd

ISBN 0 7088 3445 0

Reproduced, printed and bound in Great Britain by
Hazell Watson & Viney Limited,
Member of the BPCC Group,
Aylesbury, Bucks

Futura Publications
A Division of
Macdonald & Co (Publishers) Ltd
Greater London House
Hampstead Road
London NW1 7QX
A BPCC plc Company

Contents

Acknowledgements   6
Introduction — Christmas Day   9
Declan   26
Anna   69
Polly   121
Robert   155
Gus and Lewis   206
Casualty   251
Stacey   264
Kristie   302
Appendix 1   334
Appendix 2   336

Acknowledgements

Many people have helped to make this book possible – too many to be thanked by name. Our foremost debt, as we acknowledge in the Introduction to this book, is to the parents of the children who are featured in *Children First and Always*. Without their permission – and their willingness to talk so frankly about their experiences – the concept of the book as an authentic portrait of Great Ormond Street would have been impossible. We are grateful also to the many other families who talked to us while their children were in hospital; their children are not named in the book but it was through such conversations that we began to gain some understanding of life inside Great Ormond Street. We thank, too, those parents who gave permission for us to attend out-patient clinics while their children were being examined. We are sorry that we were unable to mention all their children; it was hard to omit any child, but ultimately the need for a balance of ages and conditions meant that some children had to be excluded.

The second broad category of people whose help we must acknowledge are the staff of the hospital. We spent virtually a year in their company and we will be forever grateful for the courtesy with which we were received and the patience with which busy people sought to explain complicated conditions to two non-medical and non-scientific minds. When we and the publisher approached the hospital authorities for permission to write this book we suggested that the facts be checked for accuracy by appropriate members of the staff. We did so because in simplifying complex medical procedures for a non-specialist audience it is all too easy to make inadvertent errors. We are grateful to the many people who meticulously checked our text and also for the acceptance that, apart from questions of fact or accuracy, the hospital had no right to interfere with what we wrote.

Children First and Always is an officially-authorized portrait of Great Ormond Street in the sense that we were invited to observe a year in its distinguished life. It could not have been done otherwise and the hospital, quite rightly, will share the profits from each book that is sold. But it is an independent account: although there was close consultation, the selection of case studies and the opinions expressed are our responsibility alone.

Mostly, though, this is not a book of opinions – it is a book through which hospital staff and, above all, parents describe what happened to a cross-section of children. We have tried to make it an honest account which is why we wanted to use real names throughout. Once you introduce false names or backgrounds into a narrative, readers can be forgiven for wondering where falsehood ends and truth begins. These are real lives as experienced by real people. The overwhelming majority of the hospital staff accepted this proposition and most welcomed it. In the Department of Psychological Medicine it posed difficulties because it was felt that identifying patients might affect their subsequent recovery. This we accepted totally because at no point have we wanted to do anything which jeopardizes a child's recovery; as the title says, it must be *Children First and Always*. However, it means that the large and important psychological department is under-represented in this book.

A few other departments of the hospital have also been treated somewhat cursorily in order to keep the focus of the book firmly on the children and their families. The administrative, financial, personnel and maintenance problems of running such a large institution are incidental to this account but, of course, crucial to its day-to-day management. We regret that for reasons of space it has been impossible to do more about the research activities of the Institute of Child Health or to describe some of the smaller units, such as the Wolfson Assessment Centre for handicapped children. We have also referred only briefly to the sister hospital in the group, the Queen Elizabeth Hospital for Children, but we were grateful for the friendliness with which we were received while researching the 'Casualty' chapter.

Having said at the outset that there were too many people to be thanked by name, we will now proceed to identify a few. Penny Uprichard, the hospital's public relations officer, helped us to fix hundreds of appointments, guided us through the bureaucracy and allowed us to share her office (and coffee) for the best part of the year. Betty Barchard, the chief nursing officer, nobly volunteered to read every chapter in draft form and her comments were always constructive and encouraging. But we hope that their colleagues – from the most senior consultants to the librarians in the nursing school library, from all the ward sisters to the porters – will accept that our gratitude to them is no less genuine for remaining anonymous. Finally, there is our publisher Susan Fletcher, whose original idea it was, and Richard Simon and Vivien Green, our agents; to them we are grateful for what has been the most rewarding professional experience of our lives.

DM and GM, April 1986.

The stories of the children featured in this book are all true; their real names are used with their parents' agreement and the medical facts have been checked by the staff of Great Ormond Street responsible for their care. This does not mean that another child with a similar or even identical condition would necessarily be treated in the same way as described in these pages. Each child is an individual and treatment is tailored to the condition of each particular one. Age and weight, for instance, are factors which will frequently influence the nature and course of treatment. For many of the rare conditions treated at Great Ormond Street (some of which are represented in this book) treatment is also continually evolving. Parents whose children are admitted to the hospital in the future therefore should not expect treatment automatically to follow the same courses as described in *Children First and Always*; they can expect their children to receive the very best treatment that is currently available.

Introduction
– Christmas Day

On this Christmas Day there were 113 patients in the Hospital for Sick Children as it is formally known, or Great Ormond Street as it is popularly known throughout the country and, indeed, much of the world. It is not the oldest children's hospital in the world, or even in Europe, but it is among the most renowned. Doctors come here from countries as advanced as the United States to be trained, children from Russia (and elsewhere) to be cured.

Not every child who comes to Great Ormond Street will be cured. It is a hospital for critically ill children, often suffering from rare conditions which are invariably serious and occasionally incurable. That is why, despite the best efforts to let children go home for Christmas, one-third of its beds are still full. Its doctors frequently say: 'We're the end of the line – there's nowhere else for people to go.' The hospital is therefore a place of tension, even at Christmas, since children would not be here if they were not seriously ill. And yet, overwhelmingly, it is a place of hope. Here parents are given hope and, far more often than not, most are also given the life of their child. Many conditions which just a few years ago would have crippled or killed are now being conquered; others, for which there is still no certain cure, are having their most corrosive and life-sapping effects diminished or at least delayed.

Great Ormond Street lives at the frontiers of medicine. Many doctors work jointly for the hospital and the adjoining Institute of Child Health, part of the University of London, where pioneering research is undertaken. The links between research and clinical practice have never been closer: yesterday's laboratory research is today's ward routine. Such is the pace of change that some of the children whose lives we follow in this book benefited from treatment developed here which would not have been available even a few months, let alone a few years, earlier. Other children's hospitals boast spheres of excellence, but what puts Great Ormond Street amongst the world's leading paediatric centres are not only the results produced by individual departments but the fact that such a wide range of specialist teams exist on one site. Many of the doctors are acknowledged world authorities in their areas of medicine and Great Ormond Street is thus a magnet for paediatricians from all over the world.

It was at first sight an unlikely Mecca that Father Christmas saw before him as his sledge was hauled up the driveway. Admittedly, it was a filthy day with dark grey clouds and torrential rain. Yet his view of the hospital would not have been so very different to that of parents arriving here for the first time. At 49 Great Ormond Street Dr Charles West opened a Hospital for Sick Children on 14 February 1852. Since then the hospital has grown from a single house to a sprawling site squeezed between three roads in Bloomsbury in central London. Entering the main driveway, which is usually cluttered with cars, there is a black building on the left which has clearly known better days. If you called it Dickensian, you would not be far wrong: it was erected in two stages during the Victorian era and for over half a century it was the hospital itself. At <u>one</u> point the unmistakable shape and style of the chapel juts out from this old hospital building. On the right of the drive are more modern buildings erected in the 1950s which house the out-patients' department. Straight ahead is what is now the main hospital block, completed in 1938 and housing 333 beds spread over seven floors. Two wings of the building form a courtyard around and above the main entrance and, as Father Christmas arrived, the balconies of the upper floors were filled with children and parents awaiting his arrival. The balconies enable the children to get some fresh air but, for obvious reasons of safety, the patients have to be protected; blue mesh grilles therefore envelop the balconies giving the children an inevitable if unfortunate air of imprisonment.

On Christmas Day, the faces peering through the wire mesh were smiling and happy. There is generally more laughter than tears here. Perhaps ignorance is comforting; children can play happily, unaware of what awaits them. But they are in any case astonishingly resilient, recovering far more quickly after operations than adults and displaying a spirit which constantly amazes the most experienced of nurses. The excitement of Christmas is often mingled with poignancy as parents remember other Christmasses unsullied by illness or wonder what future years will bring. Some parents are happy to be celebrating a Christmas they thought their child might never see, others fear it may be their last. But most manage to subdue any doubts or anxieties and strive to make the most of Christmas, for all the children's sake. It's not for nothing that the hospital's motto (slightly amended in the title of this book) is 'The Child, First and Always'.

Father Christmas, in fact, was late. Malicious rumour had it that he was waiting for the rain to stop, although the children doubted that a burly man who lived beyond the Arctic Circle would be unduly daunted by a spot of rain. The delay only served to heighten the sense of anticipation among the children. The excitement had been fuelled for weeks as wards vied with each other to make *their* ward the most attractively decorated of all. Television and sports stars toured the hospital, dispensing gifts and autographs. So many cakes arrived that some were given away to other needy recipients. Gifts ranged from large sums donated by businessmen to 'a few peg dollies for the Christmas clinic', as one lady, over eighty, described her gift to play co-ordinator Gail Petersen; they were in fact beautifully hand-made. Presents piled up in a room awaiting selection by ward sisters and play staff, once they knew who would be in at Christmas.

Ward playleaders worked hard in the Christmas build-up. They helped nurses to decorate the wards, and children to make cards for their parents, nurses and doctors. Every child would have a present from Santa. These have to be chosen with care – not merely to be suitable for age and sex but also not so lavish that the child will fail to appreciate what Mum and Dad have given, and nothing edible which could interfere with special diets. Many of the wards and departments had parties in the days immediately preceding Christmas. So, too, did some out-patient clinics such as that for leukaemia where parents sipped wine in the play centre where a Wendy Corner was transformed into Santa's Grotto. As the countdown to Christmas progressed, children began to go home; every child who can conceivably go home will be there. Some will go home just for the day, if necessary with a nurse.

By Christmas Eve almost half the wards were closed. Some children were moved to other wards where nursing staff could be concentrated. Most ward sisters, though were working. Some staff, including nurses, would have to walk for thirty minutes or an hour to get into work because there was no public transport. They do so because Christmas in this hospital is special. 'I was off last year and I missed it terribly,' said one sister. But on Christmas Eve there is something of a lull with darkened wards and staff departing for their own family celebrations. More than usually, the hospital becomes an inward-looking world at Christmas with its own life and rhythms. The most visible presence now are parents. At any one time there are between 100-150 staying in or around the hospital and the empty wards make it easier to find room for the extra fathers who will be staying for Christmas.

Many parents were among the congregation for the Midnight Eucharist in the chapel. Some members of this congregation carried balloons, others had tinsel around their nursing caps. The organist practised feverishly if soundlessly during the spoken parts of the service – Martin Parrott, a male nurse, had been hauled off night duty to play the organ for the first time in years. At one point a bleep sounded; it was for Kim Cecil, the physiotherapist on duty that night. It was a relaxed occasion with the Reverend Derek Bacon, the hospital chaplain, wryly welcoming unfamiliar faces. The spirit of Christmas, he said, exists every day at Great Ormond Street through 'ordinary men and women who, in what they do for others, become ever so slightly extraordinary'. Derek Bacon is a man held in immense affection and respect by hospital staff, regardless of their religion or even their lack of it. A perhaps unorthodox priest who never pushes dogma, he offered a Christmas message to his colleagues which was candid as well as appreciative: 'In all the power-seeking and empire-building, the cynicism and manipulation, in all the politicking and career-making that is Great Ormond Street, the work of self-giving goes quietly and gloriously on.'

It did indeed. The children who stayed in hospital through Christmas were ill and many required one-to-one intensive nursing. Two children on 5A, the intensive care ward, were fighting for their lives. A child had just been admitted to another ward with leukaemia. There were children, some no more than a few days old, who were recovering from operations. There were children in isolation because they lacked the normal bodily defences against infection. There were children dependent on artificial ventilators to stay alive and many more receiving intravenous infusions of drugs, nutrition or blood. There were children being sick and others with diarrhoea. It was by no means an easy night for the staff; the battles to keep children alive and to make them better are unaffected by either calendars or clocks.

Hospital days always begin early, but on Christmas Day nobody complains. On ward 2C the first child was awake by five a.m. and by six-thirty all nine patients on the ward were rummaging through presents left for them in stockings attached to their cots or beds. Parents had set alarms early in their rooms so they could fill the stockings and see their child wake up. For them and for the nurses, as much as the children, it was a thrilling moment. What nurses liked best were patients between two and eight years old for whom belief in Father Christmas was as yet unsullied by doubts instilled by playground cynics. On 5C, the renal ward, only one patient out of seven fitted into this category and this four-year-old girl, according to Sister Maggie Randell, was 'being spoilt something rotten'.

Other wards had only babies yet even here extra efforts were made. On 6A, the neonatal surgical intensive care ward, the babies had special stockings with soap and talc in them and in one cot a little woolly soft toy had been placed alongside a tiny, sleeping baby who was recovering from a major operation performed late on Christmas Eve. For wards such as 6A and Cohen, which also only had babies, the celebrations were restrained – simple drinks amongst staff and parents. There was nothing restrained about some of the other wards.

In the intensive cardiac ward, a post-operative recovery area is normally the apogee of high-tech medicine, crammed to bursting point with machines and monitors. On Christmas Day it was transformed with coloured drapes and a spread of fruit, cake and wine. As well as Father Christmas, the children were entertained by a parade of Wizard of Oz characters – staff in costume with Marc de Leval, the elegant and volatile Belgian heart surgeon, as the Tin Man and Sister Jane Jacob, a slight, dark and attractive Yorkshire girl, as Dorothy. Nursing staff in the oncology and leukaemia ward were also in fancy dress so that throughout the day children might be nursed by Andy Pandy or Danger Mouse, or a female nurse in top hat and tails, or a male nurse in a long evening gown. And on ward 2C Dave Albert, senior surgical registrar in the Ear, Nose and Throat Department, became a Dalek (courtesy of the BBC) and threatened to exterminate all and sundry with scant regard for his Hippocratic oath.

Most of the activity was confined to the morning. It was then that the bedraggled Father Christmas toured the hospital so fast that some swore there must be two of them. His helpers, ringing bells to announce his coming and rooting in the sack for presents, bore an uncanny resemblance to members of the theatre nursing staff but that was presumably an illusion induced by the magic of Christmas. In the morning, too, consultants arrived – often with their families – to visit wards rather more sedately than Santa. They talked to on-duty colleagues, nurses, parents and, of course, the children. In the neurosurgical ward surgeon Norman Grant, having exchanged his customary surgical gown and scalpel for chef's apron and carving knife, was in charge of the turkey; in the gastro-enterological ward, the wife of consultant Dr Peter Milla arrived with a turkey she had cooked at home. Everywhere small ward cookers were producing roast potatoes, sprouts and other vegetables. Wards without patients had been used as space for trestle tables which now carried cold buffets, usually prepared jointly by staff and parents. It was that sort of day because it is that sort of place: Great Ormond Street is not a hospital which stands on ceremony or formality and staff on most wards are on first-name terms with each other and parents.

One special lunch was being held in 1C, the neurology ward. Usually this closes at Christmas but this year it stayed open in honour of one patient – Christopher, a five-year-old who had spent virtually his entire life on the ward. This was to be his last Christmas here, for in the spring he would move to a residential unit in the Sussex countryside. Christopher was paralyzed and dependent upon a ventilator in order to breathe, but this did not dilute his pleasure. Nor that of the doctors, and nurses and other hospital staff who had shared so much of his life and who now shared his Christmas. The table was beautifully set with fourteen places and Christopher at the top, alongside Sister Celia Mostyn who probably knew him better than anyone.

Along the corridor in the neurosurgical ward, where Norman Grant was proving a predictably expert carver, an Indian family was experiencing a particularly joyous Christmas. Yaser, their ten-year-old son, was able to get up for the first time in ten days after his operation. He was also free of pain which had plagued him for years. Sister Lindy May wasn't sure whether or not Yaser's family – there were four other children as well as mother and father – would want to join in a traditional British-style Christmas, but they could not have been happier. True, they brought in some spices to enliven the turkey but what the family appreciated most was the atmosphere in which everyone – doctors, nurses and all the parents – joined in together. 'It has been a wonderful Christmas,' said Yaser's father. 'In fact, it will seem awfully dull next year at home.'

Some people, of course, were working. Not just the doctors and nurses, but catering staff who prepared a free turkey meal for staff and resident parents in the canteen, porters who manned the reception desk in the front hall and cleaners who ensured that intensive care wards, especially, and operating theatres remained scrupulously clean. Underneath the building a boilerman spent a lonely Christmas Day, as did Paul Turner, the telephone supervisor, who manned the hospital's antiquated switchboard for a double shift of fourteen hours. This act of martyrdom was somewhat true to form as the poor pay rates and unglamorous working conditions make it hard to attract telephonists. 'A couple of people popped down to say hello but the rest of the time I've been on my own. I got my Christmas dinner on a tray from the canteen, but it took me an hour and half to eat it. The type of calls I have been getting resemble a busy evening, fewer "business" calls and mainly people ringing in to enquire about the children. Most of them have been wishing me a Happy Christmas!' he said.

There were also laboratory technicians such as Bandula Chandraratna on duty. He volunteered to work as he is a Buddhist and he spent the day conducting various tests in the biochemistry lab. The haematology lab was also manned because there are always blood samples to be taken and tested. The life of the hospital changes on Christmas Day, but it does not stop. Chief dietitian Dorothy Francis was at her desk from eight a.m. as she has been for fifteen of the twenty-two years she has worked at Great Ormond Street. 'There has to be a senior dietitian on duty, someone who will be able to cope with any emergency that might arise. We have thirty-nine babies on special feeds today, three children who had a Christmas dinner which had to be sterilized and five other special diet Christmas meals. Normally about fifty per cent of the children who are left in the hospital at Christmas are on special feeds or diets,' she said.

Still, the day was not too busy – 'like a quiet Sunday' – which is just as well after two frantic days teaching mothers how to prepare special meals for children who were being allowed home. On Christmas Day itself two mothers rang in from home with queries: their children were ill and they wanted to know how to cope with their children's special diets. But there was time for Dorothy Francis to see each of the in-patients receiving special meals (and to give them a small present from her department) as well as organize special diets for children in a sister hospital in Hackney before joining Dr Peter Milla, the gastro-enterology consultant, Sister Patsy Stapleford and the staff of 2D for their Christmas dinner on the ward. She also made time for what has become one of her own Christmas traditions. 'One thing I always like to do on Christmas Day is to take my staff, who wash up, on average, 600 of the tiny bottles which are used in this hospital every day for babies' feeds, to the wards. Normally they don't get a chance to see the children, so I took them to 6A, the neonatal ward, and 4AB, the general surgical ward, so they could see why they have all those bottles to wash up every day!'

As the day progressed, it gradually quietened. Off-duty staff – including administrators headed by general manager Paul Cooper, as well as consultants – drifted home and Christmas became a more private occasion for the families. The hospital radio station shut down at four o'clock after six hours of special programmes and by evening many of the younger children were frankly exhausted. Older children watched television or played with brothers and sisters while their parents sat talking to each other, people who may have little in common with each other except that their children are sharing a common illness. But even that can be a comfort. Many parents with children at Great Ormond Street must grapple with illnesses of which they had never previously heard and which even their GPs have never encountered. In such circumstances it is reassuring to be cared for by specialist doctors and nursing staff, but often helpful to exchange experiences with other parents.

For many parents, Christmas had been a goal or target by when they would be home. Despite this, longer-term residents knew the staff well and made the most of Christmas in hospital, joining in the fun and savouring a rare moment of relaxation in what was probably the greatest crisis of their lives. Other parents found it difficult, even impossible, to enjoy anything about this Christmas. On the cancer and leukaemia ward, two families had seen their children admitted in the forty-eight hours before Christmas. Both families had been anticipating a normal Christmas at home; now, suddenly and traumatically, they found themselves in a ward with pale, bald children most of whom were trailed everywhere by intravenous 'drip' stands. The staff did their best to console the families and they were given greater privacy; some of the other parents also tried to rally their spirits, remembering how they had felt at the time of diagnosis. 'At the time you think you will never smile again,' said one father, 'but you gradually realize that some kind of life has to go on.'

On other wards, too, these private nightmares were endured

as parents reeled from the shock of finding themselves – or, what always seems worse to any parent, their child – in hospital. Three children were admitted as emergencies during Christmas Day, one of whom was just seven days old. The two children most critically ill in intensive care were still alive, but both would die in the next forty-eight hours. For their families, Christmas would never be the same again.

Yet for most parents thoughts of Christmas would soon turn to those about the New Year. What would it bring for them and their child? Would this be the year, for instance, when two-year-old Robert Payne finally came home from Great Ormond Street? He had spent most of his life in hospital after being born with a whole series of abnormalities. Anna Wells, not yet two, was also in hospital this Christmas; she was suffering from a rare form of cancer and her treatment was not going as smoothly as doctors had expected. Kristie McWilliam, just two months old, had become the youngest baby ever to have a bone marrow transplant at this hospital, but was it going to work? If not, she would inevitably die. We meet Robert, Anna and Kristie in the pages that follow. We share the drama as Gus and Lewis fight for life in intensive care; we reflect the struggles and setbacks of Stacey's twenty-eight operations; and we join Polly and Declan as they face critical heart and brain surgery which offers them their only chance of survival.

All these children are real children; their stories are true and real names are used throughout. Their stories need no pseudonyms as an excuse for fictional drama; there is nothing bogus about either the triumphs or the traumas endured by these families. The facts have been checked by the medical, nursing and other staff who occupy a place in their stories. By describing what happens to these eight children – why they are here, how they are treated, how their parents cope – we hope to show something of the life that goes on within the enclosed world of Great Ormond Street. Eight children out of 9000 in-patients a year cannot reflect fully an institution as large and complex as this hospital. We have interwoven the stories of the eight children with an account of a typical twenty-four hours in the life of the hospital. In this way we hope to show different aspects of the hospital's work and many of these

18

areas could equally well have been expanded to more prominent roles. There is no shortage of drama at Great Ormond Street.

Children First and Always could not have been written without the co-operation of the hospital authorities and its staff – our gratitude, along with a fuller explanation of how the book was produced, is contained in the acknowledgements. But more than anything it could not have been written without the co-operation of the parents. To them, above all, we must express our thanks. It was only possible to write about these eight children (or any of the others named in other sections) with the permission of the parents. Only then were hospital staff free to talk about these children to outsiders. No pressure was put on any parent to co-operate, but all did so enthusiastically because they wanted the wider world to know something about what goes on inside this extraordinary hospital. There was pride, too, in how their children had coped, completely understandable when you discover what they went through. The parents are very different people, but they share a profound gratitude for what the staff of Great Ormond Street have been able to do for their children. For us, as authors, it was a privilege to be allowed to enter their lives, just as it was to enjoy such access within this world-famous hospital.

We cannot conceive that it would be possible for anyone to spend much time at Great Ormond Street and fail to be moved or changed by the experience. It is humbling to see so many people coping with such spirit and resilience with such unimaginable stresses. And yet it is the underlying tension, on any day, even Christmas, which ultimately makes the achievements of the doctors so remarkable and so rewarding. In his Christmas sermon, the Reverend Derek Bacon recalled a conversation he had just had with a parent and it's as good a text for this book as it was at the Midnight Eucharist:

'One father, whose life had been turned on its end by what his family have come through here, said this to me on the day he was able to take his son home. "I'd like to take everybody in the whole world," he said, "and march them through this ward. Then we'd have no more bloody trouble."'

Derrik and Gillian Mercer
London, 1986.

6.00 a.m. *Dawn breaks and the children of Great Ormond Street begin to stir in their beds or cots. Some slumber until they are wakened by the sun, others are roused by the nurses; it varies from ward to ward and day to day. If a ward is full, the nurses are more likely to wake up the patients because they have a lot to do before the day shift arrive at seven forty-five. There's the early morning drug round which, if there are a lot of children receiving intravenous drugs, can take more than an hour. There are babies to be fed and, since on average one in three patients is under one year old, this can also take time. There are routine observations of temperature, pulse and breathing to be done on all wards and reports to be written on each patient for the nursing records. Surgical wards will be busier on days when their consultants are due in theatre, with the first children on the day's list to be washed and dressed in operating gowns. Everywhere beds must be made, nappies changed. And yet, despite these chores, it is a peaceful, almost magical time. Nurses who an hour or two before may have been yawning are revitalized by their wakening patients: no child is too young or too sick to be cuddled or stroked or talked to constantly. Few children wake up unhappy or tearful. How much this is due to their own resilience or the sensitivity of the nursing is impossible to say, but it is a tribute to both qualities. For a few precious minutes the nurses have the children to themselves. But soon the younger children will begin to ask for Mummy and by six-thirty the first of the resident parents have arrived on the wards. The tranquil dawn prelude is coming to an end; for the patients, parents and staff it will be a long and busy day, bringing sadness to a few but hope to many more.*

6.30 a.m. *'Don' Donaldson makes his way to the basement of the old hospital building to begin his day's work for the Hospital Sterilization and Disinfectant Unit – or HSDU as it's understandably known for short. Mr Donaldson is the unit's porter and almost certainly the hospital's only porter who is also a member of Equity, the actors' union. Portering being more reliable than acting, most days see him among the earliest arrivals of the day shift. His day begins with a visit to the wards from where he collects items to be returned to HSDU for re-sterilization. There are 230 separate items and ninety per cent of them can be used more* *than once. By eight o'clock he's back in the basement where the rest of the HSDU staff are arriving. Here, in far from ideal surroundings, the staff disinfect large items such as incubators or oxygen tents and put together packs of smaller equipment ordered by the wards. The range of packs is enormous – from multi-purpose dressings and plastic connectors to highly specific equipment for tracheostomies and ventilators. Anything, in fact, which needs to be sterile when used on a patient. When the equipment has been assembled in packs, it is put through the sterilizers ready for Don Donaldson to take on his travels around the hospital.*

7.00 a.m. *The canteen (or cafeteria as the catering staff like to call it) opens for breakfast, attracting not only staff but also some of the parents who are staying at the hospital. On average around a hundred parents will sleep overnight at the hospital, but sometimes the number is nearer 150 if you include people in hotel accommodation nearby. It is a far cry from the days when the main hospital building was completed in 1938. Then parents were only allowed to visit for two hours in the morning and two hours in the afternoon. Now, because research has shown that children suffer serious and long-term emotional damage if separated from their parents while in hospital, parents are encouraged to stay with their children whenever possible. Although it is usually Mum who stays, Dads have become increasingly evident. There was some official nervousness at the prospect of resident fathers – even though most couples are married, nobody uses the word 'husbands' – but they, too, are now accepted as part of the modern hospital scene. One person who is certainly not complaining about resident parents is Anne Allen, group catering manager. To her, they're extra customers and extra income, greatly reducing the net cost of her round-the-clock operation and boosting the numbers for breakfast to anything between seventy-five and a hundred customers a day.*

7.30 a.m. *A trickle of staff has been evident since six-thirty but now it gathers momentum. Domestic staff start to clean the wards and corridors, porters begin to sort the post, the first consultant is logged in by the reception desk in the front hall. In the bowels of the old hospital building Elizabeth Ogarro, the linen room super-*

visor, organizes the day's laundry. Most of the washing is done at the Queen Elizabeth Hospital for Children in Hackney, the sister hospital in the group, but there is enough to keep her team busy – especially on a Monday. Then there will be between 230 and 300 blankets, 300 and 360 towels and 400 to 500 bibs. Theatre gowns for nursing staff are also washed here, although they then need to be taken along the basement corridor to be sterilized at HSDU. One item rarely figures in the linen room's weekly laundry list – nappies. Fortunately all are disposable these days – the two hospitals get through 11,000 a week or 575,000 a year. The group is the biggest consumer of disposable nappies in London and, presumably, the country.

7.45 a.m. *The day shift nurses arrive for their morning 'report'. This is the handover when the staff nurse or sister in charge overnight briefs the day staff on each of the patients. Most of the day shift will only have finished work at nine-thirty the previous evening. It is a short break for everyone, but particularly the senior nursing staff who are more likely to live some distance away. Student nurses, who comprise a third of the hospital's 678-strong nursing establishment, live in hostels provided by the hospital. 'We couldn't staff the hospital if we didn't offer them accommodation,' says Betty Barchard, the group's chief nursing officer. They don't earn enough to rent flats in central London (see Appendix), yet it is impractical to live too far from the hospital. Housing co-operatives may be one solution to this problem.*

8.00 a.m. *In the basement an engineer throws a switch to turn off the main electrical power supply for the hospital. Fourteen seconds later the emergency generators fire into action. Or so the engineer and everyone else hopes. The generators are tested every six weeks and each time they are left running for ninety minutes. Each test must be planned and publicized with care because so many children are hooked up to electronic equipment. For some it will be pumps controlling the flow of intravenous drugs; for others artificial ventilators without which they would die. As eight o'clock approaches nurses as well as generators are therefore on stand-by, particularly in the three intensive care wards where high-technology medicine is most evident. Here, during the fourteen-second* *electrical shut-down, nurses must operate breathing equipment by hand – 'hand-bagging' as it is known – until the machines flicker back to life.*

8.15 a.m. *The first ward rounds are in full swing, usually led by a registrar with the senior house officer and the sister or staff nurse. Apart from one or two exceptions the entourages accompanying consultants' rounds later in the day are not as large as found in other London teaching hospitals. This is because Great Ormond Street does not train medical students, only the less numerous postgraduates. Another difference is that hardly any of the doctors wear white coats; ordinary clothes, it is thought, are less likely to make children nervous. Although the doctors do not wear name badges, there is one clue to discerning status: very few consultants carry a bleep. Sex is no longer a totally reliable guide since there are around a dozen distinguished female consultants at the hospital, including anaesthetists and a radiologist. But it's only two cheers for sexual equality. At the junior levels women predominate – although they are still called 'housemen' – while with registrars the split is roughly fifty-fifty. The crucial hurdle for a woman to jump is the transition from registrar to senior registrar. Even so more women hold senior positions in paediatrics than in general medicine.*

8.25 a.m. *The first patients arrive in the anaesthetic rooms adjoining the operating theatres. Surgery has expanded into worlds unimagined when the hospital building was opened in 1938 with just two theatres on the sixth floor and one on the seventh. Now there are also two theatres on the first floor but these are stretched to the limit by the number and complexity of operations performed there – including some 550 heart operations and 350 neurosurgical operations a year, most of which last several hours. For some of the theatres there are no 'recovery rooms', just a corridor in the theatre complex. Not that this necessarily affects the quality of the medical care, otherwise patients would not come from as far afield as Russia or the Middle East. By the time the surgeons arrive, the theatre nursing staff have prepared a trolley with all the appropriate equipment for the operation. There can be as many as fifty separate items for a single* *operation. The theatre sister will designate one of her staff as 'scrub nurse' which means to be at the surgeon's side, and another as the 'circulating nurse' to bring any additional equipment which may be required. For major operations consultant surgeons will be assisted by their registrar so, with at least two nurses and two anaesthetists, it can become quite crowded. For an operation to separate Siamese twins there were twenty-five doctors, nurses and technicians in the two first-floor theatres – plus a TV crew.*

8.30 a.m. *Pat Cornick and Jane Linward, the sisters in charge of the out-patient clinics, arrive to prepare for what, in terms of numbers, is the busiest department of all. Each year around 60,000 appointments are made by the medical records office, each requiring the appropriate medical notes to be in the right place at the right time. There are more than forty separate clinics, some meeting more than once a week and some only once a month. On any one day there can be a dozen doctors seeing patients either upstairs in surgical out-patients or downstairs in medical out-patients. Many children are referred to Great Ormond Street for second opinions and may never need to be seen again, but many more are seen over a period of many years. Often it is a happy atmosphere because, as Sister Cornick puts it, 'we are seeing a lot of children who are doing well'. But some clinics today will have an underlying tension and end in tears.*

Declan

Declan Carroll screamed all the way to the anaesthetic room next to the operating theatre. He gripped his mother's hand until she had to force him to let go. His sobbing haunted Mary Carroll as she and her husband, Danny, paced the streets, trying hard but unsuccessfully not to look at their watches. Would they ever see their son alive again? What was happening now, at this minute, in the operating theatre? Their minds were in turmoil as they tried to recall all they had been told in the last few bewildering days. There had been so many strange words, so many complicated tests. Mary was in a strange city, too, having been to London only once before in her life. And now her son was undergoing an operation which, even it were successful, would leave him dependent upon a small armoury of drugs for the rest of his life.

The minutes seemed like hours that July morning. If all went well, the operation should be over in four hours. Simply thinking about the operation made them shudder: as they walked, the surgeon would be cutting, drilling and sawing a hole in their son's head. He needed a hole three or four centimetres deep before he could even begin the most danger-ous and delicate task of all – the removal of a tumour tucked away underneath the brain. Depending upon the size and precise location of the tumour, the operation could leave Declan blind or without vital hormones such as those which control growth or puberty. If, that is, he survived the next forty-eight hours. It seemed a lifetime ago that they arrived at Great Ormond Street. In fact, it was just two weeks. Whatever happened now, life would never be the same again.

Nothing in their lives had prepared the Carroll family for the trauma of that day. Declan Carroll was then six years and nine months old. He was born in Bedford, fifty miles north of London but, as his first name implies, his family's roots were in Ireland. Danny and Mary Carroll grew up in County Cork where they married in 1974. It was a large wedding, not least because Danny was one of thirteen children. Mary's family by comparison was small – a mere three brothers and two sisters. For a time one of Danny's sisters lived in England and after spending a holiday with her, Mary and Danny Carroll moved to the same town, Bedford. There would be more opportunities here, they thought, and besides, Danny was tired of working on a farm.

Bedford is a town of light industry surrounded by farmland, less than an hour's train ride for commuters to London but retaining something of its old individuality as a county town. The variety of its industry has long attracted many immigrants – Asian and Italian as well as Irish – who found work relatively easy to come by. Danny got a labouring job with one of the country's largest building contractors, Mary worked as a shop assistant in Woolworth's. They are a quiet, but sociable couple who quickly settled into their new life, acquiring friends outside as well as inside the local Irish community. Each Sunday they went to mass, most summers they went back to Ireland. They worked hard so that when Declan was born they had bought a terraced red-brick house on the south side of town. Their commitment to the Roman Catholic Church and their Irish upbringing is profound, although neither Mary nor Danny had ambitions for a family as large as their own. Two, perhaps three, children would be plenty enough. Declan was the first, born on 6 October 1978, four years after they married.

Mary was then twenty-six years old. Like all of her family she was tall – five foot nine inches – and this probably helped her to have a normal pregnancy and delivery. At first, it looked as though Declan would take after her: he weighed in at eight pounds nine ounces (or just under four kilograms, as hospitals say these days). Whatever the form of weights used, it was the last time he was destined to be big for his age.

Elation soon turned to exhaustion. Mary says: 'He would never keep his feeds down – it would shoot straight out. And he hardly ever slept for more than two hours at a time. We were up so often that he slept in our room until he was two when Anna [his sister] was born. Eventually we used to take it in turns to get some sleep with Danny sometimes being booted out into the spare room during the week and me catching up at weekends.' Like all new babies, Declan was seen regularly at the local health clinic and doctors could find nothing wrong with him. He was not the first baby to leave his parents shattered: they accepted it stoically as something they would have to put up with until he grew out of it. After all, most children do.

When Declan was two months old his parents took him to Ireland to show their families. The celebrations were cut short when Declan caught a chest infection. The local doctor gave him some medicine which should have cleared it up, only to discover that Declan was allergic to penicillin. It produced such a rash and swelling that he was admitted to hospital for a fortnight. At least, though, they knew about the allergy; that wouldn't happen again. Back in Bedford, life resumed its exhausting pattern until, at ten months, a chest infection put Declan back in hospital. Two weeks of antibiotics eliminated the infection and tests revealed no other underlying problem.

For three years Declan paid regular visits to the out-patient clinics at Bedford General Hospital. His general development was normal: he walked at eleven months, talked at twelve months. He was still a poor, somewhat fussy eater and he was regularly sick. This was upsetting and frustrating for his mother – 'I tried everything, even those strained Heinz meals, to try and help him keep it down' – but his vomiting, while more violent, was becoming less frequent. This offered some respite for his mother who in 1981 had her second child, a daughter called Anna. She, luckily, proved to be a model baby, feeding happily and sleeping soundly. Family life seemed to be approaching a more equable phase. Declan had suffered no more infections and could start nursery school. He was a quiet boy, somewhat shy, but he enjoyed the games and in particular began to acquire a love of drawing.

He was then three years old. About that time the out-patient appointments ended because the hospital could find no cause for his feeding difficulties. Two new problems were beginning, however, although one would not become apparent for a couple of years. Initially, what continued to send Mary Carroll regularly to her GP were Declan's headaches. Standard tablets prescribed by the doctor had little effect and Mary grew increasingly frustrated by what she interpreted as a feeling that she was exaggerating Declan's problems. They changed GPs, but say they still found little sympathy. 'I kept saying to the doctors that there was something wrong with him. Why is he always getting sick or having headaches? They couldn't find anything wrong with him. It made me angry because it was saying I was a liar or a neurotic mum who was always calling to see them about nothing,' says Mary.

By the time Declan was ready to start infant school, the second problem was beginning to emerge. Declan was now conspicuously small for his age, barely three feet tall at the age of six. He still rode a bike with stabilizers on its wheels. His shortness made him timid, nervous during PE at school and vulnerable to teasing and bullying. Mary and Danny moved him from the local school to the more protective environment of St Joseph's, a Catholic primary school on the other side of town. His shortness was another problem for Mary Carroll to mention during her frequent visits to her GP.

It is only in the last twenty years that short stature has been recognized as a medical problem susceptible to treatment. Previously it had been regarded as one of those unalterable quirks of birth, much as people might have different colour hair or eyes. The development of growth hormone has enabled doctors to help children grow – once the problem has been identified. A common complaint among parents whose children attend the growth clinics (among others) at the Hospital for Sick Children is that local GPs took too long to act upon their concern. Such charges are often unfair, if understandable; few GPs will ever encounter many of the unusual conditions treated at Great Ormond Street. And Mary Carroll faced one particular obstacle when she voiced her concern about Declan's height: her husband Danny was only five feet four inches tall himself. 'The reaction I got was that my husband was small, so my son is going to be small,' she says.

Declan did not appear to be growing at all, though. His sister Anna, aged four, was two years younger but three inches taller. He was also tiring more easily, flopping on the sofa when he came home from school and riding in a push-chair to the shops while his younger sister walked alongside. 'There was no life in him,' says Danny. 'He wasn't interested in what was going on.' What alarmed Danny and Mary even more, however, were his headaches. For the last year these had been getting much worse: more frequent, more intense and longer-lasting. Sometimes Declan would wake up screaming or complaining of flashing lights. None of the tablets prescribed by the doctors seemed to have any effect at all. After one week, when Declan had suffered headaches every day and spent most of a Sunday being sick, Mary and Danny decided they had had enough. 'We got so angry at nothing being done that we insisted on going to the hospital. It was the best thing we ever did,' says Danny. And so began a week that was to change their lives.

On the Monday, Mary took Declan to see Dr Arthur Ferguson, consultant paediatrician at Bedford General Hospital. If there was a hero in this story, said one of the Great Ormond Street doctors later, it was Dr Ferguson. He had known Declan as an out-patient. Now he weighed and measured him. There was a chest X-ray, too. He asked Mary to return later that day so that Anna could also be measured. Then he told Mary to return the next day with her husband and both children.

On Tuesday Declan was photographed and the family told to wait for an hour. 'We were glad people were listening to us and taking us seriously, but we had no idea what was to come,' says Danny. 'Dr Ferguson returned and said he had been in touch with Great Ormond Street and arranged for Declan to be admitted as an emergency case the next day. He didn't say what he thought was wrong. We said we had been worried about the headaches, but he said he was more concerned about Declan's height. When he mentioned Great Ormond Street we knew there was something wrong; we didn't know it was so serious. All we knew about Great Ormond Street was that it was a children's hospital, nothing more than that, so we were more uneasy than alarmed.'

In fact, Dr Ferguson suspected more than he told. Declan was admitted to Great Ormond Street for investigation into growth failure, headaches and vomiting. 'I think he needs a fairly urgent scan,' wrote Dr Ferguson in the letter which the Carrolls brought with them to London. The significance of his suggestion would become clear to Declan's parents before the week was out. They arrived at Great Ormond Street on the Wednesday, forty-eight hours after seeing Dr Ferguson, and were admitted to ward 5D. It was a confusing time for Mary and Danny. They had only been to London once before and the size of the hospital, as well as the capital, seemed daunting. 'I couldn't work out why they had barricades around the hospital,' says Mary. Actually these were the blue safety grilles around the balconies on which children play. The seriousness of the illnesses treated at the hospital was to prove a greater shock – 'we didn't realize that such problems could exist' – but ward 5D provided a gentle introduction to the realities of Great Ormond Street life.

5D, on the fifth floor of the hospital, was presided over when Declan arrived by one of Great Ormond Street's legendary characters, Sister June McElnea, known to one and all as Sister Mac. She was one of the longest-serving sisters, having notched up twenty-two years at the hospital, but was then working her last two weeks on the ward before a transfer to a less taxing role in charge of emergency admissions. She would miss her ward and the frequent contact with families. Patients whom she had nursed as babies now came back with their wives or husbands. One girl sent a postcard: 'Wish you were here. Glad I'm not there.' The kindly Sister Mac was a reassuring person for the nervous Carrolls to meet on their first day at Great Ormond Street.

The ward was not what Mary and Danny had expected. For a start, it was smaller – just six beds in an open section plus three individual cubicles. It was not immediately obvious what was wrong with the other children and their ages varied enormously. Some were babies, some in their teens. There was none of the elaborate monitoring equipment with which they would become familiar on other wards. Nor did any of the patients have wires or tubes running into their bodies though that, too, would soon be familiar. 5D is a complex ward to get to know because it deals with a wide range of problems. The turnover of patients is high with many, like Declan, coming in for investigations. Often they then go home while the doctors await the results of tests and consider their next move. As it was a Wednesday when Declan arrived, some children were occupying beds as 'day cases' for particular investigations while the normal occupants of the beds went to the playroom. What most of the patients have in common are endocrine problems. What most parents have in common is that they have never heard of endocrine problems.

The details of endocrinology will remain beyond most parents, but in simple terms they involve the ways in which bodily hormones control human life and development. Man's physical and mental activities, his ability to grow and his ability to reproduce are all controlled by a highly complex system of hormones. These are produced largely by a network of glands scattered around the body from the head to the sexual organs. Most children in 5D are there because doctors suspect they may have too little or too much of particular hormones. This is why so much of the ward's work is taken up by investigations. Failure to grow, for instance, could be a consequence of insufficient growth hormone. Or it could be a sign that a child's parents are not feeding him properly. Only clinical tests can establish the answer.

For all the patients these begin with being weighed and measured: Declan was 17.1 kg (37.7 lb) and 103 centimetres (three feet four inches). Many of the tests were routine: his temperature, pulse, breathing and blood pressure, taken every four hours, were normal and stable. His eyesight and hearing appeared to be fine, although the former would later be checked more thoroughly by a specialist. 'A healthy, pleasant boy but a bit timid and pale,' wrote the first of the many doctors who saw him that week. Declan finds it hard to remember his feelings as the seemingly endless tests and questioning began. Certainly he was not feeling ill and ward staff recall him being alert and co-operative. 'Somewhat angelic-looking,' said one. Doll-like cuteness can be deceptive, though. Student nurses arriving on 5D are warned against judging a child by its height. It can be very upsetting for a six-year-old to be treated like a toddler, just because he is so small.

The nurses encouraged Mary and Danny to help Declan settle by feeding and keeping him occupied. They both stayed in London (as did daughter Anna) in 'the Home from Home', a large house a quarter of a mile away which had been refurbished by a charity to enable families to stay together while their child is in hospital. The companionship of other parents – on the ward as well as at the house in the evenings – eased their adjustment to hospital life. And they began to appreciate that Great Ormond Street was not just another children's hospital. 'You would see an ambulance come up the driveway and out would come an incubator containing a tiny baby. They were so small. It doesn't seem right,' says Mary.

Mary and Danny Carroll are warm-hearted people and they were genuinely moved by what they saw and heard. Nor will they ever hear a word said against nurses. 'They always made time to explain things, even though they may have been through it with us already, and they always did their best to make us feel at home,' says Mary. Declan was not a difficult patient to nurse – not that he relished either the tests or the hospital food. 'Only had jelly for dinner but enjoyed a packet of dolly mixtures!' noted one nurse on his second day. Nurses were told to keep a record of what he ate and to discourage 'junk food'. But they found it easier to overcome his shyness than his feeding habits. Declan responded particularly to the efforts of Helen Mitchelhill, then the ward playleader. She soon discovered his flair for drawing and she later succeeded in enticing him to the playroom with other children. At other times, if there was a lull between the tests, the family would go for a walk in a nearby park. Such interludes were rare: there always seemed to be another test.

His limbs were checked for their reactions and muscle sensitivity, samples of his urine and blood sent for analysis in the biochemistry laboratory, his chest X-rayed. The hospital staff wanted to observe Declan during one of his headaches yet, as is often the way, since arriving in hospital he had not experienced any of the headaches which plagued him daily the week before. From the beginning, though, the doctors seemed most concerned about Declan's growth.

His wrist and hand were X-rayed; this enabled radiologists

to establish a 'bone age' which in Declan's case turned out to be the equivalent of a child three and a half years old – more than three years younger than Declan. His height would also have been about average for such an age. Other tests now sought to work out why Declan had stopped growing. Insulin (and other drugs) were injected into a vein in his arm in order to stimulate the production of hormones such as cortisol and growth hormone; blood samples were then taken over a ninety-minute period in what is known as an 'insulin tolerance test' to enable doctors to find out whether or not certain hormones are being made properly. It is not a pleasant procedure for the patient, nor is it without risk. Patients are starved overnight and denied any fluids other than water during the test. In effect, the test lowers the blood sugar which, unchecked, can cause convulsions. Patients must be kept awake at all times and a doctor must stay with them throughout the test to counter any sign of danger. Declan became drowsy, sweaty and his heart rate jumped from 86 to 110. The results of the test would later show that the production of at least four hormones, including growth and cortisol, was seriously impaired. But why? The answer, as suspected by Dr Ferguson in Bedford, was provided by a scan.

A CT scanner is one of the most expensive, coveted and campaigned-for items of medical technology; the one at Great Ormond Street cost £400,000 in 1984. 'CT' stands for compu-terized tomography, which may not necessarily clarify matters for the layman. Essentially, it is based on the principle that different elements of the head, such as brain, fluid or tumour, absorb X-rays at different rates. By directing a narrow beam of X-rays through the head from a variety of positions on an arc, the scanner's computer can calculate the differing absorption patterns in a particular layer or 'slice' of the head. The results are converted into visual form for interpretation by the radiolo-gists.

All this was not so much above Declan's head as all around it. He was lying on his back on a trolley. Behind him was a large machine with a circular hole in the middle – 'it looks like a Polo mint,' a doctor on the ward had told him. Once Declan was secure, the trolley slid him backwards until his head was in the centre of the hole. Declan, like many children, was nervous of the machine. He was therefore mildly sedated to ensure that he kept still during the scan; it doesn't hurt, but movement negates the results. Once Declan was lined up correctly by the radiographer, the scanning process began. The X-ray beams are sent through two narrow slits in the casing of the 'hole'. Behind these slits, hidden within the casing, the X-ray machinery turns a complete circle to complete a single scan in anything between two and eight seconds. In all, twelve or thirteen separate scans are normally taken of each patient, each scan portraying a different horizontal slice or layer of the head. As each scan is completed, the table slides forward one centimetre to position the head for the next 'slice'.

The CT scanner at Great Ormond Street is under great pressure, with twelve or more patients a day. Though used to scan the abdomen and lungs as well as the head, it has brought the most dramatic improvements in the detection of brain tumours. For example, it will reveal liquid cystic tumours which do not show up on normal single-shot X-rays. Declan's first scan on the Thursday was still unclear, however. On one of the layers there appeared to be a slightly darker mass which could be a tumour, but the doctors could not be certain. They decided to repeat the scan in the afternoon, this time injecting him with a radio-opaque 'dye'. The dye enters the blood stream to highlight blood vessels – and tumours.

This time the radiologists were in no doubt: the darker mass, clearly visible now, was a tumour inside the head which was 'almost certainly a craniopharyngioma'. The news was broken to the family on Friday morning just two days after Declan had arrived at Great Ormond Street and four after his mother had taken him to see Dr Ferguson in Bedford. Declan would have to return to the hospital in nine days' time to have an operation on his brain to remove the tumour. There would then be further tests and the possibility of drug therapy lasting several years, perhaps forever.

'It was a terrible shock. We knew there was something wrong but we weren't prepared for a tumour. It was very hard to take in. When they first tell you, it doesn't hit you for about an hour or so. Then it's such a shock that you can't take it in.

You keep saying to yourself it can't be true, why did this happen to us? We haven't done anything to anybody to deserve this. We spent nights and days afterwards just crying,' says Danny.

The trauma of such a diagnosis is shocking enough even when parents know their child is seriously ill. But psychologists recognize that sudden or unexpected shocks normally induce greater stress than bad news which people have anticipated. Thus it was for Mary and Danny. Within a week Declan had gone from a short boy with headaches, who was nonetheless mostly well enough to go to school, to a boy who needed brain surgery. The rest of that grim Friday passed in a blur. Doctors came and went, including one of the neurosurgeons who would be involved in the operation. The nurses did their best to comfort parents who were becoming more distraught as the news sank in. There is little privacy for grief in Great Ormond Street so it was something of a relief for the Carrolls when they could leave for home.

Danny was glad he had not driven to London since he was sure he'd have been unable to concentrate. All the next week, back at work, he found his mind wandering. Declan went back to school for the week, mainly to pass the time more quickly. 'We told him he had to have an operation on his head because there was something inside which had to come out. We wanted to explain without frightening him,' says Mary. 'Our faith was a great help to us at this time. We saw our priest and they held special masses for Declan before we went back for the operation.'

They arrived back at Great Ormond Street on the Sunday evening. The operation was set for Wednesday. This time Anna stayed with one of Mary's sisters in Bedford and the Carrolls were found a room in the old hospital building above the chapel. Declan went back to 5D where there were the usual checks of height, weight, temperature, pulse, breathing, blood and urine. Declan seemed well, if slightly pale and still very quiet. The next day there would be tests more specifically related to the diagnosis of craniopharyngioma. Mary and Danny had scarcely taken in this term when it was first used. All that they could fasten upon at that shattering moment of diagnosis was the word 'tumour'. Now they were ready for a fuller explanation.

Craniopharyngioma is a tumour which exists underneath the brain, very roughly inside the skull on a horizontal line behind the bridge of the nose. A tumour is a swollen mass of tissue and craniopharyngioma can exist in either solid, calcified form or mostly liquid cysts. Whatever the form – and sometimes it can present in both forms – craniopharyngioma is a 'benign' tumour. This means that it will not spread and develop secondary tumours elsewhere in the body. That's the good news. The bad news is its location, not merely difficult to remove in the sense that any brain operation is risky, but dangerously close to some of the body's most vital organs. The tumour grows in an area close to the optic nerves, the hypothalamus and the pituitary gland. As it grows, the tumour exerts pressure which can damage these organs. The consequences of such damage depend upon the precise location of the tumour, but they commonly include loss of eyesight, delayed growth and puberty, uncontrolled urine output and convulsions. A lack of cortisol hormone is potentially lethal since it renders the body unable to cope with physical stress such as illness. So fundamental are the functions of the pituitary gland that it is sometimes known as 'the master gland'.

Craniopharyngioma is primarily a disease of childhood, although it has been diagnosed in people over sixty years of age. The most common symptoms are headaches and vomiting (because the tumour increases pressure within the brain), deteriorating eyesight (because of damage to the optic nerves), delayed growth (because of damage to the pituitary gland which produces growth hormone) and uncontrolled urine (also because of damage to the pituitary gland). Ordinary skull X-rays can be sufficient to show the tumour, but a CT scan will provide confirmation. These days the response is almost always surgery because damage will inevitably increase as the tumour grows. What nobody knows in advance, however, is whether or not surgery will succeed in removing the entire tumour. Either way further damage to those crucial internal organs is almost inevitable. At least the surgery would give Declan a chance, something denied some children with malignant brain tumours. Declan was lucky; Mary and Danny tried hard to believe it.

Before Declan was transferred to the neurosurgical ward he faced one more day of tests. The ophthalmic registrar checked his eyesight; there had been no deterioration in the past week and, indeed, it was virtually normal. The growth department did a more precise measurement to establish a base-line for any later treatment. Neither of these tests troubled Declan, something which could not be said of the 'water deprivation test'. For seven hours he was unable to drink any fluid. Every hour he was weighed and his urine was collected for analysis. This would establish the extent to which he lacked a pituitary hormone which enables the body to absorb water. Too little of the hormone produces too much urine and uncontrollable thirsts, symptoms of a disease known as 'diabetes insipidus'.

Nurses have known sufferers try to drink water from flower vases or even lavatories in order to quench their thirst during a water deprivation test. Patients are therefore monitored closely and the test is aborted if weight loss exceeds four per cent. Declan became thirsty, but not excessively so, and the results suggested a partial form of diabetes insipidus. Past experience suggested that an almost inevitable side-effect of the operation would be total diabetes insipidus. The doctors wanted to know now so that drugs could be given to control urine output before and during the operation. Likewise the results of the insulin tolerance test, performed the week before, enabled Declan to be given cortisone steroids to overcome a shortage of cortisol caused by the effect of the tumour on the pituitary gland. The development of such steroids was a crucial factor in reducing the risks of this type of brain surgery. Cortisol is essential to enable the body to cope with physical stress, such as an operation. If Declan came through the operation, cortisone* would

---

*Cortisol and cortisone are virtually identical. Cortisol is the chemical name for the substance which should be produced by the adrenal gland; cortisone is a closely related chemical which for many years was more convenient to be taken in tablet form to compensate for a lack of natural cortisol. More recently cortisol itself has become available in suitable form to be given to patients.

number among the drugs he would need for the rest of his life.

On the eve of the operation Declan moved to 1B, the neuro-surgical ward. The thought of brain surgery unnerves many people and, for all they had been told, it was still something of a shock for Mary and Danny to see children with so many tubes attached to their bodies. One corner of the ward is designated as a 'recovery room' for intensive care after operations, but often there are more children requiring such nursing than beds available. Seriously ill children will then be found in the open section of the ward to which Declan was directed on arrival from 5D. It is a ward where, from time to time, children will die or where parents learn that their children will die.

The death of a child is invariably painful. A fatal diagnosis can be equally unsettling. What do you say to parents if their child has an irreversible brain tumour? Intensive care imposes intensive pressures on hospital staff. 'I love my work but there are times when we're all tired, emotionally as well as physic-ally,' says Lindy May, the senior of the ward's two sisters. So why do they do it? Naomi Warren, the second sister, says: 'Obviously, it's very sad when someone dies, but more often you see a child before an operation, nurse him afterwards and then see him up and running about. You see the complete process, whereas if it was just intensive care, you would only see patients who are critically ill. We can get to know families better and there are a variety of ages and conditions for us to nurse.'

It is certainly to the credit of Lindy May and Naomi Warren that 1B exudes a relaxed and welcoming atmosphere, despite its stresses. They are an attractive team: Lindy is in her late twenties, tall and dark with a warm contralto voice; Naomi is in her mid-twenties, petitely pretty with the enviable quality of looking younger than her years. They were both on duty when Declan arrived from 5D. One of their tasks was to prepare Declan and his parents for the next day's operation. In this they were not alone. Mary and Danny were also seen by an anaesthetist and Norman Grant, the consultant neurosurgeon who would be in charge of the operation the next day. Mr Grant is the senior of the hospital's two neurosurgical consult-ants, a quietly spoken Scot who was appointed a consultant at the age of thirty-five in 1969. He tries to see all parents before major operations to answer their questions and to tell them the risks. Mr Grant says:

'There is nearly always a fraught forty-eight hours after the operation so I think parents have to have a pretty frank picture presented to them. I run through it from my point of view. Starting from the simplest end I tell them about convulsions because there is a high incidence of epilepsy after cranio-pharyngiomas, no doubt related to the prolonged retraction on the brain. I tell them that's not so much a complication as an expected side-effect. I tell them that the sense of smell is likely to go, certainly on the right side if that's where we are operating. If the eyesight is already compromised, I tell them there is a risk of making that worse. I tell them of the proximity of the carotid artery and other major arteries to the brain and that while we aim on the conservative side – we would rather leave a bit of tumour than produce damage – occasionally an artery can get damaged. In simple terms, that amounts to having a stroke from which the patient may or may not recover. I say that at the extreme of the bad end one might lose a child from the bleeding at the time of the operation.'

This harrowing message left Mary and Danny feeling numb. It usually does. The ward sister – or a senior staff nurse – normally goes through it again, answering questions which some parents are too nervous to ask a consultant. Sister Warren told Mary and Danny Carroll what they should expect after the operation – the wires, the tubes, the monitoring devices and the pain. She said there would be a nurse with Declan twenty-four hours a day for the critical two days after the operation. And they discussed what they should tell Declan. 'I don't think you should tell children anything unless you are sure it is going to happen. They have got to be prepared but there is no need to frighten them unnecessarily,' says Naomi Warren.

Declan therefore knew that his head would be shaved for the operation; he knew that he would be given a general anaesthetic for an operation that would last several hours; he knew that when he woke up he would have various wires and tubes attached to his body; he knew he would be given various drugs;

and he knew that he would have to lie in bed for several days. Somewhat surprisingly in these circumstances, after initial restlessness Declan slept soundly. This was more than could be said for his parents. They had been comforted by other parents in 1B, including one woman whose child had come through the same operation. While reassuring, this did not dilute the impact of Mr Grant's message. 'We knew he could be left blind or that he could die,' says Mary. Their stomachs churning, they went to the hospital chapel to pray before they went to bed. They did not sleep much that night.

Declan was set to leave the ward at eight o'clock. Mary and Danny arrived shortly after seven to find him bathed and dressed in a white surgical gown. Normally, sedatives given as a 'pre-med' will calm nerves but this is rarely possible before neurosurgery; sedation may affect vital neurological signs and increase pressure within the brain, making it more difficult for the surgeon to operate. So Declan's pre-medication at half past seven was simply to dry up secretions; it did not staunch his tears or his parents' anguish. Mary went with him when he was wheeled on a trolley twenty yards down the corridor to the anaesthetic room. At the door she said goodbye. Mary remembers this as the worst moment of all: 'He was screaming and gripping my hand so tight he wouldn't let go. We didn't want to show him that we were worried. We wanted to calm him down a bit but there was nothing we could do. It really hurt.'

In fact, distressing though the memory remains for Mary and Danny Carroll, Declan's sobs soon subsided under the experienced care of Dr Angela Mackersie, one of the hospital's consultant anaesthetists. She is normally responsible for neurosurgical operations and today she was assisted by Dr Kate Grebenik, a registrar. In Britain, unlike the United States, all anaesthetists are doctors and, in the next four hours, the partnership between anaesthetist and surgeon became clear. It is not just a question of putting a patient to sleep and then waking them up after the operation is over, although these are critical moments. 'It's a bit like being an airline pilot,' said one anaesthetist. 'Take-off and landing are the two most obvious danger points, but in between you need constant awareness for even the smallest changes in vital signs.'

Dr Mackersie adds: 'Generally, the smaller the child, the more unstable they are, but craniopharyngiomas are among the most complicated cases because of the associated endocrine problems whatever the age.' Norman Grant, the surgeon, is in no doubt that the anaesthesia can make or break the operating conditions. He says: 'Ideally one wants the brain as slack as possible so that you can retract it without using a lot of force and ideally one doesn't want a lot of pressure in the veins because, if you cut one, everywhere floods with blood and you can't see anything.'

Dr Mackersie's first task was to prepare Declan for his operation. It took around twenty minutes of concentrated work by both anaesthetists. Reassurance and a small dose of gas rapidly stopped the crying and enabled them to insert a 'drip' line into a vein in each foot; one would be used for blood, the other for anaesthetic drugs or dextrose to prevent dehydration. His breathing was controlled artificially via a tube inserted down his throat. A small plastic tube was inserted into an artery to provide constant measurement of his blood pressure, then a catheter was inserted to collect urine in the knowledge that the tumour had caused partial diabetes insipidus. Other wires monitored temperature and heart-rate. Finally, before he was wheeled next door to the operating table, his head was shaved.

Under the lights, his shaven head looked extremely white. His eyes and mouth were covered by tape. The table was tilted at an angle of perhaps ten or fifteen degrees to raise the level of Declan's head. This would reduce pressure in the veins and give the surgeon an easier angle at which to work. What Mr Grant* and Henry Marsh, his senior registrar, had to do this morning was a craniotomy – an operation which cuts through the skull. Essentially, it involves cutting a flap in the forehead of the skull and then easing down beneath the frontal lobe of the brain in order to reach the site of the tumour. The telltale CT scan pictures were clipped to a light-box so Mr Grant knew where it was. But it would probably take at least ninety minutes before he was in a position even to see the tumour.

---

*Surgeons who are Fellows of the Royal College of Surgeons, such as all consultants, are called 'Mister' rather than 'Doctor'.

Norman Grant would make his flap on the right side of the head because for most people the left side of the brain controls speech. For cosmetic reasons, however, he made his first cut above the hairline. It adds twenty minutes or so to the length of the operation but it leaves the forehead unscarred. The cut went virtually the width of the head. The surgeons then injected a fluid either side of the cut, causing the flesh to bulge. The resulting tension in the scalp reduces bleeding and also separates the layers inside the scalp. The skin is clamped either side of the cut and then, on the forehead side of the incision, it is peeled back across the entire length of the cut until it rests over the lower half of the face. This reveals both sides of the front of the skull. It was now time to make what Mr Grant called 'a trap door' into the brain.

This trap door or flap has to be cut level with the floor of the front part of the skull so that the surgeon can later see between the brain and the floor. He begins by drilling holes into the skull with an instrument which, for all its delicacy, still bears a disconcerting similarity to drills used by weekend handymen at home. The registrar sucked away the blood as the shuddering drill made two holes a couple of inches apart. Mr Grant then sawed a crescent-shaped flap between the two holes, except for one end on the side of the skull which remains uncut. The sawing took just over five minutes, producing a high-pitched whirr and foetid burning smell as the saw gets hot. The uncut side of the flap was then cracked so that it could be turned back, with a muscle acting as a hinge; the flap cannot be cut off totally because it would lose its essential blood supply.

The surgeon could now see the dura, a fibrous bag which separates the brain from the skull. Here, too, a flap was made so that the brain was at last visible. It is pink in colour and criss-crossed by distended purple veins and arteries. Well over an hour had passed and the surgeon was still nowhere near the tumour. In fact, his real difficulties have yet to begin. He has to get into a narrow cleft underneath the frontal lobe of the brain. To do so he must gently 'retract' the brain which means squeezing it back progressively with clamp-like instruments in order to gain access to the site of the tumour. By the time he has done so the cleft will be three or four centimetres deep. With Declan submerged under surgical sheets, by now splattered with blood, it was difficult for a layman to work out where all this space had come from, let alone exactly where the surgeon was now working.

For the latter stages of the operation Mr Grant uses an operating microscope with an in-built light. Such microscopes have played an important role in reducing the risks of brain surgery; smaller surgical tools, improved anaesthetics and the use of cortisone steroids have all helped too. Looking down the microscope reveals almost an underwater scene, although here it is not water but cerebral spinal fluid which the surgical registrar sucks away. But there is also some blood, and one snag with the operating microscope is that even a small volume of blood can swamp the surgeon's field of vision.

This is where the anaesthetist can assist the surgeon. By using a drug called Labetalol to lower the blood pressure, the anaesthetist not only reduces bleeding but also enables the surgeon to retract the brain more easily. Reducing carbon dioxide also decreases inter-cranial pressure, thereby creating more space for the surgeon. Dr Mackersie tried both ploys on Declan but the brain remained tight. A drug called Lasix was used to reduce the fluid in the brain but this, too, produced little immediate effect. The surgeons simply had to be patient, gradually pulling up the frontal lobe and sucking away the fluid as it came. By removing the fluid around the brain in this way, the surgeons reduce the size of the brain and create an opening. But the more they squeeze, the less blood reaches the brain. If blood pressure has already been reduced, there is a danger that the part of the brain being retracted will not recover from the loss of its essential blood supply. Trying to get the right balance is a skilled process.

In addition to helping the surgeons, Dr Mackersie had three worries of her own: excess fluid loss caused by diabetes insipidus, blood loss and high temperatures. The urine catheter showed how much fluid Declan was losing, so Dr Mackersie could replace this with a dextrose-saline solution through one of the drips into his feet. Through the second of the two drips she transfused blood. Blood loss poses a particular danger in paediatric neurosurgery since children's heads form eighteen per cent of their total bodily surface area compared to nine per cent of adult's bodies. 'Children having neurosurgery therefore lose much more blood in proportion to total volume than adults,' says Dr Mackersie. 'If they lose too much it is a major, and in some rare cases, a potentially mortal, problem. We allow them to lose approximately ten per cent of total blood volume before giving them a transfusion.' Such a transfusion is virtually inevitable during a craniopharyngioma operation – the surgeon's gowns as well as the sheets were stained with blood and some had also splashed onto the floor. If temperatures rise, as they often do in such operations, cold fluids would be transfused among other measures to return it to normal. High temperatures now could cause serious complications later.

Meanwhile Norman Grant was approaching the area of the tumour. 'It's very unusual not to get down to the tumour. It has happened, sometimes because the head is not in a good position causing the veins in the brain to become distended, despite everything the anaesthetist can do,' he says. No such problem arose today: he could see the tumour lying next to the right optic nerve. But could he see all of it? One difficulty of craniopharyngioma is that you cannot always see the entire tumour. Another is that the tumour tends to stick to neighbouring structures such as optic nerves or the pituitary gland. Together, these difficulties pose considerable dangers.

For all the precision of the CT scan, a surgeon will never know until this moment whether or not he will be able to remove the entire tumour. Parts of the tumour could be hidden behind the optic nerve and if he tugged too hard, the surgeon could damage or destroy a patient's eyesight. On the other hand, failure to remove the tumour would mean extensive courses of radiation and the possibility of more craniotomies with all the consequential dangers of brain damage.

After the difficulty which Norman Grant had experienced in gaining this first sight of Declan Carroll's tumour, he was therefore relieved to see it mostly visible. These tumours can vary in size from that of a pea to a tangerine and vary in substance from a cyst to a calcified crust. The area where Mr Grant was working was about one centimetre in diameter.

Declan's tumour was partly cystic so that when Mr Grant inserted a needle into it, he was able to suck away a yellowy-brown fluid rather like engine oil. Removing the tumour capsule itself was trickier. Gentle retraction made space while the surgeon snipped and pulled at the capsule. One small chunk was put in a jar for analysis by the pathologists; in some brain tumours this is a crucial moment of discovery – is it malignant or benign? – but with craniopharyngioma the laboratory analysis serves essentially to confirm rather than to establish the diagnosis.

Most of Declan's tumour came away from the optic nerves and the carotid artery quite easily, but the capsule had partially covered the stalk of the pituitary gland. Rather than leave any of the tumour Mr Grant removed the stalk, too. It seemed likely that a few fragments remained out of sight at the point where the optic nerves cross, but the surgeon was well-satisfied. 'The basic rule is that if you can't see the point where the tumour is sticking, don't pull on it. Otherwise you might cause even greater damage. In this case it was pretty satisfactory because most of the tumour came out cleanly. The most difficult part was getting there in the first place,' says Mr Grant.

It was two hours after the operation had begun, and another ninety minutes before it would be complete. Dr Mackersie gradually increased the blood pressure to ensure that there was no internal bleeding before the surgeons sewed up one layer after another. As the clamps were removed, blood oozed from the wounds before the stitches went in. Additional drill-holes were made into the 'trap door' of the skull so that this could be sewn back in place with thick, black thread known as sutures. Finally, the scalp was pulled back across the forehead. Thinner thread is used here for these are the only stitches which will later be removed. Before the wound was finally closed a plastic catheter or tube is inserted to drain away fluid. Mr Grant's work was over.

The operation had lasted just under four hours. It was time for a sandwich and a cup of coffee in the corridor before the afternoon's surgical list began. The atmosphere in the theatre had been quietly professional, almost casual to the outsider.

But although Dr Mackersie, for instance, had time to chat, her eyes never left the bank of monitors which recorded heart rate, temperature, breathing and blood pressure. And her work with Declan was far from over. She now inserted a line into a neck vein to provide constant read-outs of his central venous pressure. A tube was passed through his nose into his windpipe so that Declan could be attached to a ventilator machine in the ward and his breathing controlled artificially until the next day. A vacuum pump was attached to the fluid drain in his head. Finally, Dr Mackersie took samples of blood and urine to see how they had been affected by the operation. Then she accompanied him back to the ward. Dr Mackersie or another anaesthetist continued to keep a close eye on Declan throughout the afternoon and night. She did so because she knew that, in many ways, his most critical time was yet to begin. So, too, did Sister Lindy May. 'It's the first twelve hours after the operation that are most dangerous,' she says.

To most parents, though, the operation appears the major hurdle. Mary and Danny were no exception. Mary's mother and brother had flown to London to be with them; it was the first time either of them had left Ireland. The nurses advised them to leave the hospital and get some fresh air rather than to wait on the ward. Even so, the minutes dragged, says Mary. 'I was looking at my watch the whole time. I wanted to go back but there was nothing I could do, so we just walked and walked until it was about half past one. As we turned back into the hospital entrance we met a ward sister who said: "I've got good news for you – the operation is over and it's gone well."'

Declan had returned to the open ward. His head was swathed in bandages pinned together by large safety pins. This, though, was the least of the surprises that awaited his parents. From head to toe Declan had ten wires or tubes connected to his body and he was surrounded by electronic monitors. 'We couldn't see that much of him at all,' says Danny. 'The nurses had tried to prepare us, but it was still a terrible shock to see him like that. It wasn't a pretty sight and it upset me a lot.'

At the top of his head, poking out from the bandages, was a vacuum drain exerting gentle pressure to pump fluid from the surgical wound. A naso-gastric tube drained the stomach via his nose to prevent vomiting. Declan was still being ventilated artificially, his breathing controlled by a machine delivering forty per cent oxygen at twenty breaths a minute, so also in his nose was the ventilator tube. A tube (or 'line' as it is known) into a vein on the right-hand side of his neck gave constant readings of venous blood pressure. These readings were shown on the screen of a large monitor alongside Declan's bed, as was the heart rate from a wire taped to his chest. A rectal thermometer provided a similarly continuous reading of temperature which, like blood pressure and pulse rate, can be a warning sign of trouble.

Of the remaining four tubes or lines, one was a catheter to extract urine, one primarily to check blood pressure and two were used to add fluids. The arterial line into the right wrist provided constant measurement of blood pressure but it also enabled samples of blood to be taken; these samples would be analysed for blood gases from which the doctors could check if the ventilation was correct. Lines also led from veins in each foot. One was being used to infuse a dextrose-saline solution so that his body received some basic fluids; the other transfused blood to replace what he had lost during the operation. The bags of dextrose and blood hung from 'drip stands'. In fact, although the term 'drip stand' is still used, you rarely see fluids dripping into intravenous lines by gravity alone as is common for adults. For children the volumes to be infused must be so precise – and often so minute – that the fluids pass through electronic pumps whose monitors flash when all is well or bleep when they need attention. Despite their essential role, many of the pumps have to be bought with money given privately because the National Health Service budget cannot afford them!

The battery of monitors and the profusion of lines reflect the intensity of nursing care required after a craniopharyngioma operation. Nor is it just high-tech care. At least one nurse would stay with Declan constantly for the next twenty-four or forty-eight hours, depending on his progress. Some problems can be anticipated. The damage to the pituitary gland would almost certainly mean he had lost his ability to concentrate urine. Fluids would then pass straight through his system, raising the danger of extreme dehydration. For this reason the specific gravity (or diluteness) of the urine was tested and a detailed chart maintained to measure how much fluid went into his body and how much came out. Initially, this would enable the staff to increase fluid input to keep Declan 'in balance' but soon it would provide the basis for prescribing appropriate volumes of a drug to control urine output. Another specific danger from the operation is damage to eyesight. Sometimes poor vision will have existed before the operation as a result of compression by the tumour on the optic nerves. Sadly, it is not unknown for children to lose their eyesight altogether after the operation.

More general dangers stem from the disturbance to which the brain has been exposed during the craniotomy. So every fifteen minutes a torch was shone at Declan's eyes to see if (or how) the pupils responded to light. Arm and leg reflexes were also checked – again, initially, every fifteen minutes. There is little respite for the patient. Declan was fully ventilated, which kept him still – no bad thing given all those wires – but made him vulnerable to mouth and body sores. He was also unable to cough so that every half-hour a nurse had to suck out secretions from his windpipe which might cause chest infections or vomiting.

Yet all these hazards are minimal compared to the overriding danger that a patient might die as a result of increased pressure within the brain. For all the parental relief that the operation is over, the following forty-eight hours are critical. 'You are nursing to catch problems before they arise,' says Sister Lindy May. Everything is interrelated. Increased intracranial pressure produces higher blood pressure and a slow pulse. There are dangers of convulsions and strokes as well as death. High temperatures can also prove fatal: anything above thirty-nine degrees* will require prompt treatment, perhaps by using cold fluids, fanning or even surrounding the child with ice. If the temperature remains too high for too long, the proteins of the brain substance can become clotted and the brain dies.

---

*Normal temperature is 36.8 Celsius or 98.4 Fahrenheit.

So many dangers and so much activity seemed to Mary and Danny to intensify their sense of helplessness. There was nothing they could do but watch and hope and pray. After an hour or so nurses told them that Declan would be able to hear their voices, even though he could not see them. So they sat next to their son and told him how well he was doing, perhaps as much to convince themselves as Declan. Yet it was true. The neurological arm and leg reflexes were good and by tea-time both eyes were responding well to light. Temperature was high, at thirty-eight degrees, so an electric fan was placed next to him. This did not reduce his temperature, but it prevented any further increase. Neither his slight fever nor a lower blood pressure concerned the doctors unduly. Their only worry was some bruising around his right eye. It appeared to be the result of damage during the operation and as the swelling increased the eye began to close.

Despite this, after their nightly visit to the chapel, Mary and Danny managed to get some sleep that night. 'We were still worried because we knew that the first forty-eight hours were critical, but the worst hadn't happened. We were grateful for that,' says Mary. The next day Declan's eye looked even worse – 'as though he'd had a fight with his shadow and lost,' said one doctor – but otherwise the news was encouraging. Best of all, the first of the tubes came out. He was weaned off the ventilator during the morning and by mid-afternoon was off it altogether, although for a couple of hours he breathed through an oxygen mask. His temperature fell to 37.2 and while his blood pressure remained low, it was stable.

Declan, though, was feeling slightly worse. The previous day he had been sedated; now he began to notice the pain of what he had undergone. He resisted attempts to keep his mouth and eyes free from infection and was restless when his parents left him to have a meal. He was, in short, tired. Who wouldn't be if every fifteen minutes for twenty-four hours someone had shone a torch in your eyes or told you to flex your legs and arms? Relief, albeit mild, was in sight: after twenty-four hours these observations became half-hourly, after forty-eight hours they were hourly. At seven o'clock on the evening after the operation Declan began to drink water so that in the early hours of the next morning one of the intravenous lines into the feet was removed. Next to go was the naso-gastric tube followed by the wound drain and the lines into the neck and wrist – all on the second day after the operation. 'That was the best thing of all – to see the tubes coming out one by one, day by day,' says Danny.

The critical forty-eight hours after the operation had passed. And by day four only the urine catheter remained from the plethora of tubes, and the monitors had also been wheeled away. Declan was looking much better, his eye was less swollen and he was now talking normally. He began to sit out of bed on the balcony overlooking the hospital driveway. After some reluctance, he began to eat solid foods, displaying a relish for brown bread which would have gratified those nurses on 5D who had fretted over his liking for 'junk food'. In the first few days after the operation his intake of fluids had been strictly controlled. Now he was allowed to eat and drink as much as he liked. In this way the doctors would be able to establish the extent of his inability to control his urine output. A drug known as DDAVP had been given to Declan since the day after the operation to help control his urine; it was now a question of finding the right dose. Detailed fluid balance charts were supplemented by analysis of the urine and another water deprivation test. Declan hated this test, saying he would protest to the police unless he got a drink. He didn't get a drink, but he got some reward: once the test was completed the catheter was removed.

The next day – one week after the operation – he celebrated his freedom from wires and tubes by going for a walk outside the hospital with his father. It was one of the few hot sunny days in a poor summer and Danny's mood matched the weather. A wiry man who reminded one ward sister of a jockey, he was not used to being cooped up all day. His employer, the building firm of George Wimpey, had been very understanding and given him time off with full pay. Danny now took Declan out for a long-promised treat: not brown bread this time, but a hamburger.

Danny and Mary endured one final shock before Declan left ward 1B – the removal of stitches from his head wound. 'We had no idea it was such a long scar going right across the head, virtually from one ear to another,' says Mary. The first thing which Declan did was shuffle to the playroom to see for himself in the mirror. The second thing was to put the thread used for the stitches in a jar which he still keeps at home. . ·

Eight days after the operation Declan returned to 5D. He was happier and more outgoing than before, joining in games with the playleader and responding with interest when a teacher showed him a computer. 'He seemed a different boy,' says Alice Wheaton, who had taken over as ward sister from Sister Mac. The games helped to pass the time during a long, rather anti-climactic week of testing. The fine weather also enabled them to escape to the local park, even if the sunshine did prompt wry reminders that this week should have been the start of their summer holidays. Instead of travelling to Cork, Mary and Danny merely commuted to and from St Pancras railway station. One of them was always with Declan but they did not want their daughter, Anna, to feel too neglected. What they still had to come to terms with, however, was the nature of the drug treatment now facing Declan. He might have passed the period of most acute difficulty, but new problems were looming.

The scale of these problems – and the nature of the drug therapy required to combat them – was established by repeating many of the tests to which Declan had been subjected before his operation. There was another insulin tolerance test, another CT scan and yet another water deprivation test. This time the effects of water deprivation were more severe: Declan became extremely thirsty and the test was cut short after he had lost seven per cent of his weight in fewer than five hours. He now had no control over his urine output, in other words total diabetes insipidus.

A new test sought to discover whether he was releasing any growth hormone; like several others this required Declan to be starved of food overnight. His urine was collected for analysis as well as being measured for volume. He was weighed daily and the detailed fluid charts were continued. The results of these tests showed that Declan lacked all the functions controlled by the pituitary gland. Without artificial hormones he would not grow or achieve the sexual changes of puberty; without drugs he would be unable to control his urine; without cortisone he would have convulsions because of low blood sugar. Without help, one way or another he would die.

'The responsibility on parents to administer the drugs properly is very considerable,' says Dr David Grant, the endocrinology consultant who took over responsibility for Declan Carroll from his surgical namesake. 'It is very important that parents know what to do if there is any drowsiness, vomiting or illness. They have to give their child extra steroids and get medical attention quickly. We have lost patients because we are so dependent upon their parents once they leave the hospital. The greatest danger is hypoglycaemia, caused by low levels of sugar in the blood which in turn occurs if patients cannot make cortisone. Therefore cortisone steroids have to be increased in times of stress such as illness or infection in order to prevent serious and possibly fatal collapse.'

The dangers are apparent from research studies into craniopharyngioma and, occasionally, on 5D itself as children return after encountering fresh problems. One study by Dr Grant and a colleague at Great Ormond Street summarized the experiences of fifty-nine patients between 1960 and 1980.* Of the fifteen children who had died, eight died unexpectedly between three months and eight years after the operation – beyond, that is, the period of so-called maximum risk. The cause of death was given variously as gastro-enteritis, lung infections or sudden collapse, but these can all produce potentially lethal hypoglycaemia. Nine other children required emergency hospital treatment because of hypoglycaemia. Poorly controlled diabetes insipidus (control of urine) was thought to have contributed to five deaths, possibly by causing a blood clot in the brain. Some of the deaths may have been unavoidable, but the authors suggest that 'inadequate homes' were responsible

---

*Other findings from the research showed the average age at time of diagnosis to be six or seven, that one in three children required more than one operation and roughly forty per cent required post-operative radiation. Improvements in surgical technique may mean that better results are now achieved. (*Archives of Diseases in Childhood*, 1982.)

for some unnecessary deaths. They conclude: 'The attendant risks of hypoglycaemia or sudden collapse place a heavy responsibility on the family and call for careful long-term medical supervision.'

The dangers of endocrine failure and the importance of reacting to symptoms of hypoglycaemia such as drowsiness and to infections are therefore hammered home to parents. One day's diarrhoea or vomiting, they are told, may mean that their child has not absorbed the drugs, rendering them vulnerable to serious, potentially irreversible collapse. If in doubt, they must seek help: phone Great Ormond Street or go to your local hospital. Sister Alice Wheaton regards reinforcing what doctors say as one of her prime duties. 'Some parents are a bit over-awed by doctors and medical terminology. I think Mr Carroll probably was, to some extent. It's our job as nurses to make sure they really understand everything. I always go through things again in simple English and tell them to write down a list of the questions they want to ask. Nothing is too silly. Then we teach them how to administer the drugs. If the child is old enough, we teach them.'

It was not just a question of the odd pill to swallow each day. When Declan Carroll went home, exactly one month after first arriving at Great Ormond Street, he took with him three separate forms of drugs – a nasal spray of DDAVP to control diabetes insipidus, hydrocortisone to replace his lack of cortisol and thyroxine to supplement the thyroid gland. These drugs had to be taken not only every day, but in some cases at particular times of the day. Even the very hour mattered at first. And everywhere Declan goes, an emergency supply of the drugs has to accompany him. He wears a Medic-Alert bracelet, just in case he is ever in an accident. As if all this were not enough, in due course growth hormone will have to be injected three times a week to make sure he grows.

'We know that he will be on medicines the rest of his life and that life will never be the same again. It is a huge responsibility but we'll learn to live with the worry about the pills. The main thing is we've still got him,' says Mary. Declan had sailed through the recovery period without many of the worst complications. The post-operative CT scan showed no evidence of any tumour so there would be no need for further surgery or radiation. His eyesight was fine, once the bruising over the right eye disappeared. Relief over Declan's progress was intensified when another child whose parents they had befriended in the hospital died after an identical operation. 'We felt terrible about this and we still keep in touch. His parents had been encouraged by how well Declan was doing, but he didn't make it. It made us realize how lucky we have been,' says Mary.

They also realized quickly how much Declan had changed. He was more alert, more daring: a promise of a new BMX bike was enough to persuade him to cast off the stabilizers from his old one. He played constantly with his sister whereas previously he had been too tired after school. Indeed, when he came home from hospital he was so active that for the first time Mary felt obliged to rein back on his energies. One problem which many parents face after the serious illness of a child is how to be caring without being over-protective. This is intensified for Mary and Danny because Declan's lack of height still leaves him vulnerable in playground rough-and-tumbles. For the first term back at school he stayed inside at playtimes – unless accompanied by a teacher or Mary – and missed some of the games lessons. A keen football fan, he was not allowed to head a ball.

Anxiety about accidental injury was a lesser worry than fear of his first illness. 'We dreaded his first cold,' says Mary. Three months after leaving Great Ormond Street, Declan was admitted to his local hospital for three days because he was vomiting his various tablets. He also had one epileptic fit, after which the Bedford hospital, in consultation with Great Ormond Street, increased his daily dose of anti-convulsant. By then the local hospital and GP had been briefed fully by Great Ormond Street about the nature of Declan's problems, and the rare drugs which he required had become familiar to an initially-bemused local chemist's shop. He would continue to visit Great Ormond Street as an out-patient where he would see not only Dr Grant but Professor Michael Preece, the head of the growth department.

On each visit he is weighed and measured with great precision by the growth department – not just overall height but sitting height since the spines of boys can grow at different rates to their legs. Folds of skin are also measured by calipers. Declan was hardly growing at all although, ironically, he was putting on weight. The somewhat gaunt youngster who had first come to Great Ormond Street was now rather plump, more a side-effect of lacking growth hormone than the result of steroids. Mary now bought clothes broad enough for an eight-year-old even though in height he was more like a short four-year-old. Dr Grant was delighted by Declan's progress, but it was clear that he would need growth hormone.

In the 1960s the then newly-established Department of Growth and Development at the Institute of Child Health adjoining Great Ormond Street became one of the first places in Britain authorized to conduct clinical trials in the use of growth hormone. As the use of the hormone was seen to be effective, the department began to acquire responsibility for some in-patients as well as rapidly expanding its out-patient clinics. Then, in 1985, doubts arose about the safety of this natural hormone when three children in the United States developed a fatal disease after being treated with it. American and British experts think that the hormone may have been contaminated, rather than being dangerous in itself. Although this was difficult to prove, the natural growth hormone, which had been obtained from bodies during post-mortems, was withdrawn.

The sudden decision dismayed parents whose children were receiving the hormone but, happily, a genetically-engineered growth hormone waited on the horizon. It would be available in time for Declan to begin his treatment eight months after his operation. Any delay is undesirable since it is hard to make up lost growth, but it would have taken around six months to establish the baseline growth pattern before treatment starts. The new artificial hormone costs three times as much as its human predecessor and in some areas of the country there have been disputes over who should foot the bill. Yet without such treatment children such as Declan could never be normal-sized adults. Without additional hormone treatment at the age of twelve or thirteen he will almost certainly be unable to enjoy ordinary puberty and a subsequent normal adult sex life.

'It is almost impossible to have had a craniopharyngioma without some endocrinological damage,' says Professor Preece. Such damage can have psychological as well as medical implications. The diagnosis and immediate treatment are shocking enough. So, too, is the burden of care entailed by life-long dependence upon various drugs. But problems of growth and puberty can pose particular stresses upon children and their families. A short child can be teased or bullied at school. This can be difficult in a primary school, but dangerous in a secondary school where the potential tormentors are so much bigger. Adolescence strains many family relations, even when there has been no disturbance to normal puberty.

Psychological stress is thus linked in varying degrees to endocrine damage. Research into craniopharyngioma in particular has shown that family life, educational attainment and adult sexual relationships can all be affected for the worse. Some of the survey samples were small and in no area was deterioration inevitable. Nevertheless one study concluded: 'The need for a craniotomy is a stressful event for anybody, especially for children or adolescent patients. Even though it is clear that in most cases there is no evidence for decrease in cognitive function, it is clear that in many patients severe emotional, social and familial problems arise or are intensified.'*

Any serious or life-threatening illness imposes (or increases) psychological stresses upon the patient, the family and those who care for them. This is why Great Ormond Street pioneered a system called the 'psycho-social round' to discuss psychological and social problems. The system began with a psychiatrist attending ward rounds on 2AB where children with complex metabolic disorders are nursed. It evolved into separate meetings to discuss non-medical matters, sometimes the work problems of staff as well as the psycho-social problems of the families. The concept was adopted by the oncology and plastic surgery wards which, like 2AB, tended to see

---

*Source: research report by Galatzer et al. in *Child: Care, Health and Development*, vol. 7 (1981).

patients frequently over long periods. Gradually, it has spread to most of the hospital, although not all wards view psycho-social meetings with equal seriousness.

Some meet for an hour or more each week, meticulously discussing each in-patient, ventilating any staff worries and thrashing out strategies for patient care; others will gather fortnightly and discuss only a few patients; a few wards go for lengthy periods without any psycho-social meetings at all. At some you will find doctors, the ward sister, other nurses, psychologist, social worker, playleader, teacher, chaplain and speech therapist. At others doctors never attend. Although some surgeons take such matters very seriously, on the whole surgeons are less likely to regard psycho-social discussions as part of their own role than physicians. Some ward sisters were also initially hesitant about the meetings, fearing that the presence of outsiders might dilute their authority. Most now welcome the meetings as an opportunity to pool information, an outlet for staff anxiety or, best of all, a means of obtaining specialist help for particular problems.

At their best, the psycho-social meetings are invaluable. For one thing, they ensure that everybody knows what's happening. Parents may talk more readily to the playleader or social worker than the 'authority' figures of doctors or sisters. Beyond the sharing of information, the meetings can help nurses understand and therefore manage patients and their families. Richard Lansdown, the chief psychologist of the hospital's Department of Psychological Medicine, sees an important role in interpreting what parents are doing or saying. 'If one can come to some understanding of why they may be rude to people, fly off the handle or go very quiet or whatever, this can help quite a lot in terms of ward management,' he maintains.

Psycho-social meetings can act as a safety-valve for staff anxieties, particularly if a ward is going through a difficult phase such as a run of deaths. Student nurses frequently find it helpful to talk about their emotional responses when confronted by parental grief. 'I always say that if they feel sad, they ought to be sad. It's not unprofessional to be sad; it's unprofessional to do your job badly. You can do your job well and still be sad. Some parents actually appreciate it if a nurse is showing some degree of emotion, providing she doesn't collapse in floods of tears,' says Richard Lansdown. Such discussions take place fairly regularly on 1B, the neurosurgical ward, but neither of the two wards where Declan stayed had well-established psycho-social meetings at that time. The sisters, social workers and psychologists say they would like the meetings to become a more regular – and prominent – feature of ward life. However, each ward has evolved its own responses to the very different problems and pressures posed by their highly-specialist areas of medicine.

For 5D the psychological and social implications of problems such as growth failure or delayed puberty are obvious – so obvious that a psychiatrist and social worker have always played a prominent role in the ward rounds and out-patients clinics of the Department of Growth and Development. But the complexity of the ward – with three consultants – has made it difficult to establish regular psycho-social meetings which would involve nursing staff in such discussions. For 1B the pressures are often more critical and immediate: many children will be diagnosed as suffering from malignant tumours from which there may be no chance of survival.

To help these families the efforts of the ward social worker, Jenny Gray, are buttressed by Jane Watson, its home liaison officer. She was ward sister until a back injury left her unable to cope with the rigours of nursing. 'I had always felt that children with cerebral-spinal malignant disease and their families do not get sufficient support. They have to go to University College Hospital for radiation but no one had any responsibility to see them through it. So I approached the nursing officer and the consultants with the idea of liaising between the two hospitals,' she says. The job has become much more than this, thanks to the commitment of time and emotional energy which Jane Watson has given. So although Jenny Gray sees the 1B families initially, Jane Watson usually becomes the prime point of contact for the families whose children are the most critically ill. Many of the children will die. She helps them to prepare for death and is sometimes with them when a child dies. 'Emotionally, it's very draining,' she admits.

Jane Watson's appointment is an undoubted success: nobody on 1B can now envisage managing without her. But her role is confined to the children with malignant tumours requiring radiation at University College Hospital. Other families will be seen by social worker Jenny Gray, but her direct involvement usually ends when the patient leaves hospital or transfers to another ward. Hospital social workers can liaise with their local counterparts, health visitors or GPs, but only if the families wish them to do so. And some families, in the euphoria of coming through a risky operation, may not always realize what still lies ahead of them.

'The diagnosis of a tumour is a very devastating and shocking event for any family,' says Jenny Gray. 'It is human nature to think that the operation to try and remove the tumour is the most important event, but post-operatively it is always a very stressful period, until parents know how their child will recover. If the child recovers well, the parents usually feel relieved, but unfortunately being diagnosed with a tumour is like beginning an obstacle course of trauma, despair, uncertainty and hope. This is often felt much more acutely by parents whose child is being transferred to another hospital for radiotherapy treatment than by those returning home.'

Originally Jane Watson's appointment was seen as an experiment, designed to pave the way for other home liaison sisters; families can be forgotten if Great Ormond Street and a local hospital each assume the other is looking after them. But plans to appoint additional home liaison sisters have fallen victim to spending cuts. With insufficient money to keep all the wards open within the hospital, this is perhaps inevitable. With few funds for community nursing in many areas it means that there can be little support for families once their child goes home. Yet although craniopharyngioma is not a malignant tumour, it is a disease with the probability of long-term medical, social and psychological consequences.

At first, Mary and Danny Carroll understandably basked in feelings of relief that Declan had avoided the worst pitfalls which await victims of craniopharyngioma. Then the scale of their own responsibility for his future care began to sink in. Mary decided to learn how to inject Declan with the growth hormone to avoid dependence upon doctors; when he is older, Declan could do it himself, much as a diabetic injects insulin. A year earlier the very thought of this would have made Mary and Danny tremble. Now they were coming to terms with unheard-of problems with quiet determination. And unlike some Great Ormond Street patients, Declan has the chance of leading a virtually normal life, albeit with the help of drugs and hormones.

'We know that he'll be on some drugs for fifteen years and others for life. We know it won't be easy and we know we'll be worried every time he is sick. We don't want to wrap him in cotton wool but one of us has to be around to keep an eye on him, just in case. The teachers at his school also know that they've got to be around. But never mind, we have got him – thanks to Great Ormond Street – and he's already a different, livelier boy. His energy wears me out,' says Mary.

Declan now scampers round the house, grinning impishly, whereas once he lay strained and exhausted on the sofa. He does not remember much about his time at Great Ormond Street, except for the injections. 'I hated them. I said I would call the police if they didn't stop,' he says. Not that he bears the nurses any grudges: each time he returns for a clinic, he always runs off to the wards to see them.

Mary and Danny are grateful that Declan does not remember much of his ordeal. It is not something that they will ever forget. But the fear of his death is receding, their new optimism crystallized in Declan's preparation to take Holy Communion: 'There was a time when we didn't think we would see that day,' says Danny. They began to look forward, rather than back, planning an Easter holiday at home to thank everybody for the messages and prayers which sustained them during their private nightmare. They wanted to show the family how well Declan now was. His hair had grown to cover the scar and he appears emotionally unscarred, too. With luck, the growth hormone will have begun to work by the time of the family reunion. 'What we're looking forward to now is to see him shoot up and slim down. He's been that height for so long,' says Danny.

So the Carrolls planned for the future – and came to terms

with its constraints. As they did so, they remembered the boy who died from craniopharyngioma when they were in Great Ormond Street. 'We thought about his family a lot on Christmas Day,' says Mary. 'We thought about what they must have been feeling on that day and we thought, we've been very lucky.'

Postscript: one year later

He has continued to do well, visiting Great Ormond Street only as an out-patient to check on the progress of his growth hormone treatment. Now full of energy, he is able to play football and all the other sports at school.

9.00 a.m. *A time for departmental meetings. In an office underneath the Department of Psychological Medicine, Donald Hooley, group supplies manager, meets his senior staff to discuss the provision of everything from paper-clips to plasters, chairs to copying machines.* Most of the items that the hospital buys come through Mr Hooley's department, including those 575,000 disposable nappies. Storage space in the wards and departments is limited so the eight storekeepers are kept busy putting together consignments for frequent deliveries around the hospital. Most of the operation is now computerized so that there is a running check on stock positions as departmental orders are processed. Not all requests will be granted, 'One department has put in an order for Anglepoise lamps,' says Mr Hooley. 'Well, unless they can convince me there's a special reason for them, they'll have to manage with the ordinary lighting like everyone else. Often departments don't know what they want, but our buyers should be able to advise them because they know what's available. It's also our job to know about things like quality, delivery, durability and maintenance costs as well as the best purchase price.'

The economics of demand and supply are not entirely absent from the weekly meeting of the radiology department under the chairmanship of Dr Isky Gordon. Radiology is a capital-intensive speciality, so much so that if the department were to be razed to the ground by fire it would cost £4 million at 1986 prices to replace all the equipment. And that was excluding the Nuclear Magnetic Resonance scanner then under construction at a cost of £1.5 million. The high costs reflect the high sophistication needed to diagnose the rare and complex illnesses frequently encountered at Great Ormond Street. Radiology plays a vital role in the diagnosis of illness whether it be based on sophisticated radio-isotopes and CT scanners or the relatively routine X-rays and ultra-sound scans. The images produced by any form of test will be the subject of a written report by one of the consultant radiologists and, where necessary, discussed informally with the appropriate clinical team. They are also reviewed at weekly meetings between the specialist medical teams and the radiologists who thus acquire their own areas of specialization. If a diagnosis is not clear, the radiologists will advise the medical teams on what, if anything, should be done next. 'There are times when we have to say that we cannot do anything more,' says Dr Gordon. 'The more unusual or difficult cases are often discussed at our own weekly meeting, but we also discuss broader questions such as how to prepare children for X-ray procedures.' By the time the meeting ends queues have begun to form for X-rays or scans as the in-patients are joined by referrals from out-patient clinics. Portable ultra-sound X-ray machines are being used in wards and operating theatres; like most of the hospital's medical support services, this is available twenty-four hours a day, seven days a week.

9.10 a.m. Betty Beech, director of nursing services, goes to see a ward sister who is today saying goodbye to a long-term patient. The child, a five-year-old boy has spent virtually his whole life on the sister's ward but is now moving to a specialized residential unit in the country. The move has taken a great deal of planning and the boy should do well there; but Betty Beech knows that the sister will be very distressed to see him go. She was a sister here herself once and has been associated with the Great Ormond Street group since 1957. She believes this background as a working nurse is essential for her present managerial role in which, in effect, she is what used to be called Matron with day-to-day responsibility for nursing care in the hospital.

Back in her office she sees a regular flow of nursing officers and grapples with the management problems of finance, space allocation, noise caused by rebuilding the cardiac block and a seemingly perpetual shortage of staff for the high-dependency nursing in the hospital. As an overall nursing manager in a hospital which is a collection of highly-specialized empires, she sometimes faces problems trying to make them converge, but says firmly: 'The specialization is good for the children and good for the ward teams.' Her worst feelings are those of frustration when she just cannot find enough nursing staff: 'Having to close wards because of lack of funds is terrible.' Often she has to ask nurses to work an extra shift or do without an extra nurse they really need. 'I go up to thank them but I know that's just a placebo – it isn't what they really need.' Yet amid the fights against cutbacks and the battles to upgrade wards and services, Betty Beech tries not to lose sight of smaller details which may help a child in hospital. Thus she will be discussing today an order for new theatre gowns; she'd like *them to be made of a print fabric which she feels would be less forbidding than the present all-white gowns.*

9.20 a.m. *A child dies on 1A, the intensive cardiac ward. It is not unexpected and the doctors and nurses have done their best to comfort the parents. The nursing staff prepare the body for the mortuary; babies are usually carried down in a nurse's arms so as not to attract undue attention. At the mortuary underneath the adjoining Department of Histopathology Ken Humphrey, the chief mortician, has already been alerted by the ward staff. If a coroner is involved in a child's death the department acts as a mortuary for a wide area of London and it is frequently involved in post-mortems either for research or at the request of the coroner. But Mr Humphrey gives a lot of his time to try and help bereaved parents. 'My role is to guide them through the formalities such as registration of a death, where to go, what forms they need and I give them advice about funeral arrangements.'*

9.30 a.m. *Anne Ralph arrives with paints, paper and crayons in the medical out-patient department. She is one of the hospital's playleaders and through the play activities which she provides she hopes to reduce the children's anxieties while they wait for their appointments. In addition to her play table there are also activities designed for older age groups, such as a snooker table, a Wendy house, slides, a rocking horse, model cars and toy garages. Toddlers (or young brothers and sisters) usually play happily but for older members of the family, waiting can be tedious. The sisters do their best to keep the appointments flowing, but it is an uphill struggle; doctors are often delayed by emergencies on wards, patients often arrive late to avoid the rush-hour and obtain cheaper fares.*

9.32 a.m. *Fire alarms sound – luckily in the old hospital building which since 1938 has been used for offices, not patients. The only patients decanted onto the pavement of Great Ormond Street therefore are those who had just arrived for the first lessons of the day at the hospital school. They join technicians, administrators, secretaries, fund-raisers, cleaners and a few doctors. Some clutch carrier-bags or files full of papers, just in case it isn't a test or false* *alarm. Dr John Wilson, the neurology consultant, is not a man to waste time; he puts his papers on a brick wall and dictates notes into a miniature tape-recorder. Five minutes later the all-clear sounds.*

9.40 a.m. *Tim Mossman answers his bleep and reports to one of the biochemistry laboratories. He is senior scientific officer in the Department of Biomedical Engineering; it means, among other things, that he's the person whom people call when machines break down. This time it is a machine used as part of a regional screening programme to detect diseases in new-born babies which is faulty. He has already been to 1A where one of the monitors was playing up and to one of the sixth-floor operating theatres where a pump wasn't working. If equipment cannot be repaired on the spot, it is taken back to his department's overflowing offices on the hospital's fourth floor. Here the engineers carry out repairs and adapt or construct equipment for paediatric use. As much as half the monitoring equipment used in wards is bought from privately-donated funds. Often parents will raise cash for specific items, but otherwise Tim Mossman will advise what can be bought for particular sums. An intravenous pump which controls infusions, for instance, costs around £1000; there are now roughly a hundred in the hospital, all fulfilling essential roles yet hardly any bought with National Health Service money.*

9.45 a.m. *Mackayla, a seventeen-month-old girl, arrives from South Wales with her parents at the genetics clinic to see Dr Michael Baraitser, the consultant. She suffers from a condition called multiple exostoses which produces lumps on her legs. It is a rare condition, seen perhaps once a year at the clinic, but one which runs in Mackayla's family – her mother and her maternal grandfather are among the sufferers. Mackayla's parents want to know the chance of any future children being similarly afflicted. It's a high risk, says Dr Baraitser. 'Anyone in the family who has got it has a fifty-fifty chance of passing it on.' But, he adds, the chance of the condition posing serious health problems is very small indeed; the lumps can be removed, which is what Mackayla's attractive mother has had done. 'There is no right or wrong decision,' Dr Baraitser tells the parents. 'In many ways if* the risk was high for a serious condition it might be easier for you to make up your mind about having another child. We never tell people what to do. All we can do is to leave you with the facts.'

Mackayla's parents were among ten families seen by Dr Baraitser during this clinic. The children ranged from a three-month-old baby to a burly eighteen-year-old. In one case a mother had miscarried a Down's Syndrome foetus and wanted advice about the likelihood of having another such child. Several of the children had rare combinations of abnormalities such as broad hands and feet, high arches, widely-spaced eyes, loose joints and arms shorter between hands and elbow than is normal. Dr Baraitser, accompanied by several colleagues, measures and examines the children. They sometimes take photographs and usually withdraw to another room to discuss their findings. For the last few years Dr Baraitser and Dr Robin Winter from Northwick Park Hospital have been building up a computer database for dysmorphic syndromes – unusual facial features or unusual combinations of malformations – to aid diagnosis. But he is still sometimes defeated by what he encounters in clinics. One such case was Jennifer, a fifteen-year-old. Her parents were not thinking of having another child; like many families who come to the twice-weekly genetics clinics, they simply wanted to know what was the problem which made their child different. Dr Baraitser could not give them a diagnosis, but said that they had excluded a large number of genetic conditions and that this should be of some comfort; it made the problem less likely to recur in Jennifer's own offspring.

One in forty children is born with some kind of abnormality. A minority of conditions or syndromes can now be detected by pre-natal screening and this area occupies much of the research effort of the genetics department. Family counselling involves detailed preparation, tracking elaborate family histories before either of the two consultants, Dr Baraitser and Dr Marcus Pembrey, are able to offer advice to families in the clinics. 'It is easy to play safe from our point of view by erring on the side of high risks,' says Dr Baraitser. 'If the parents go ahead and have a normal child, people will be delighted. But how many people will we have put off by saying the risks are high?'

10.00 a.m. *More departmental meetings. Paul Buxey, group works manager, meets his senior staff to review problems and to discuss new projects. Forty-three people are employed in the works department at Great Ormond Street, among them boilermen, plumbers, carpenters, electricians and engineers. Their work ranges from replacing light bulbs to million-pound building projects. It costs £950,000 a year just to keep the hospital and associated buildings in basic running order. The weekly departmental meeting will review the cycle of ward closures for spring-cleaning, maintenance and, if there's enough money, up-grading. It is also a time to discuss problems. A cold winter, for instance, will make it difficult to shut down any of the four boilers to carry out repairs. And if it is either too hot or too cold, there will be complaints from the wards or offices.*

Also at ten o'clock Betty Barchard, the group's chief nursing officer, meets Betty Beech, the director of nursing services. They are frequently in informal contact, but the formal meeting is a chance to take a more strategic view of problems. Usually these centre upon money – or the lack of it. For the last year or so thirty of the hospital's 333 beds have been closed because there has not been enough money to pay for nursing staff and the problem is getting worse. It is exacerbated by the trends towards more specialized and intensive nursing which require not only more nurses overall but a higher proportion of trained staff. In 1980, for instance, there were on average 124 intravenous injections to be done each day; three years later the figure was 456 and each injection can take two nurses up to twenty minutes to perform. Since then the trend has accelerated still further with sometimes more than forty patients being 'specialled' – having a nurse with them all the time, twenty-four hours a day. 'My main job is to ensure that the nursing budget is sufficient to provide the proper standard of care,' says Betty Barchard. It's a job which takes her to many committees, but she has devised her own form of therapy after particularly bureaucratic days: 'I escape to the wards.'

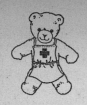

Anna

As soon as Janet Wells knew she was pregnant, she cut out her glass or two of wine at weekends and the odd cigarette after meals. The gesture was essentially symbolic. Neither of her occasional indulgences was medically significant, but Janet was taking no chances. Her first baby had been planned with care. Janet and husband Glenn had waited to start a family until they were settled into a house of their own and Janet was established as a teacher at a local school in Kent. Initially, their preparations seemed blessed by good fortune: Anna Wells was born five and a half years after her parents married and ten months after Janet came off the pill. It was an easy, happy birth. Mother and child were soon discharged home. Then their luck ran out. Within a fortnight Janet and Glenn Wells knew that their daughter had been born with cancer.

The statistics of cancer in children offer no comfort if your child is the victim. If anything, the rarity makes it more difficult to bear. On average there are around a hundred new cases a year for every million children; of these, eight will have neuroblastoma, a cancer of the nervous system. Among them was Anna. Months later Janet said: 'Just occasionally I see a pregnant woman and wonder if she'll have a healthy child. I don't wish her any ill, but I do still wonder why *me*! In retrospect we think about how much we prepared to have a baby and how we did all the supposed proper things during pregnancy, and yet this happened. It seems so unjust.'

Although cancer is rare in children, it now causes more deaths between one and fourteen years of age than any other illness because deaths from fatal illnesses such as polio and diphtheria have declined. Yet the outlook for children discovered to have cancer has improved substantially over the last twenty years. Doctors prefer to talk about survival rates rather than 'cures', if only because it will take a generation or more to measure the long-term effects of current treatment.

But just over half the children suffering from cancer can now expect to live for more than five years after diagnosis. This overall figure, however, disguises significant differences in survival rates for different forms of cancer – from eighty per cent for Wilms' tumour to fifteen per cent to acute myeloid leukaemia. And among the cancers with the bleakest prognosis is the form diagnosed in three-week-old Anna Wells – neuroblastoma. Here the average survival figure is just twenty-five per cent. Or, to put it in more human terms, just one child in four will be alive five years after diagnosis.

New procedures at Great Ormond Street would boost Anna's chances to fifty-fifty, perhaps slightly more. But the road to the Hospital for Sick Children was a bumpy one for her parents, even after the initial shock of learning that their baby had cancer; like most people, they scarcely knew that babies could have cancer. Events propelled them from hope to fear with unnerving speed. At Great Ormond Street, for instance, Anna was to develop a rare complication which perturbed – and baffled – the specialists, threatening her life and causing her stay to extend beyond that of any other comparable patient. It was not exactly the childhood envisaged in the plans laid so meticulously and lovingly by her parents.

Janet and Glenn Wells live in Staplehurst, a village straddling a main road south of Maidstone in Kent. She teaches in the local primary school, he works as an engineer for British Telecom. They are a contrasting couple whose temperaments would complement each other well in the ordeal which awaited them. Janet was twenty-eight when Anna was born, a tall, slender woman with shoulder-length brown hair who regards herself as a bit of a worrier yet who, to others, seems enviably calm and thoughtful. Glenn is two years older, a burly man well suited physically to the centre-back's position he occupies in a village football team. He is more of an extrovert than his wife, blunter and decisive where Janet will want to talk things through. 'It rarely happens that we're both down at the same time,' says Glenn. 'In fact, we try to pull each other up. But if I'm down, I tend to react by being a bit sharp whereas Janet has a more caring attitude. You could say it starts from me being not particularly romantic.'

Certainly their first meeting was not romantic. Glenn was a friend of one of Janet's flat-mates when she was at a teacher's training college in south-west London. She says: 'Usually when you meet someone for the first time, you make a special effort. But Glenn had seen me wandering about the flat with my hair in a mess for a long time before we ever went out with each other. He was a friend first.' She had been brought up in Hertfordshire, north of the capital, whereas Glenn is much more of a Londoner. He was born in Edmonton and still follows the fortunes of the local team, Tottenham Hotspurs, with a true fan's fervour. They moved to Kent when Janet, having spent one summer as an airline stewardess, was offered a job as a teacher in Maidstone. It was what she had always wanted to do.

By the time Anna was born Janet had moved to a school in the village of Staplehurst, nine miles south of Maidstone. She and Glenn bought a house on a new estate just off the main road to Hastings. It was a quiet and prosperous corner of England in which to establish roots: they were surrounded by pleasant countryside, the coast was half an hour away, London and their families less than two hours. It all seemed too good to be true, especially when Janet conceived within a month of coming off the pill. She continued working until she was six months pregnant and took maternity leave so that she could return to the classroom a year later. Physically, the pregnancy was uneventful but Glenn says they both worried a lot: 'We had planned it so much, when we'd have this baby, that our worry was that something would be wrong.'

At the time they put it down to the normal anxiety of a couple awaiting their first child. Certainly their fears appeared groundless when, at noon on 2 April 1984, Anna was born at Maidstone General Hospital. She weighed 3.6 kilos (a fraction under eight pounds) and it was, Janet recalls, a 'marvellous, fantastic' moment. She looked well, a little pale and sleepier than most babies, perhaps, but nothing to prevent her return home. 'I had no reason to suppose that the baby wasn't all right. I hadn't had another baby to judge her by. She seemed extremely content, still sleeping a lot but quite alert in her waking times. The first noticeable sign that something might be wrong was after about a fortnight when she began to flop half way through a feed, slightly breathless. Then a pot tummy began to develop. At first we didn't think anything more of it but then, at two and a half weeks, veins were appearing in the tummy and it was getting very big. It all developed very quickly, just a matter of days,' says Janet.

Within hours of taking Anna to the local health clinic (where she was due for a routine check) Janet had been referred first to her general practitioner and then to a hospital at Pembury, twelve miles away near Tunbridge Wells. Anna was three weeks old. She immediately began an intensive round of tests. Temperature, pulse and breathing were normal. So, too, were a bone scan and chest X-ray. But an X-ray of her abdomen revealed a greatly enlarged liver and spleen. Pembury's provisional diagnosis was a liver disease. Blood samples were taken to test how the liver was working, but before the results were complete Anna was on the move again – to the larger King's College Hospital in the London borough of Southwark.

She had been at Pembury for just two days. They were two days in which the lives of her parents were turned upside down. Days when puzzlement about a large tummy was transformed into fear that Anna might not survive at all. The first hint of the seriousness of Anna's condition was the X-ray technician saying: 'I'm going to special care with this.' Then came the dreaded words from a doctor: 'Would you like to sit down?' Glenn, characteristically blunt, asked the doctor if they should prepare themselves for the worst: 'I expected him to say no, it's not that bad, but he didn't – he said yes.' It was the only time in Anna's life when Janet avoided contact with her, as if to insulate herself from too much grief should the worst indeed happen. 'The day that we were told I didn't want to go and see her at all,' she says. 'It had become a nightmare.' The one consolation for Janet and Glenn was their own closeness and the support of their families. Janet's sister, Helen, had arrived with her two sons just before Anna was rushed to Pembury. She shared the trauma from the start and, along with both sets of grandparents, stayed in constant touch throughout.

Anna was transferred to King's because only a large hospital would have the facilities to undertake the wide range of tests required to confirm the Pembury diagnosis or to produce an alternative. All this time Anna's stomach was continuing to grow. When she arrived at King's her girth measured forty-three centimetres or 16.93 inches. She needed outfits designed for ten-month-old children, although their dangling legs and arms were twice the length of Anna's own limbs. Of the many tests to which Anna was subjected two were crucial. The first was an ultrasound 'scan' of her abdomen, similar to the kind undergone by many women in pregnancy; the 'mixed echoes' it produced suggested a tumour might be causing the swollen liver and spleen. The second key test was to establish the level of Vanillyl Mandelic Acid (VMA) in the urine; in Anna's case, this was twice the normal level. The two tests brought a new diagnosis – neuroblastoma. A biopsy of the liver, in which a sample of the liver tissue is extracted under anaesthetic by a needle for laboratory examination, confirmed the diagnosis. Anna had cancer.

A tumour is literally a swelling but it is usually taken to mean a lump caused by a collection of cells. There are two types of tumour – benign and malignant. The latter are cancerous because they not only invade and destroy the tissues in which they arise but are also capable of producing secondary growths away from the original or primary tumour. Three possible forms of tumour had been mentioned to Janet and Glenn shortly after Anna arrived from Pembury. Yet the precise diagnosis – a kind of neuroblastoma known as stage 4S – was presented as not only the best of the three but potentially better news than prolonged liver disease.

Neuroblastoma develops in the nerve cells which run from the abdomen to the skull along the line of the spinal cord. It is overwhelmingly confined to children, just as stage 4S neuroblastoma almost always occurs only in children under six months old. Unlike all other forms of neuroblastoma, a 4S tumour usually disperses spontaneously without any intensive treatment with drugs. A week earlier neuroblastoma in any form would have shattered Anna's parents, not that they had ever heard of it. Now, reacting to the curious way that hospitals distort the values of the outside world, they were elated. 'We were quite singing,' says Janet. 'We'd lived through the news of a liver disease, and what that might entail in terms of four-hourly feeding and weekly hospital visits stretching before us for years. Then it was a liver tumour, one of three possibilities, and we'd got the best of the bunch. If the consultants tell you it's good news or better news, you believe them.'

In Mountbatten ward, though, Anna was less happy. The doctors wanted to let the growth of the liver continue naturally until the tumour exhausted itself. But as the liver continued to grow – her girth increased to fifty-two centimetres – this put pressure on her diaphragm, causing her to breathe in short, uncomfortable gasps. She was given oxygen as well as vitamins and blood plasma. The swollen liver was also pressing on her stomach, making it difficult for her to eat more than two tea-spoonfuls of feeds at a time. The deterioration in Anna's condition prompted talk of a pressure-relieving operation which would allow her liver to expand into a bag outside the body until it began to shrink in size.

This unappealing prospect helped to reconcile Janet and Glenn to a ten-day course of radiation on her abdomen in the hope that X-rays would attack the tumour. Radiation is not universally accepted by doctors as a proven benefit but, coincidentally or not, Anna's stomach began to decrease after the radiotherapy. She had survived her first crisis – so, too, had her parents. Janet lived in King's with Anna throughout her stay. Her feeling of rejection, experienced fleetingly at Pembury, was swiftly forgotten: 'I was very positive because I felt the doctors had answers – they knew what it was and how to deal with it.' She was to learn, however, that there are few certainties with illnesses as rare as neuroblastoma.

After seven weeks in King's, Anna went home. She had just started to smile and for the next ten months she gave her parents and doctors much to smile about. 'This beautiful little girl' (as one registrar wrote after a check-up) became a model patient. Out-patient visits passed uneventfully, even encouragingly. Anna's stomach continued to shrink and the various tests showed no fresh signs of disease. She was feeding well and put on weight steadily. Janet still found it difficult to relax totally; many first-time mums become anxious about the responsibility of motherhood and Janet had more to worry about than most.

Looking after your own, sick child, she found, is very different from a class of thirty, however skilled you are as a teacher. But a tendency to worry is not Janet's sole or predominant trait: she is also practical and positive. She kept a diary of Anna's diet to help her concentrate and to keep herself occupied. She told herself that it was silly to worry unduly: if the doctors were happy, why shouldn't she be pleased?

At six months Anna began to sit up, at eight months she was crawling. All seemed decidedly normal and so, after the autumn half-term holiday and when Anna was seven months old, Janet went back to work. She was just in time to organize her school's Christmas play, something she would miss one year later. 'It was always my intention to try and carry on working, while keeping an open mind about whether or not it would work – for either of us,' she said. 'In fact, we found it worked really well from day one.' Anna spent the days with a neighbour, Penny, who soon became more of a friend than a child-minder. Janet and Glenn began to settle into a routine. He started work at eight o'clock so that he could finish at four in time to meet Janet from school. Then they'd both go and collect Anna. One hurdle remained to be cleared before Anna could be regarded as 'cured': a liver biopsy roughly one year after the initial diagnosis of cancer. For this she would return, briefly, to King's as an in-patient. A date was set eight days after Anna's first birthday.

'We were obviously anxious about the biopsy. When it was getting near I noticed, as she sat in her chair in the kitchen, that her left eye didn't look right. It was squinting and the lid was heavy. We couldn't believe it, two weeks before this appointment after being so well, but I certainly didn't link it with anything being wrong. I groaned and thought "Oh dear, that's another thing she's got to go through, to get her eye put right". But it turned out to be the first signal.'

Another sign that all was not well was a slight nose-bleed from her left nostril. Neither problem dimmed the welcome Anna received when she returned for her biopsy. 'Here's our star patient,' said one nurse. Her pallor had gone and she displayed no signs of any liver disease. Cardiac and respiratory systems were normal. The biopsy was performed under local anaesthetic, but the results would take some days to come through. Just one abnormality was detected upon examination – slight swelling and bruising on the left-hand side of the face. A skull X-ray showed nothing amiss, but Janet had reported the apparent squint and the nose-bleeds so an ophthalmologist (an eye specialist) was called in. He examined Anna and found that, although her vision was normal, the globe of her left eye was slightly higher than the right. The ophthalmologist thought there could be an obstruction under the eye which was lifting the eye upwards and forwards. In order to establish this one way or the other Anna needed a CT scan – a technique which involves a narrow beam of X-rays being directed through the head from a succession of positions. A computer produces an image which indicates the differing pathologies of, say, brain, skull and tumour as well as their location.*

At that time King's did not have its own scanner, so Anna went to the fourth hospital which had figured in her short life – Guy's Hospital near London Bridge. Here, the CT scan provided incontrovertible evidence that the ophthalmologist's fears were justified. The 'obstruction' pushing the left eye upwards was a tumour. It was on what is known as the left orbit – the socket containing the eye, close to the left nasal cavity. The good news was that the brain was normal; the bad news was that the neuroblastoma had not merely failed to disappear spontaneously but had spread. Anna was one of the minority of 4S neuroblastoma patients whose disease progresses to stage 4. The consequences for Anna Wells were sombre: her chances of surviving until she was six years old were now reduced to one in four, perhaps one in three.

Janet and Glenn were initially unaware of this grim prognosis. But they were told it would be better if Anna was now referred to the Hospital for Sick Children in Great Ormond Street. Despite its world renown, parents are not necessarily overjoyed by such news. In time most come to be grateful to the skills and commitment of the staff; many parents devote much of their time to raising funds for the hospital. But at the time of their first visit fear and anxiety usually predominate.

_____

*See pages 35-6 for more on CT scans.

As in Anna's case, they have probably been referred to Great Ormond Street because their child is seriously ill. This is cause enough for worry, even without the problem of adjusting to yet another hospital. 'My heart sank at the news, to be honest,' says Janet Wells. 'I would have preferred to stay at King's where we knew the people.'

Anna was transferred to Great Ormond Street because it is a specialist centre for childhood cancer – one of twenty in the United Kingdom Children's Cancer Study Group. The centres co-operate closely so that treatment 'protocols' are based on the experiences of patients in every centre rather than simply those in one hospital. The collaboration needs to be close since the boundaries between treatment and research are often blurred. Survival rates have improved dramatically, but many forms of treatment remain experimental. Anna Wells, for instance, would benefit from one research project which was still in progress when she first arrived at Great Ormond Street.

Anna was admitted to ward 3AB – two adjoining ten-bedded wards staffed by the same team of nurses and therefore regarded as a single medical unit. It is here that most of the children suffering from leukaemia and other forms of cancer are treated. Even for parents like Janet and Glenn Wells who knew their child had cancer the ward can provide something of a shock. Virtually all the children are bald – a side-effect of one of the drugs used to combat the disease. Most have tubes leading from their bodies to 'drip' stands from which bags of liquid drugs or blood are pumped via machines which flash lights and occasionally bleep. Everywhere these children go, the drip stands will be wheeled beside them. Not all the children, though, will be well enough to leave their beds. A few will be feeling sick, another side-effect of drugs. Others will be crying – so, at times, will some parents. The ward is noisy, cluttered with equipment and crowded with people. Even if you have been told all this, the first sight of 3AB can still be a shock, as Ian Botham discovered when he visited the ward before his epic walk from John O'Groats to Land's End.

The ward is widely regarded within the hospital as a difficult one. Nurses on other wards talk about the pressures of knowing that on average half the children they care for will die. And yet it is also a friendly, even happy ward – once you overcome the initial shock. It closes round the parents and becomes a world where others understand their anguish. In the world outside, parents often feel alone, forced to cope with an illness which not even their local GP will know much about. Here there are not only specialists but other parents to provide companionship and support. The ward policy treats parents as part of 'the team' and their frequent visits for different phases of treatment establish them on first-name terms with the staff. 'At first you don't think you'll ever laugh or smile again,' said one father. 'You can't understand how the other parents can be joking with each other and the staff. But as you get to know people and come to terms with the situation, you realize that it helps keep you going. Life has to go on.'

A patient as young as Anna Wells is perhaps lucky. She will be unaware of the trauma endured by her parents. Anna settled quickly and happily into one of the four individual cubicles which were then on each ward. 'A delightful child – alert, lively and interested,' wrote one of the doctors after the initial examination. Janet slept in the cubicle with her while the doctors began an exhaustive series of tests. These were intended more to assess the stage of the disease than to confirm the diagnosis of neuroblastoma; this would be crucial in determining the form and length of treatment. But even before the tests were completed Janet and Glenn were left in no doubt that the diagnosis was much more serious than they had anticipated.

Candour is a hallmark of Great Ormond Street. The side-effects, the risks and the chances of survival are invariably spelt out with numbing frankness. Parents often find this unnerving, even brutal, but most come to appreciate the openness; it establishes credibility and trust. What parents tend to find more frightening is the discovery that on many occasions even these doctors – specialists at one of the most famous children's hospitals in the world – do not have answers. 'Everything was "if" or "might be". It was always "we are trying this",' recalls Janet Wells. Many illnesses are too rare for certainty: doctors are frequently working at the frontiers of medical knowledge. This is one reason why the hospital is linked to a research centre, the Institute for Child Health, which is part of London University. Many doctors have dual responsibilities – for patients in the hospital and research in the Institute. Among them is Dr Jon Pritchard, the oncology consultant who was in charge of Anna Wells.

Jon Pritchard is a softly-spoken, rather intense figure whose charm is matched only by a reputation for taking endless time with parents; hospital porters who log consultants in and out of the main entrance each evening say that Jon Pritchard or Mike Dillon, the renal consultant, are invariably the last to leave. Like many specialists at Great Ormond Street, Dr Pritchard has a worldwide reputation in his field – not that you would know this from his poky office. (Visitors from abroad are generally amazed by the conditions in which this renowned hospital and its staff function. Jon Pritchard's office is not conspicuously worse than most and better than some. At least he does have a room to himself, however antiquated and inadequate it might be; Dr Dillon shares a smaller room with two other consultants.)

Jon Pritchard became interested in oncology (the study of cancer) when working as a general paediatric registrar at the Alder Hey Hospital in Liverpool in the 1970s. 'I came to realize that cancer was a relatively common cause of death but that not much seemed to be available in terms of treatment,' he says. 'It's still a bogey word. Most people who come here have never heard of anything but leukaemia.' Dr Pritchard joined Great Ormond Street initially as a lecturer in haematology but as the case load increased he became a consultant in 1978 at the age of thirty-five. He took over the responsibility for oncology which enabled the existing haematology consultant, Dr Judith Chessells, to concentrate on the leukaemia patients. They were later joined by a third consultant, Dr Hilary Blacklock, who is responsible for the bone marrow transplant programme and who was to play a significant role in Anna's story.

Dr Pritchard's appointment coincided with significant changes in the treatment of childhood cancer. Until the 1960s, surgery and radiotherapy were the only available options. Both are still used. But many tumours cannot be removed by surgery without damaging other vital organs. Or the cancer may simply have spread to too many places to be cured by one-off excision. Radiation is similarly limited to specific sites and can also cause damage unless it is strictly controlled. During the 1960s doctors therefore began to combat cancer with drugs which would circulate throughout the body, attacking tumour cells wherever they might have spread. At first the drugs were used separately but later, as two in particular were seen to have an effect, they were tried in combination; it was the beginning of the form of treatment now known as chemotherapy.

Other drugs were tried and a third was added to the cocktail. Progress was slow, however, and for many tumours 'success' was initially measured in months rather than years of life. Then, in the late 1970s, a drug called cis-platinum was shown to be active against many cancers. There were now four drugs and in 1979 these were put together to form the basic treatment of the 1980s which is known by the acronym OPEC. This OPEC has nothing to do with oil; it originates simply from the first letter of each of the four drugs within the treatment protocol.

Chemotherapy has significantly improved the survival chances of many children with cancer. Some cancers, notably forms of leukaemia, are treated with chemotherapy alone whereas for others, such as Wilms' tumour, it is used to attack secondary deposits after the primary tumour has been removed by surgery. The results are impressive, but they have not been achieved without some cost. The drugs have to be very powerful in order to have any effect on the cancer cells and, unfortunately, they also act against other healthy parts of the body. Cis-platinum will damage the kidneys and hearing unless it is strictly monitored; other drugs will almost certainly cause vomiting and the loss of hair. The baldness is temporary but it makes many children (and parents) acutely self-conscious. Another temporary side-effect can be more serious. The anti-cancer drugs affect the white blood cells reducing the body's ability to fight off infections; measles or chicken-pox caught at that stage of treatment can be fatal. In the longer term there are also doubts about future fertility, but most parents have more immediate concerns, particularly if their child suffers from a form of cancer more resistant to chemotherapy. Among these is the cancer afflicting Anna Wells – neuroblastoma.

The initial diagnosis of neuroblastoma had been indicated by the higher levels of Vanillyl Mandelic Acid (VMA) in the urine and confirmed by a biopsy. This enables internal cell tissue – sometimes including a sample of the tumour itself – to be extracted and thinly sliced for examination under the microscope; pathologists can then interpret certain cell structures or patterns as characteristic of specific diseases. But as well as occurring at different parts of the body, neuroblastoma can exist in differing degrees or stages of severity. Basically, the staging of the disease is determined by the number of organs affected by tumours. Patients are therefore subjected to a series of tests to establish the stage of the neuroblastoma since this will determine the form of treatment. These tests also establish a base line upon which to judge whether or not a patient is responding to treatment.

Blood samples are analysed to provide a 'count' of different types of cells. A radio-opaque dye is injected into a vein so that bone scans will reveal any secondary tumours. An ultra-sound scan, similar to those often undergone in pregnancy, can be another useful test. And the bone marrow, from where the body derives its blood cells, is checked for the presence of cancer cells. Not all the tests undertaken on Anna Wells were discouraging. No tumour cells could be seen in the bones, skin or the bone marrow. But the evidence of the CT scan – which was shown to Anna's parents at Great Ormond Street – was conclusive. Anna's stage 4S version of the disease had not disappeared spontaneously as happens in roughly three cases out of four. Why this sometimes happens, nobody knows – no more than anybody yet knows why or how neuroblastoma occurs at all.

What Jon Pritchard and his colleagues did know was that Anna was now suffering from the more aggressive stage 4 neuroblastoma. This means that the original primary tumour, which had caused her liver to expand, had spread and could be expected to spread again without intensive treatment. Usually there is more than one secondary tumour. There was no sign of this in Anna so there was a possibility that the new tumour might be treated locally. However, the location of the new tumour adjacent to the eye made surgery virtually impossible and radiation a hazardous option. Experience in any case told Jon Pritchard that the odds were against secondary tumours being confined to one place. 'We decided to work on the assumption that there were other tumours, as yet undetected,' he said.

For Anna therefore it would be chemotherapy alone, to be administered in a series of perhaps eight courses. At the time this was about the average number of courses*; six tended to be the minimum to have any effect, ten the maximum without causing excessive damage to the kidneys or hearing. In Anna's case the doctors had one other procedure at the back of their minds: a final dose of an exceptionally powerful drug called melphalan combined with a form of bone marrow transplant. A research programme into the effects of these procedures would produce interim results by the autumn. In a summary of Anna's case written on 1 May – eight days after arrival at Great Ormond Street – her chances of surviving for five years were put 'in the region of thirty per cent'. Anna's parents, the summary added, were 'extremely shocked'. Janet remembers their feelings with stark clarity:

'I felt resentment, almost, when the doctors here told us that the outlook was far worse than we had been led to believe. I felt – how do you know? How can you be sure? We were told they would have to run tests to find where else the cancer might be because it was unusual if it was just in the head. They suspected it might be elsewhere in the bone or bone marrow. The news seemed to get worse and worse. Slightly above average chance of a cure, said Jon Pritchard. Which was really good, a lot better news than some people get, but still a bigger blow to us than we'd been expecting. We had in our minds a definite cure before we came here, just a bit of a nuisance having to have more drugs but no question about whether she would live or die. Now it was *if* she gets over this hurdle, then you might keep her, but if not, it's bad news I'm afraid. If she

---

*Treatment of cancer is still evolving. A few months after Anna's chemotherapy, a shorter but more intensive 'protocol' was introduced at Great Ormond Street based on research evidence from overseas.

didn't respond to treatment, we were talking about a fatal situation.

'It is weird coming to terms with cancer in children at all. Yet we had a pleasant picture painted for us for a year with talk about a ninety or ninety-five per cent chance of a cure. Then we were hit with a wallop of bad news. We lived with the illness for a year but we had thought the really grim part was over. Through all the check-ups it looked so good. Now it was a question of whether we were going to have Anna alive or not. A cure seemed much less likely. It was an incredible shock and scared us a lot, but in retrospect we were very pleased they did tell us everything. Psychologically we could give ourselves a bottom line. It would be easier to live with things getting better than to have false hopes.'

Within a fortnight Janet and Glenn had gone from optimism to despair. It was the lowest of low points. They tried to rally their spirits by looking forwards rather than backwards to hopes which had been dashed. Janet, priding herself on being 'sensible', devoured books to find out as much information as possible about childhood cancer. Their positive approach received its greatest boost by the way in which Anna responded to treatment. 'All those feelings of resentment towards the doctors went as soon as Anna's treatment seemed to be working. But initially you've got to take it out on somebody,' says Janet.

Parents react differently to the trauma of having a child who is critically, possibly fatally ill. Some will find solace in religion and many turn, in desperation, to faith-healers. But for others, like Glenn Wells, illness shatters all faith: 'If you look around 3AB, you think that if there is someone up there, He's not doing a very good job.' General practitioners are frequently blamed for failing to recognize warning signs. This is often unfair – childhood cancer is so rare that a GP may never encounter it and many symptoms can be those of less serious childhood illnesses – but, as Janet Wells said, parents have got to take it out on somebody. Sometimes, they take it out on each other – blaming the other side of the family for 'causing' the illness – although Dr Pritchard tries to convince them that this, too, is unjust. The pressures on parents (and marriages) are immense, however rational and resilient they might be normally. What is remarkable – and humbling – is that most cope so well with problems which are unimaginable to anyone who has not known and loved a potentially dying child.

Richard Lansdown is the psychologist attached to ward 3AB. He says: 'I've been struck by the extent to which the same kinds of problems arise for 3AB parents. What's different is the way people cope with them. The overwhelming problem is uncertainty. That screams out at you – parents often say: "It would be so much easier if I knew he or she was going to die, but I don't." Another problem is isolation. This is partly because parents are so wrapped up in their problems that for many of them the hospital becomes the centre of their life. So what was the centre of their life – their family, their locality, their church, their club or whatever – isn't any more and so they cut themselves off from other people. One father said to me: "I get cross when people ask me how my daughter is and I get cross when they don't ask me." He was so wrapped up with his daughter that he couldn't really cope with other people. Whatever they said was wrong. So people cut themselves off and also, of course, the public cut themselves off from our parents because there is so much anxiety about cancer and leukaemia. People shuffle their feet and don't know how to speak or what to say.

'A third common problem, which is not only for 3AB parents but many others, is the danger of overlooking the sibling so they get left out. "I am sick and tired of making allowances for my sister," one girl said. "Why doesn't someone make allowances for me?" This is associated with the danger of spoiling the sick child. Again it's something parents know about, but which they find very difficult to do anything about. This doesn't apply just to 3AB parents, of course.

'Then there's anger which seems to me to come through more strongly than guilt. Sometimes it's anger at themselves – why didn't I take him to the doctor sooner? – although this could be transferred guilt. Sometimes it's anger at a doctor. Sometimes with their husband or wife. Sometimes it's with God. There's an awful lot of anger around. A further generalization is that parents often feel de-skilled. One day they were mother and father of a child and they were entirely responsible for the child, apart from education. The next day the child is being looked after by nurses and doctors and the parents are visitors to the hospital. Their skills as parents are no longer important. This is one reason why we have parents in the hospital doing so much for their kids.'

Janet Wells was one of about 125 parents resident in the hospital on Anna's first night at Great Ormond Street. Some were in rooms above the chapel in the old hospital building, some in four-bedded rooms on the main block's fifth floor, some on camp beds in waiting-rooms, some in waiting rooms and some, like Janet, in cubicles on wards alongside their child. Nobody pretends that the accommodation is adequate, let alone comfortable. But Great Ormond Street had never been designed for parents. Even visiting was restricted when the main hospital block opened in 1938.*

Although Janet and Glenn Wells did not have another child to care for, they did both have jobs. When Anna had first been unwell, Janet had still been on maternity leave. But now she was a working woman again. As the Great Ormond Street prognosis sank in, Janet's first instinct was to give up her job. All the things which had once been important to her (and Glenn) no longer seemed to matter. 'Anna's illness changed us fundamentally inasmuch as we are no longer at all materialistic. Where we used to plan everything, we now live from day to day. Every day must be enjoyed,' she says.

However, the pessimism – or realism – that underlay this new-found hedonism was also an argument to retain her job, if possible. If she quit and Anna were to die, Janet would have lost both her daughter and her livelihood. Her ability to carry on teaching would obviously be affected by Anna's progress, but it was aided by the nature of the treatment. Chemotherapy is administered in a series of courses lasting anything between three days and a fortnight. It is not always necessary for each of these courses to be carried out at Great Ormond Street or any of the other specialist cancer centres in Britain. Alternate

---

*See Kristie's story for more about parents' accommodation.

courses can be provided by local hospitals following drug protocols laid down by Great Ormond Street. Such 'shared care' is
virtually essential, given the pressure on the twenty beds of
ward 3AB. It was also the means which enabled Janet Wells to
keep working, at least for a while. Alternate courses of Anna's
chemotherapy would be administered at her local hospital,
Maidstone General, where Janet would sleep and from where
she commuted to and from school while her own mother stayed
with Anna during the day.

The chemotherapy began even before the initial tests were
completed. The various drugs were infused via a vein into her
foot. She was sick three times after the cis-platinum and had
two nose-bleeds, but otherwise remained cheerful – so lively, in
fact, that a nurse noted: 'Anna is very lively so the IV (intravenous) line is very likely to be pulled out and needs looking at
every hour.' It established a pattern which would be followed
for each of Anna's four courses of chemotherapy at Great
Ormond Street during the summer. Janet stayed with Anna,
sometimes in a cubicle, sometimes in one of the parents' rooms
scattered around the hospital. Only the cis-platinum ever
caused any distress, although Anna (like most children) cried
when doctors took blood samples from her veins. Anna was too
young to be affected by the sudden loss of her brown hair and
the nursing notes are sprinkled with remarks about her 'cheerful' manner. Janet, too, was feeling more cheerful – partly
because she fought depression by keeping busy but mainly
because Anna's progress was encouraging.

Initially, this was because things did not get worse. When
Anna returned to Great Ormond Street in June, an ophthalmic
registrar could detect no deterioration since the original examination six weeks earlier. In July the ophthalmic specialist
was talking about an improvement; by October vision was
judged to be normal in each eye, with perhaps a small
squint to be followed up locally. A CT scan in July was
equally bullish. This ws examine in the regular meeting on
Thursday afternoons at which the radiologists discuss their
findings with the oncology team. Their verdict on Anna:
'no apparent orbital deposit'. Bones and the bone marrow
were checked – since this is where neuroblastoma most

commonly spreads – but were clear of cancer cells.

The chemotherapy was evidently working and the prime worry for Dr Pritchard and his team from the battery of tests performed on Anna was that her kidneys were no longer working at full efficiency. This side-effect of the drugs confined the chemotherapy courses to eight and would later reduce the dosage of the high-intensity drug called melphalan. 'We obviously don't want to convert her from a child who has neuroblastoma to a child who needs a kidney transplant,' says Dr Pritchard. Nevertheless Anna was withstanding the chemotherapy better than many children and her chances of five-year survival were edging up from one in three or four to one in two. The worst option facing her parents – that Anna would fail to respond to treatment at all – had been overcome. They had cleared the first hurdle faced by all parents of children with cancer: Anna was in 'remission'.

This means there is no clinical evidence of cancer remaining within the patient and he or she can be discharged from hospital. Yet this very moment of success is also, cruelly, when they learn to dread another word – 'relapse' or the moment when a patient is hit by a recurrence of the disease. Fear of relapse comes to haunt all parents – and children – because if, or when, it occurs there is as yet no treatment to stave off death. The tension is almost palpable when families return to hospital as out-patients for check-ups. They sit and wait while blood tests are done which will determine whether or not their child remains free from disease and perhaps alive.

Janet and Glenn Wells were already learning to live with the fear of death. It wasn't easy and for a time Janet began to suspect that she, too, was suffering from cancer. She found it helped that she had a life beyond that of being simply Anna's mum. Or, at least, she did at Maidstone where she would arrive in the evenings laden down with books to mark or work to prepare for the next day's classes. They were sustained not merely by their own closeness – 'We always talked a lot when things were bad,' says Glenn – but by friends and family. 'There was never any embarrassment over Anna having cancer,' says Janet. 'People always wanted to know how she was. They would stop me in the street and ask. Sometimes it would take forty-five minutes just to go down the road to the shops.'

The summer passed with visits to Great Ormond Street or Maidstone every two or three weeks. There was no possibility of a holiday and even a few days in Bath with Janet's parents were marred when Anna developed a high temperature. Mostly, however, Anna appeared very well. She walked at thirteen months and began to acquire a vocabulary which startled hospital staff. How many other eighteen-month-old children could remember doctors' names or identify a stethoscope? How many other children, though, would have had so much opportunity to acquire such medical terms? And although her courses of chemotherapy were drawing to a close, Anna had not seen the last of hospitals. Her longest and most perilous admission was about to begin.

For three years a European study had been in progress to compare the effects of two forms of treatment for neuroblastoma. Half the children had been treated with OPEC chemotherapy, half with OPEC plus a final dose of a drug called melphalan. In October 1985, just as Anna was completing her eighth and final course of OPEC, members of the European Neuroblastoma Study Group met in Venice to consider the preliminary results of the study. The Group was at that stage run from Great Ormond Street and one of its leading members was Dr Jon Pritchard. He says: 'It seems that OPEC is better than the previous form of chemotherapy but that the high-dose melphalan patients are doing significantly better compared to those who had no further treatment after OPEC.'

The rationale of melphalan is that it is an extremely powerful drug which mops up any cancer cells which remain at the conclusion of normal chemotherapy. For even when a patient shows no sign of the disease – as in the case of Anna Wells – doctors can never be a hundred per cent sure that *all* the cancer cells have been destroyed. This 'belt and braces' policy was explained to Janet and Glenn Wells one Saturday morning in October when they drove to London to discuss Anna's future treatment with Dr Pritchard. If they agreed, Anna could be the first Great Ormond Street patient to benefit from the new policy under which all neuroblastoma patients achieving remission will be offered the additional course of melphalan. Previously, in the interests of research into a then unproven hypothesis, she would have had only a one-in-two chance of being offered melphalan. Now, said Dr Pritchard, it had been established that melphalan improves chances of survival by around two years. There were, however, some snags.

Melphalan is a powerful drug given in a single, large dose which can cause prolonged sickness and painful mouth sores. These can be unpleasant enough, but melphalan also attacks the bone marrow, a soft substance inside the larger bones where the body manufactures its blood cells. These cells provide crucial defences for the body against infections and bleeding, yet so devastating is the effect of melphalan that it erodes the ability of the bone marrow to produce cells for six to eight weeks. During this time patients are acutely vulnerable to potentially fatal complications. In order to minimize the period of greatest risk, patients at Great Ormond Street now have some of their bone marrow removed before the melphalan is administered. It is given back to them the next day after melphalan has been flushed through the system. In theory, this procedure – known as a bone marrow autograft, not a transplant from one patient to another – should reduce the period of low blood counts to between two and four weeks. 'It is not in itself a treatment,' says Dr Pritchard. 'It's a rescue procedure.'

So the hazards as well as the benefits were spelled out for Janet and Glenn Wells. The extent to which parents are left to make decisions is a delicate one. In Anna's case the potential gains seemed well worth the risks to her parents. But it is not always so clear-cut. At what point do parents decide their child has suffered enough? If chemotherapy has failed to get a response, should parents let doctors try unproven drugs? How can parents choose if, as happened in one case, one option would leave their son sterile and the other leave him impotent? Parents will vary in their desire to take such daunting decisions and Jon Pritchard, himself the father of two teenage children, tries to protect them from subsequent anguish:

'You try not to make them feel that they are actually taking the responsibility of deciding because they might afterwards wonder whether their decision was the correct one and blame themselves if their child dies. I often use the phrase: "If it were my child . . ." This makes it clear that you mean what you say. But effectively the parents do make the decisions. We would put the case, say, for further treatment or against further treatment to them and they would be able to assess the facts for themselves. A decision is thus arrived at which is greatly influenced by what the parents think. So if they said they didn't want to go through more chemotherapy, I certainly wouldn't say to them that they are not giving their child a chance. But we phrase our discussions in such a way that we hope they don't feel that they are the only people making a decision and that they've got our support, whatever they decide. Obviously, the day-to-day medical and nursing problems have to be dealt with by hospital staff, but explanations are always given to parents. They are consciously part of the team and they have a right to understand what's going on.'

This perception of the parents' role – and sense of teamwork – meant that Jon Pritchard was accompanied when he saw Janet and Glenn Wells by Jean Simons, the medical social worker attached to the oncology unit. Many families will be unaccustomed to social workers and perhaps rather disparage them. Dr Pritchard therefore explains that Jean sees *all* families whose children have cancer so there is no stigma about her help being confined to 'problem families'. By no means all social workers in the hospital have either Jean Simon's status within their teams or her ability to draw upon additional resources such as the Malcolm Sargent Cancer Fund for Children.

She is in her mid thirties, brisk and bright yet a comfortingly good listener; each day she visits her wards talking to families while, during out-patient clinics, the door of her office is left symbolically open to encourage callers. She regards her job as part practical help over matters such as travelling expenses, part emotional support. The latter – which sees her working closely with psychologist Richard Lansdown – can be taxing because it will inevitably involve helping some people to come to terms with the death of a child. Even when treatment has been effective, she says, the fear of death can never be completely forgotten. Yet parents are usually most shocked by the initial diagnosis of cancer. She adds:

'At the beginning there is often a bereavement-type reaction in which people are shell-shocked by the news. The fact that they are on a ward where, among other things, the children have no hair brings home the diagnosis. I try to make sure that they understand what's involved in their child's treatment. Sometimes parents want medical information, sometimes practical help, sometimes advice about what to tell their children. Our attitude is the hopeful side of realism, but not excessively so. We always say to parents – tell your children the truth. Obviously what you will tell a three-year-old will differ from what you tell a twelve-year-old but, from one year old, they have to be told something appropriate to their age. We want to create an atmosphere where people feel their questions are being answered and we encourage them to talk about their own feelings, not to bottle them up.'

Jean Simons became a familiar presence on the ward when Janet Wells arrived with Anna for the final phase of her treatment. It was mid-November and if all went well Anna would be home for Christmas. The 'A' side of 3AB was closed for building work. Ironically, this work was designed to create two sterile cubicles for bone marrow transplant children, yet it had caused so much dust that Anna's admission had been postponed for a week. Infection-laden dust could be fatal to Anna.

Because of the building work the 3AB team had taken over ward 3C, also on the third floor but on the western wing of the hospital. Anna was shown into cubicle number four. It measured just fifteen feet by seven feet six inches. Yet it was larger than many cubicles because it included a sleeping area for a parent. Janet was grateful for the extra two feet or so of space, even though the need for Anna to be nursed in 'isolation' meant she could not sleep alongside her daughter. The isolation is designed to minimize the chances of a patient picking up an infection during the time when the normal bodily defences have been laid low. Only the parents and essential medical staff could enter the cubicle – and Anna could not leave. Thus began a routine which became all too familiar to Janet Wells.

Each time she went into the cubicle she put on a plastic hat. She changed into shoes which had to stay inside the cubicle. Once inside, she put on a gown. She washed her hands with disinfectant. If she took anything inside the cubicle, it had to be sprayed with disinfectant. She had to scrub the floors, walls and windows daily. Drip stands, trolleys and bed linen were changed daily. There was only one departure from the absolute insistence on maximum precautions: Janet, as the resident parent, did not have to wear a mask.

Everyone else, from the doctors to Glenn, did so; once, mothers were similarly constrained. But masks not only lose their effectiveness after an hour or so, they prevent children seeing lips moving and this has been found to impede the development of speech. In any case, since mothers are the people who usually spend by far the greatest amount of time in the cubicles, they are also the least likely to import dangerous infections. It is a small concession to normality in an otherwise impersonal regime in which it becomes hard to distinguish the individuals beneath the masks and gowns.

In one sense this hospital admission was much like any other: it began with a long line of people asking questions or offering information. There was the houseman taking a full medical history, a nurse weighing and checking blood pressures, a dietitian explaining that children in isolation receive 'sterile' meals specially-prepared in ultra-hygienic conditions. Dr Hilary Blacklock, as the consultant in charge of the bone marrow transplant programme, went over, again, the procedures involved and the subsequent risks, including infection. Some children had died because of infections, she told Janet. Dr Blacklock added: 'I have to tell you this, not because we think it is very likely, but it is something you have a right to know. You should then put it to the back of your mind and concentrate on the positive aspects, for example, the reason why the autograft is being done – that the benefits to a number of children have outweighed the risks.'

All the visitors were greeted by a friendly (and much-repeated) 'hello' from Anna. All remarked how well she looked. She certainly had little opportunity to become bored – and no need at first for the reading and painting books which Janet had brought to the hospital. If the succession of visitors was not distraction enough, there were the inevitable tests to check for bacteria or viruses which might cause infections, or to monitor the effects of treatment. Urine and stools were collected for analysis, her nose and throat swabbed, her chest X-rayed and blood tested. No fewer than six different laboratories were involved in Anna's case at one time or another: biochemistry, haematology, histopathology, microbiology, renal and virology. Some of these are housed in the neighbouring Institute of Child Health. Here, too, is an Imperial Cancer Research Fund laboratory which was to play a key role by 'cleaning' Anna's bone marrow in a revolutionary technique developed by the lab's director, Dr John Kemshead.

Anna's big day was Thursday 14 November. She had been 'nil by mouth' since midnight and was given a pre-medication sedative at nine-thirty – forty-five minutes before leaving for the sixth-floor operating theatre. There she faced two separate operations. First, her bone marrow would be 'harvested'; secondly, a silastic or plastic tube known as a Hickman Catheter would be inserted into a vein leading to her heart. Anna was given a general anaesthetic and then lifted onto the operating table. She lay on her stomach, her head wrapped in metal foil to prevent her getting cold. (Children's heads form a larger proportion of the body's total surface area than in adults and consequently are a major site of lost bodily heat, particularly if, like Anna, children have lost their hair.)

At ten forty-five the bone marrow harvest began. In charge was Hilary Blacklock, whose elegant clothes were for once hidden under surgical gowns. She is an attractive, black-haired New Zealander who was thirty-six when she was appointed to take charge of the hospital's expanding bone marrow programme in 1984. Assisted by Dr Peter Coates, her registrar, she inserted a needle into Anna's pelvis, just above her buttocks. This area is a rich source of bone marrow but not too close to any arteries or nerves. Chubby toddlers (and overweight adults) can make it difficult for doctors to find the bone beneath the layers of fat, but there were no problems with Anna. The marrow was drawn up through the needle into a syringe: it was red, like blood but thicker so that it oozed rather than flowed. Dr Blacklock and Dr Coates worked quickly and deftly. By moving the skin around, they could take marrow from different sites and different depths via the same surface hole. The syringes were passed to a nurse who recorded the volumes extracted and emptied the marrow via a filter to remove clumps of cells into a bag.

Dr Blacklock wanted to remove between ten and twenty per cent of Anna's blood volume – a figure calculated from the body weight of 11.5 kg (25 lb). She knew from experience that this should yield enough cells for the autograft to work quickly when the marrow was restored to the patient. After twenty minutes eighty-two millilitres of marrow, roughly one-fifth of a pint, had been removed. Dr Blacklock paused while the haematology laboratory hurriedly counted the cells. She was hoping for at least 300 million cells per kilogram, but the news from the lab was better: over 400 million cells per kilogram. More marrow was then taken in an attempt to shorten the days in hospital until the harvest ended forty-five minutes after it began with a final volume of 132 millilitres.

For stage two of the morning's work in the operating theatre Dr Blacklock was replaced by Keith Holmes, the senior surgical registrar. His task was to insert the silastic tube under the skin of the chest and into a large vein known as the superior vena cava that leads to the heart. The Hickman Catheter, as it is known, enables blood and drugs to be given and blood samples to be extracted without doctors forever having to insert needles into the tiny veins of often distressed children. When the catheter is not required it can be capped so that a child can be as active as his or her general health allows. More often than not half the children on 3AB have Hickman Catheters and parents are trained how to change the dressing at the point where the catheter enters the chest. The thought of this tends to unnerve parents, but most learn the skills quickly. Janet Wells was also upset by the thought of the catheter being inserted at all. 'I know it's a small operation which will make life a lot easier for Anna afterwards because she hates needles,' she said the day before. 'But it's the first time anyone has had to cut into her body and I just don't like the thought of it. I know it's silly.'

Surgically, it was not a particularly difficult procedure. Anna virtually disappeared underneath the green surgical sheets. Just a small area of the chest, about six by three inches, was left visible. This was covered by transparent plastic film so that the skin would not be touched. Keith Holmes made two incisions: one near the neck where the catheter would enter the vein, one above the right breast where it would emerge from the skin some distance away from the vein, again to try and avoid infection. He then pushed what looked like a skewer from one hole to the other, crinkling the skin in between, and used this to thread the catheter underneath the skin towards the vein. At one point this vein splits in two: one branch leads to the heart, the other to the arm. A chest X-ray showed that the surgeon had found the correct vein and that the catheter was in the correct place, just above the right atrium of the heart. At twelve twenty-five, the operation was over.

Janet went to meet Anna upstairs where she would have been pleased to know that her first words were 'Mummy, Mummy'. Anna was not distressed and seemed oblivious to the tube which now came out of her chest. It was through the catheter that the melphalan was given at seven that same evening. The dose was only two-thirds of the normal volume because tests in the renal laboratory had shown that Anna's kidneys had been affected by previous chemotherapy. Ninety minutes later Anna began to be sick but, after all the warnings about possible side-effects, the surprise was that Anna was not worse. So far she appeared to be tolerating the drug very well. Her temperature, pulse and breathing were recorded every four hours and all were stable. That night Janet slept better than she had done for some days. At least something was happening now. The waiting had been worse.

The next morning, at eight-forty, Anna received her bone marrow back. While outside her body, however, it had been 'purged'. This process, one of several ways of removing tumour cells from marrow, had been developed over the previous five years by one of the Imperial Cancer Research Fund laboratories now housed in the Institute of Child Health adjoining the hospital. The scientific procedures are complex but, in simple terms, they involve the use of antibodies which can identify tumour cells in normal bone marrow. These are called 'monoclonal' antibodies because they only recognize the cancer cells and not any normal healthy bone marrow cells. The appropriate antibodies for a particular kind of cancer are initially linked with minute magnetic beads, so small that they look like powder. These are then added to the bone marrow in which tumour cells are present and the antibodies seek out the cancer cells. In this way the tumour cells become coated with the magnetic beads. The mixture is then pumped through a system of magnets which attract the beads with the antibodies bound to any tumour cells in the marrow. The entire process takes up to five hours because other intricate procedures are involved not only to prepare the marrow for this magnetic 'purge' but also to ensure that the normal cells are not damaged.

In Anna's case no cancer cells had ever been found in her bone marrow, but the purge would make doubly sure that the marrow was clear. It was returned to her via the Hickman line, flowing through the blood until finding its home in the marrow spaces. Infusing marrow into the body can cause a reaction, although this is far more likely where a patient receives another person's marrow. Nevertheless Dr Ian Sanderson, the oncology registrar, remained with her for the hour that the marrow was being infused. There was no reaction at all. Anna sat up in her cot, smiling at faces which peered in through the cubicle windows. She was alert and well. Now the waiting would begin.

Doctors warned Janet and Glenn that her blood would take a fortnight, perhaps longer, to recover. Glenn came to the hospital at weekends, usually staying with his parents, and worked during the week. His employer, British Telecom, was understanding and granted him five days' compassionate leave to be taken whenever he wanted. His wife had left an array of meals in the freezer. All were neatly labelled – 'teachers are terrible ones for labelling everything' – yet few were eaten as friends invited him to their homes for supper. Each evening he would talk to Janet on the phone and then pass on any news to family and friends. One way or another he was too busy to mope or fret, not least because he had another little task on his mind – moving house.

It was not an ambitious move, hardly more than across the road, but it still required the same amount of packing as a move across the country. Moving house while their only child was critically ill in hospital may seem odd, even mad, but it was a calculated decision by a couple who were by nature planners. 'We felt we should have something else to think about,' said Glenn. This positive, bold gesture certainly kept Glenn occupied up to and beyond moving day on 21 November. Several weeks would pass, though, before Janet saw her new house and longer still for Anna.

Janet was also keeping busy. She arrived at Anna's cubicle shortly after eight o'clock each morning in time to prepare a breakfast of toast or cereal. To reduce the risks of infection other parents had to leave the small ward kitchen while this was prepared and, as with meals cooked by the dietitians, sterilized plates and cutlery had to be used. After breakfast there was the cubicle to clean, the linen to change and Anna to bath. If a mother (or father) cannot be resident this would be done by nurses, but most parents are grateful to do something for their child. It also helps to pass the time in what can be a long day. The isolation was particularly frustrating when visitors came. Grandparents and other relatives were unable to do more than wave or blow kisses through the window. Nor was the narrow and cluttered corridor outside the cubicle door the most relaxing or private of places for Janet to talk. Anna was rather clinging, frequently crying when Janet left the cubicle. This was made worse as hospital life began to undermine her usual sleep pattern so that Janet required all her teaching skills to keep her occupied.

'I read to her and we also have painting books. She likes to draw with felt pens, not crayons any more, and she enjoys puzzles. Her concentration seems amazingly good for a child her age,' said Janet. There were other distractions. Hospital equipment proved popular whether it be blood pressure pumps or foil containers. And there was television. Janet worried that Anna was watching too much television – endless videos of Postman Pat – but it did not seem to staunch the flow of conversation. 'Hat on' Anna would say as anyone came into the cubicle. 'Who's that?' she would ask – and usually knew the answer. 'Pass the clamps,' said Anna brightly as Janet strove to learn how to change the dressings on the Hickman Catheter.

Playing with hospital equipment is not merely condoned but frequently encouraged. Children in 3AB, for instance, are shown a teddy bear with a Hickman Catheter before one is inserted in them. There is also a book of photographs showing a child before and after the Catheter is fitted. A playleader thus fulfils a role in ward life beyond the simple provision of entertainment. Most wards at Great Ormond Street have a playleader and 3AB, given the emotive nature of its illnesses, is generously endowed with play equipment by outside fundraisers. But playleaders do not enter isolation cubicles unless a child is clearly near the end of its tether through frustration. Janet – and Glenn at weekends – were effectively on their own.

Janet tried to leave the claustrophobic atmosphere of the hospital at least once during the day, if only to buy groceries at the local supermarket. Like many parents she would sometimes prepare simple meals in the ward kitchen as a change from canteen food. Otherwise she was with Anna all day until she went to sleep in the evening. If Glenn was in London, they might go for a meal or see friends but weekday evenings were usually spent chatting to other parents – sometimes way into the early hours. It may be hard to imagine that anyone could be worse off than the parents of a child with cancer, but one place that you are likely to find such people is Great Ormond Street. Time and time again, parents say they are helped by sharing their troubles with others. Some will find encouragement, some consolation. Almost always there will be sympathy and understanding. 'I almost feel guilty that I should be helped by hearing about other people's problems,' says Janet. 'It's not that you wish anyone ill. It just helps to put your own problems in perspective.'

Initially the boredom was balanced by encouraging news from the front. None of the possible side-effects of melphalan materialized, except for the expected depletion of blood cells. Once Anna's temperature rose and once there was a slight infection in her urine. But there was nothing in the first ten days that the doctors could not tackle readily through antibiotics. 'After all that we had been told, it's a pleasant surprise that she has been so well,' said Janet at that time. The doctors, too, were pleased and were privately beginning to anticipate the time when Anna's cubicle would be available for the next patient.

Janet and Glenn asked lots of questions, keen to understand as much as possible. And they tried, without complete success, to adopt a phlegmatic attitude to the results of the daily blood tests which were recorded on a yellow chart which hung outside Anna's cubicle. These figures can mesmerize parents as they wait anxiously for a rise in the 'counts' of blood cell constituents which previously meant nothing to them. Each day the counts for such arcane terms as haemoglobin, platelets and neutrophils are scrutinized and pondered. Dr Hilary Blacklock is not entirely convinced that it is a good thing for the figures to be so readily available to parents. 'It's a mixed blessing because they understandably get anxious, if there is a fall or the count doesn't rise. However, if we stopped making the figures so available, parents would still ask for them or fear we were hiding something,' she says.

Hilary Blacklock assumes responsibility for children after they have had a bone marrow transplant or autograft. Other doctors such as Jon Pritchard remain involved but for the transplant and the period afterwards when close supervision for any complications is required, Dr Blacklock is in charge. Her background is in haematology, which is the study of blood diseases, and she works for the Institute of Child Health as well as the hospital, thus epitomizing the close relationship between research and its clinical application in the wards. Anna Wells should have been one of her less taxing cases. She had received her own bone marrow back so it was highly unlikely that her body would reject the marrow as can happen in transplants when a sibling or parent is the donor (see Kristie's story). It was just a matter of time before her blood recovered from the effect of melphalan.

The first sign that this comforting scenario might be overly-optimistic came twelve days after the melphalan. Ironically, the day had begun well with the weekly conference to discuss all bone marrow transplant patients hearing that Anna's white cells were beginning to reappear in the blood; these cells include the neutrophils and lymphocytes with which the body fights infection. The other area of potential risk to Anna was bleeding. This is because melphalan also reduces the number of cells called 'platelets' which help the blood to clot. Platelets are minute – normally around 300 million per millilitre of blood – but crucial in preventing bleeding. If there are too few platelets, a patient could bleed to death. However, this is usually a lesser worry for the doctors than infections as severe bleeding can usually be prevented by platelet transfusions, just as patients often receive 'normal' blood or red cell transfusions.

At first, then, there seemed nothing unusual about giving Anna platelets. At the time doctors were more immediately preoccupied with prescribing antibiotics to combat a high temperature. Then, at twenty minutes to nine in the evening, twelve days after the melphalan, Anna began to shake from head to toe in a reaction against the platelets. Steroid and anti-histamine drugs soon ended Anna's adverse reaction, but if there was a moment that changed the nature of Anna's treatment this, in hindsight, was it. At the time it seemed more odd than alarming. 'We have seen this reaction against blood transfusions before with children who have had bone marrow autografts,' said Hilary Blacklock. Drugs would be given to Anna before platelet injections to prevent any further reactions. But the donor platelets did not produce any improvement in the daily counts. There was not even much rise one hour after the platelets had been given. Dr Blacklock decided to try and find out whether an antibody was keeping the counts low.*

Samples of Anna's blood were analysed not only at Great Ormond Street but other specialist laboratories elsewhere in London. This confirmed that Anna had developed an antibody which was reacting against platelets. In other words, there was something in her body killing off most of the platelets she was

---

*The normal range for platelet counts is 150-400 million per millilitre which is expressed, in the standard international units, as $150\text{-}400 \times 10^9/\text{litre}$ of blood. Severe spontaneous bleeding usually only occurs below $20 \times 10^9/\text{litre}$. This text will use the accepted shorthand of giving platelet counts as, say, twenty — without the mathematical formula.

being given. The next task was to identify the antibody. If this could be done, it should be possible to establish which types of platelets would not be destroyed by it. There were no quick or certain answers: the doctors and scientists were operating at the frontiers of medical knowledge.

Hilary Blacklock said at that time: 'We don't fully understand why some patients make platelet antibodies and the current state of the art in platelet matching is not good. We've got to sit it out until the laboratories come up with some answers and hope that serious bleeding does not occur until her own platelets start to come through. I'm sure they will, but it may take some time.'

It was a discouraging message for Janet and Glenn. Janet was in tears the night Anna had her first reaction against platelets, but worse was to come. Eight days later Anna began to break out in tiny purple spots called petechiae. They covered most of her body and face; in the whites of her eyes they appeared as pools of blood. The spots stood out more because Anna was now very pale. In themselves the petechiae – which are tiny blood blisters – were distressing but not particularly serious. Yet they had not been caused by bruising so their spontaneous appearance emphasized the danger which now faced Anna. What the doctors had to prevent was more serious internal bleeding caused by a knock or fall, particularly to the head. That could be fatal.

Anna's case was discussed in detail at the regular weekly bone marrow transplant conference. Afterwards several doctors came to the ward and peered through the window at Anna and Janet. 'I was already feeling low and when they were standing outside I had this terrible fear that they didn't know what to do,' says Janet. 'When they told me that Anna was building up an antibody to platelets I became very upset. A day or so before they had been saying it would soon be time to think about going home. Now we were back at square one or perhaps worse off than ever.'

In her distress, Janet turned first to her mother – 'She is very calm and I didn't want to scare Glenn until I had sorted myself out a little. I knew that I couldn't settle his mind any more than I could settle my own.' Comforted by her mother and Liz Sappa, one of the ward sisters, she then contacted Glenn at work and he came to join her that evening. Other visitors included Hilary Blacklock, Jon Pritchard and Ian Sanderson, all of whom answered Janet's questions and told her what they were doing to tackle the problem. They would try to find a donor whose platelets matched those of Anna and in the meantime pre-medication drugs would prevent a re-action against unmatched platelets. Other drugs, including steroids, would be tried in the hope of blocking the production of the antibody. Anna's head would be protected from acciden-tal bruising by a hat which would act like a crash helmet and her cot would be padded. There were no guarantees that the treatment would work or that serious internal bleeding might not occur. But the doctors wanted to get across two points. Firstly, although they did not understand why the problem had occurred, they did have a number of options to deal with it. Secondly, they were confident that, eventually, Anna would produce so many of her own platelets that they would neutral-ize the antibody.

'It is the fear of the unknown that is most frightening,' says Janet. 'All they could say was "we *think* it's this" or "we *think* we can get it under control". It seemed that they didn't *know*. You can handle whatever they tell you so long as you know what is happening; if you don't know, it's unnerving and the waiting becomes much harder to take.'

The activity as much as the explanations cheered Anna's parents, particularly as Anna appeared to be responding to the treatment. Their days increasingly revolved around the daily count of platelets detected by machines from samples of Anna's blood. When Anna arrived at Great Ormond Street her platelet count had been 188. After dropping down to seven, counts of seventeen would brighten her parents' day, even though this remained below the critical point of twenty at which doctors consider there is a serious risk of internal bleed-ing. 'The chart with the figures is like a lifeline you hang on to,' said Janet. Imagine, then, the euphoria when the count shot up to thirty-four – and imagine, too, the gloom when this turned out to be 'machine error'. It was really no more than eleven.

Through all this trauma Anna looked remarkably well, especially as the bruising began to fade. She was sleeping soundly and eating heartily, with a newly-discovered taste for Weetabix, throughout the day. Her pulse, temperature and blood pressure were stable and, as one nurse recorded, she was 'as usual, bright and cheerful'. However the prolonged period of isolation in her cubicle was beginning to pall. 'Her main aim all the time is to get out of the cot and onto the floor. This has been a problem because she risks banging her head on various pieces of equipment,' said Janet. This increased the pressure on Janet who now had to keep Anna safe as well as occupied. She knew that when she left the cubicle, Anna was often whiney and restless.

Janet also recognized that she herself was on a knife-edge, outwardly calm and positive but inwardly anxious and finding it hard to concentrate. Books which she had brought with her remained unread. Time dragged and the cubicle, for all the friendliness of the nursing staff, seemed like a prison. Christmas, which meant a lot to Janet, was looming. Cards from children at her school reminded her of home. Her family was close and Christmas had always been the target by when they wanted to be home. Anna would be twenty months old this Christmas so it would be the first she could begin to understand and enjoy. With a week or more to go, the ward was being decorated and more than one Father Christmas had toured the hospital. Janet explained that one of them would bring her presents. 'Lucky,' said Anna. If they were really lucky – and Anna continued to make her steady, if slow, progress – there was a chance that they could spend Christmas Day away from the hospital with Glenn's parents. It was not what they had wanted six weeks ago, but better than nothing. Yet once again, good news was followed by bad.

On 23 December Anna suffered her worst crisis yet. Glenn was with Anna that day, the first of his Christmas holiday, because Janet had gone to see her own GP in Staplehurst. She had been unwell herself the previous day and she also needed a sick note for the local education authority. As soon as Glenn went into the cubicle, he could see all was not well. 'She was sitting in a chair looking very listless and very, very pale – her lips were almost white. I called in one of the doctors and then another doctor came to have a look. Then it all began to happen.'

Anna was listless and pale because the haemoglobin in her blood had dropped alarmingly. This is the protein in the red blood cells which transports oxygen around the body. She was given blood, plasma and platelets but at first her condition continued to deteriorate. Her temperature and pulse rate were high. And, most critically of all, she appeared to be bleeding internally: her stools were almost black, indicating a high blood content. The blackness meant they had been exposed to acid which in turn suggested she was bleeding in her stomach. Drugs were prescribed to combat the presumed gastric irritation in the stomach. Electronic monitors were squeezed into the cubicle to provide instant checks on pulse rate and blood pressures, other observations were performed every thirty minutes. At lunchtime, the afternoon shift of nurses were told Anna needed close supervision. One nurse was assigned to stay with Anna at all times. This, then, was the scene which Janet encountered when she returned to the hospital. Later she and Glenn saw Jon Pritchard who did not disguise the gravity of the situation. 'We are very worried,' he said. Later he said: 'I was worried for Anna's life that day. We weren't sure whether she would get through the day or night.'

Anna, in fact, recovered fairly quickly. Within twenty-four hours her temperature was back to normal and so were her stools. But the next crisis might not be so easy to control, particularly if the bleeding occurred in the head. Here there is less 'free' space for the blood to occupy so cranial bleeding can cause greater harm by permanently damaging the brain. 'In addition to not making platelets, Anna has the extra problem of the antibody greatly shortening the lifespan of transfused platelets,' said Dr Blacklock.

Microscopic examination of Anna's bone marrow had shown that very young platelets were beginning to appear, although the process was clearly slow – too slow, the doctors now thought, for comfort. The antibody, which by now had been identified, was a virulent presence effectively destroying roughly two-thirds of the platelets supplied by blood donors.

But as a result of the various tests, it became possible to identify platelets which – in terms of their proteins – partly matched
those beginning to be made by Anna herself. At that time,
however, only one potential 'matched' donor had been found
by the North London Blood Transfusion Centre which supplies
blood to Great Ormond Street. On Christmas Eve, of all days,
this donor was asked to come to the transfusion centre where
she was attached to a machine known as a cell separator which
concentrated the platelets from her blood. It was the first, and
in many ways the best, Christmas present Anna was to receive.
Her platelet count after the transfusion was eighty-nine!

Glenn stayed in the hospital on Christmas Eve – sleeping in
an empty cubicle on another ward – so that he and Janet could
be with Anna when she woke to receive her presents. There
were plenty of toys and books with the promise of the main
present to come when she returned home – a swing for the new
garden. It was a happy day. More than six weeks had passed
since they had arrived, longer than the worst forecast and a
bumpier ride than anticipated. But by now at least they knew
most of the other families and the staff. There was wine to help
wash down the turkey and everyone did their best to forget
their worries, for one day at least. 'It was the first year Anna
really understood Christmas and she loved it,' said Janet.

By Boxing Day, however, the platelet count had dropped
below twenty. Anna would need some more matched platelets.
Yet the rules established for the safety of blood donors do not
allow a donor to be used more frequently than once every three
weeks. The doctors clearly needed another donor. Further tests
done at the transfusion centre showed that Glenn was the next
closest match, not perfect, but closer than Janet who in any
case was still slightly unwell. And so, on 27 December, Glenn
Wells reported to the cell separation unit at University College
Hospital, half a mile away across Bloomsbury, to donate his
platelets. He returned, carrying two bottles of platelets in a
Marks and Spencer shopping bag. Did he worry about dropping them? 'Not really, but I did think that if anyone mugs me,
he's going to have a hell of a shock when he finds what's in the
bag.'

Again, the matched platelets produced an immediate

improvement in the count – this time to 116 – but, again the improvement was short-lived. The search for additional compatible donors was intensified. The antibody remained active, defying the steroid therapy which doctors had hoped would block the spleen where antibodies are generated. Another drug, Azathioprine, was therefore added to the daily cocktail to try and reinforce the impact of the steroids and suppress the antibody's production. There were divisions among the doctors about this new form of therapy, some fearing that the Azathioprine – an 'immuno-suppressant' – could reduce the white blood cells without necessarily boosting the platelets. But Dr Blacklock was convinced by previous experience that the drug was worth a try, although it would take three weeks to have any effect. During this time Anna would remain at risk.

Then, at last, Anna had two strokes of luck. First, more donors were found so that matched platelets could be given twice a week until the drug began to work. Second, over the weekend after Christmas, her white cell count began to improve, not dramatically but steadily. It was a flicker of light in what had become an unexpectedly long tunnel.

The white blood cells could have been stimulated by the steroids or maybe what Hilary Blacklock had consistently said would happen had done so: that the white blood count would eventually increase and that this would precede the appearance of Anna's own platelets. Dr Blacklock had also come to the view that, now the stomach bleeding was under control, the unmatched platelets Anna was receiving each day might be doing more harm than good. 'The unmatched platelets seem to be providing the protein which stimulates the antibody and the reaction destroys her own platelets in a kind of 'innocent-bystander' effect. It may also have slowed down the recovery of her white cells. We will therefore give her only platelets from matched donors twice a week. Anna herself is now quite well, so it is a question of treating the patient rather than the platelet count,' said Dr Blacklock.

Janet and Glenn Wells were not too downcast as they digested this news and contemplated the New Year. They knew it might mean another three weeks in hospital while the doctors waited to see whether the new drug would work. They were told that Anna had already stayed in hospital longer than any other patient who had received a bone marrow autograft. But the alternatives which the doctors had considered would have been worse. One possible course involved a risky extraction of the plasma in Anna's blood to remove the antibody while another would have meant an operation to remove the spleen.

The New Year brought an unexpected bonus: the improvement in white blood cells meant Anna no longer had to stay in complete isolation. After seven irksome weeks grandparents and other relatives could go and see Anna. They had to wear gowns in order to lessen the chance of infection but not masks or hats. Anna was puzzled by this and astonished when, a few days later, Janet said: 'Would you like to go for a walk?' 'Outside?' she replied with a look of incredulity that was both sweet and sad. In no time at all, though, she was constantly on the move, making up for eight weeks of confinement in a cubicle. The next step in Anna's progress was to leave the cubicle altogether and move to a bed in the open ward. She began to play with the other children and banged happily in time to the music when teachers organized a singing session in the playroom. As the white blood count improved, she began to venture further afield – to the cafeteria for lunch, to the park or to the shops.

Anna was now twenty-one months old and in the last two months had grown up considerably. Physically she outgrew all the clothes with which she arrived at the hospital and developmentally, too, she zoomed ahead. She was able to tackle tasks, such as cleaning her own mouth to prevent sores, which were originally beyond her. She could feed herself and drink from a normal cup. She walked more steadily and her communication, always impressive, doubled – her mother always reminding her if she forgot to say 'please' or 'thank you'. She put on weight, largely because of the steroids, but the bruising had disappeared by the New Year. The slightly puffy cheeks, bald head and alert blue eyes made her 'look like an infant Buddha', said Hilary Blacklock as Anna regarded her intently during an examination.

In mid-January Anna's platelet counts began to stay above

twenty on days when she did not receive matched platelets – not by much, but previously they had always fallen much lower between transfusions. Whether the increases were due to the effect of the new drug added after Christmas or whether it would have happened anyway, was impossible to prove. So again, thoughts began to turn to going home. Anna was no longer being nursed intensively. Once a day a sample of her blood was taken – a routine task for a child with a Hickman Catheter and one which Janet could do herself. And so, on Saturday 18 January, Anna left hospital sixty-seven days after she had arrived. Her destination was not – yet – the new home she had never seen, but Edmonton to the home of her father's parents. From there Janet would bring in each day a sample of Anna's blood and the doctors would see whether the platelets continued to increase. Eight days later she finally returned to Staplehurst, arriving at her new home nearly eleven weeks after she left the old one.

Three days later she was back at Great Ormond Street, although only for the first of her out-patient clinics. Dr Blacklock examined Anna while a sample of her blood was analysed, paying particular attention to her chest. 'At this stage we are worried about the possibility of a virus infection in the lung because although the white blood count has recovered, not all their function has returned to normal,' Dr Blacklock told Janet. The platelet count was twenty-nine, the same as the previous test forty-eight hours earlier which greatly pleased Dr Blacklock. She said: 'We have made considerable progress in the last month. The numbers may not be huge but the count is being maintained. She is out of the immediate danger area, although she is still at risk from bruising.'

Dr Blacklock suggested that Janet should be slightly cautious about letting Anna mingle too freely with other children, just to guard against infections, particularly measles. But so long as the platelet count was holding up, the drugs could be slowly reduced, beginning with the steroids. Looking further ahead, Dr Blacklock said they would not know whether or not the antibody was reacting against her own platelets until tests could be done when the count reached one hundred. Nor were they sure whether the antibody had been suppressed permanently. Tests would also be needed to check lungs and liver functions. Janet listened thoughtfully, then asked: 'But you're still confident that it's working?' 'Oh yes, it will come right in the end.'

Anna was cheerful and chatty. A wispy stubble was beginning to grow on her head. She faced three months or so of visits to Dr Blacklock's clinic before switching to the oncology clinic of Dr Pritchard. 'I won't look forward to coming back to the out-patient clinics,' says Janet. 'We had almost a year of them at King's but this time it will be worse. You live in fear of a relapse and you know that at the moment there's nothing they can do if that happens. Some parents say they would do anything. If you get this far, maybe you do want to carry on. I don't know. We have always felt that there was a very fine line between what you are prepared to let happen to your child and what is not acceptable. So far they have only been using drugs they know about and have always told us about possible side-effects. I don't know whether we would want them to try out new drugs which might only prolong Anna's agony. It's hard to say at this stage. That's why we'll help the Neuroblastoma Society* in the hope that in the future they may be able to help children who get into remission and then relapse. To give them some hope.'

At the moment, if children with neuroblastoma do relapse there is no known successful treatment. OPEC and melphalan have given children such as Anna hope where there was none ten years ago, but Jon Pritchard believes they are interim stages in the evolution of still more successful forms of treatment. Some parents coping with a relapse will want to try further chemotherapy or be willing to contemplate experimental drugs. Others will settle for 'symptomatic therapy' which involves drugs to minimize pain prior to inevitable death. 'Relapse is a huge shock but after the initial tears parents somehow bring themselves to face up to death, often because there has been an underlying preparation for it. They

---

*A charitable group formed by parents which helps to finance research into neuroblastoma: its address is Woodlands, Ordfall Park Road, Retford, Nottinghamshire.

have lived with the possibility that it might happen,' says social worker Jean Simons.

If relapse is a tragic time for the family, it is difficult, too, for the hospital staff. 'It can be difficult to maintain a delicate balance between getting to know the families well enough to attend to their individual needs and not getting to know them so well that there is a sense of personal loss if a death occurs,' says Dr Pritchard. The pressure on nursing staff is particularly acute since they will have spent more time with the children and families than the doctors. 'Nurses shouldn't try to keep a stiff upper lip,' says Pat Carter, the senior ward sister. 'We have a lot of children on the ward who are very sick and who will die. We feel terrible about this, naturally, and if you cry it shows sympathy with the parents. Nurses must not feel guilty if they cry but they must remain able to help others.'

Pat Carter was appointed ward sister at the age of twenty-three in 1978, although it was four years later that it became wholly dedicated to cancer and leukaemia. Some sisters doubted the wisdom of concentrating so many 'difficult' illnesses on one ward. The pressure would be too much, they argued, and a high turnover of staff nurses reflects the pressure. More intensive chemotherapy, however, requires more specific expertise than was necessary in the 1970s – not merely among nurses but supporting staff such as ward pharmacist Angela Bowman – so it is unlikely that the trend to specialization will be reversed. One consequence of greater numbers and more intensive treatment is that Pat Carter is now supported by two general ward sisters and one sister in charge of intravenous infusions through the ubiquitous Hickman Catheters.

A weekly 'psycho-social' meeting* discusses the problems of staff as well as those of parents. Doctors as well as nurses, social workers, teachers and psychologist attend so that information can be pooled and problems shared. The teamwork is strong enough to withstand the regular changes of registrars and 'senior house officers' as the junior doctors are

---

*See pages 57-9 for more on psycho-social meetings.

called. It is helped, perhaps, by the greater maturity of house-men at Great Ormond Street compared to most other hospitals; all must have a minimum of five years' experience after qualifying and many, such as Dr Hamish Wallace, the houseman who looked after Anna Wells, have held locum registrar posts elsewhere. The staff are helped, too, by evidence of success as children return to the ward, lively and well after an out-patients' clinic five or more years after treatment. The 3AB team is also well-supported by charities. To some extent it needs to be: private funds (or 'soft money' as they are known) finance not only extras such as play equipment and televisions but most of the essential monitoring equipment which controls the flow of drugs into the patients. In this 3AB is typical of the hospital as a whole but what is more unusual is that two of the team's three registrars and one of its social workers, Jean Simons, have their salaries paid by charities and not by the National Health Service.

The extra resources underpin the teamwork and ease the burdens on individuals, although a spate of deaths still exerts a heavy toll. 'We all get very sad if a child dies but we all know and keep in touch with some wonderful families. İt sounds corny, but you feel privileged having met the children and the families and you hope that perhaps you helped them in some way. That keeps you going, as well as the rewards of seeing the children who recover,' says social worker Jean Simons.

In fact, children rarely die on the ward. If a relapse occurs, most go home. This does not necessarily distance the staff from the emotional strain, especially for those among them who must help parents prepare for a child's death. Or even, if the child is old enough, to answer the child's own questions. 'Care doesn't end just because there is a relapse. It's important for us to convince parents that we are still with them,' says Dr Pritchard. In the frontline of this harrowing work are Jean Simons, chaplain Derek Bacon and psychologist Richard Lansdown. Richard Lansdown says:

'If the child is old enough, I like to begin by trying to find out what he or she thinks is going to happen after death so we've got a framework for discussion. With younger children I very much emphasize the importance of not being separated because what this is what children roughly under the ages of five or six most fear. What we try to do is give the message that they won't be separated; while they are still on this earth, mummy and daddy will still be with them all the time. Many children have a concept of heaven; they perceive going there as another kind of journey. They've gone from infant school to junior school, so they've gone from home to hospital and will go from here to heaven. That's for many of them, not all. Anyway we try to establish what the child thinks.

'The next point, terribly important but emotionally hard, is to establish what the parents really think because quite often they haven't come to terms with the fact that a child is probably going to die. I try to explore what they think, not in the head but in the guts. Not what doctors have told them or read in books, but what they feel deep down. Then we can get on a wavelength and we can discuss practical points such as whether the child is going to be at home or in hospital, what they are going to say to the child or siblings. I'm always asked – should we tell a child that he's going to die? My answer is no, you should never tell a child that he is going to die but if a child asks a straight question, then what is the closest to the truth? And that is yes, you may die very soon – we hope you won't, but you may die. I have never known a child upset by that reply. It often comes as a sense of relief because they now know that everybody is being honest. Nobody is keeping anything from them.

'Then there are what may seem to some parents very mundane matters but which in retrospect are very important, such as planning what to do with the child's clothes and toys, whether you are going to have a cremation or burial. If that can be planned in advance, it makes it much easier when the time actually comes. One of the very few predictions I actually make is that probably the worst time is going to be between three and six months after the death. Just after, there is so much to do and people will be rallying round, inviting them out and so on and people get buoyed along by this. Then after about three months much of that support is gone and they are just left with emptiness.

'I never pretend that life is going to be the same, because it isn't. It has changed for them already, so no false promises about getting over it because they won't; one never gets over the death of a child. But at least one can come to terms with it and life can get back to some semblance of normality. People can lead a life again where they are looking forward to tomorrow instead of dreading it.'

Janet and Glenn Wells have lived with the fear of their daughter's death for most of her life – and it would never entirely leave them. 'We have had to come to terms with the possibility of losing Anna. You've got no choice but to face up to that possibility. We would like to think that after this Anna will be all right because you need to think like that. But you've got no promises so every day must be enjoyed because every day is very important. If it continues and continues for her, then that obviously will be superb, but you don't know that so you have to live for each day, try to fit as much in as you can *now*. We used to plan, plan, plan – sometimes for years in advance as we did having Anna – but that's all gone out of the window,' says Janet.

In those distant days of planning Janet and Glenn wanted to have more than one child; now, they're not so sure. 'At the moment we don't feel we would want another baby,' says Glenn. 'If we lost Anna, I think we would just turn to ourselves and say – right, they've taken the thing that we wanted most from us, let's get on with our life and make the most of it. There is no way you could replace her with another child. People say leave it a year or eighteen months, but I don't think our feelings will change.'

Maybe time will soften these feelings of a couple ideally suited to be loving parents. Neuroblastoma is not an inherited disease, but there is no guarantee that it could never occur twice in one family – and however remote the possibility, it is not something which Janet and Glenn Wells can contemplate. Who can blame them? Yet their resilience is buttressed by realism as well as hope, as Janet explains. 'Living with uncertainty is not going to be easy, but getting to this stage at all for us is better than we feared. At the end, if Anna did have a relapse, we have done all that was possible to give her a

113

chance. So have the doctors and all the staff here and there's nowhere better for her to have been. We will be going home hoping for the best with a slightly better chance than average. To us, that's wonderful.'

Postscript: one year later
She has celebrated her third birthday and now goes to play-school three days a week. Although she has had a couple of bad coughs, Anna has had a happy year with check-ups at the oncology clinic reduced from three times a year to twice a year. She went on holiday abroad for the first time.

10.10 a.m. *In the histopathology department Professor Brian Lake is reviewing the results of tests carried out on one of the electron microscopes in the basement. It is one of several review meetings held between the pathologists and the various medical and surgical teams in the hospital. Histopathology is often a crucial element in establishing a diagnosis, so much so that surgeons will sometimes pause in mid-operation while pathologists examine a sample of body tissue. Such samples, known as biopsies, are also analysed to monitor the effectiveness of treatment and often they form the basis of prognosis and genetic counselling. There are several ways in which the pathologists examine specimens. In the simplest terms, it involves looking at minutely-thin slices of tissue under a microscope. The pathologists then hope to identify the cell patterns as distinctive of certain diseases. If light microscopy does not resolve the problem, electron microscopy may provide the answer. The magnification is so much greater – usually up to 20,000 times as against the 50-500 times by light microscopy, although it could go up to 200,000 times real size – that it can enable the pathologists to see what is inside the cells. The process is complex but, essentially, the image is produced by passing a narrow beam of electrons through a sample of tissue no bigger than a pin-head. The image is photographed and the negatives printed and examined.*

10.15 a.m. *There is only one place in the hospital where adults can be treated – the Occupational Health Unit – and this is where May Ryan, the nurse in charge, is checking the blood pressure of a member of staff. It turns into a more general discussion as May Ryan notices that the woman is very tired and it emerges that her department is very stretched at the moment. At the end of the conversation May feels that the woman will go away and do something about the situation. She is one of 500 people a month seen by a unit which employs three other nurses as well as two doctors who hold clinics here three times a week. In addition to a counselling and treatment service for staff, the unit runs preventive health programmes such as immunization against infectious illnesses and screening prospective staff. There are also hygiene programmes and advice on how to lift heavy objects – as useful to a nurse as a porter. The medical problems encountered in the unit* *are often stress related, says May Ryan, and can be caused by the pressure and volume of work. 'It's very difficult for people here to acknowledge that they are not coping, because their commitment to the people around them and their expectations of their own performance are very high.'*

10.20 a.m. *Robert Pike, appeals co-ordinator, meets two record producers who want to produce a single from which some of the profits will go to the hospital. There don't appear to be any snags with this proposal, but Robert Pike has to be careful; the hospital's name could be very useful commercially to manufacturers of children's products so he must be sure it is not misused. It was only in 1981 that hospitals regained the right to raise funds directly and Robert Pike's job has been to develop the charity attached to Great Ormond Street. The hospital has become very dependent upon private donations for medical equipment as government funding has not kept pace with the increasingly expensive nature of its specialized medicine. More than eighty charitable or commercial organizations are thanked in the current yearbook and their grants go to pay salaries as well as equipment and research projects. And then there are the efforts of individuals or small groups, raising money through sponsored marathons, swims, parachute jumps or other equally daunting stunts. Many are parents of patients, but not all. Anyone asking directions from Reg Bates, the flower-seller outside nearby Holborn tube station, will have a Great Ormond Street collection tin shaken before them. No donation, no directions. He reckons he fills a tin every two weeks.*

10.25 a.m. *The clinical biochemistry laboratories are at full stretch. There are three labs including one in the adjoining Institute of Child Health and between them they carry out 500,000 tests a year. Most of the tests are performed for the benefit of the hospital's patients; analysing body fluid (blood and urine) and body tissues for their chemical and electrolyte constituents can be a key means of establishing a diagnosis and monitoring treatment. Tests must be able to be carried out on minute volumes, perhaps no more than a single drop of blood, because of the difficulty in extracting blood from babies and small children. Like many of the other laboratories, biochemistry is split between its clinical duties for the hospi-*

tal and its more academic role in the Institute. But biochemistry also undertakes around 100,000 tests a year for the North Thames region as a whole in which each child born in the region will be checked for phenylketonuria (PKU) and congenital hypothyroidism. The department is also developing pre-natal screening tests for other metabolic disorders where families may be genetically at risk. This work, which involves the search for enzyme or chromosome defects, occupies much of the research activities of the department.

10.30 a.m. *A child arrives by ambulance from Peterborough. It's not an emergency admission, but the child was not well enough to travel by public transport. Shorter journeys are often undertaken by ambulance cars. These are driven by volunteers who are reimbursed for their petrol. Getting children to Great Ormond Street is often easier than getting them taken back to their local hospital, particularly if they are too sick for a volunteer driver. 'It's often difficult to get ambulances when the children are no longer emergencies,' says Glenys Davies, the patients' transport officer. 'The ambulance service has been understaffed and transfers to other hospitals come very low on the list of priorities. If the child lives a long way away, it could tie up an ambulance for the best part of a day.' One child had been waiting to be transferred for a week, to the mounting indignation of his parents and the irritation of ward staff who wanted the bed.*

10.35 a.m. *After waiting for patients to arrive (there are a surprising number of no-shows or DNAs – 'did not attend' – as they are called) consultant audiologist Susan Bellman sees Alexis, a fair-haired, bright and vigorous looking boy of three and a half years. Three months earlier he had meningitis and although he seems to have made an excellent recovery, he has been admitted as a day case for tests. Among these tests are checks on his hearing since one in five bacterial meningitis patients suffer some degree of hearing loss; it is therefore a major cause of deafness in children. Dr Bellman first uses a wooden puzzle into which Alexis slots cars, a house and animals. She whispers the names and tells him to put them in place. He finds them quickly and enjoys the game. She looks in his ears with an auroscope and then, using a tuning fork, asks him where he hears its sounds, left or right?*

There are other questions about Alexis's hearing at home, but Dr Bellman is already sure of her diagnosis. As he gets up and plays with a huge stuffed elephant in a corner of the room, she tells his mother that he has a moderately severe hearing loss in his right ear. This comes as a surprise to his mother, although she is obviously a caring and protective parent. Dr Bellman reassures her by saying that we only really need one ear and that the hearing in his other ear is fine. But it will be helpful to know about the hearing loss; he will need special warnings when learning to cross roads and his future teachers should be told he is deaf on one side. One child in forty has some hearing loss and one in a thousand is profoundly deaf, says Dr Bellman. Although she naturally works closely with the ear, nose and throat surgeons, her patients are referred from all over the hospital. Information about hearing loss can help build up a neurological diagnosis, children with cancer may have their hearing damaged by drugs and patients from the Department of Psychological Medicine are sometimes checked to see if a claimed hearing loss is real. Her most difficult task can be testing babies' hearing but new equipment can now get results from children who a few years ago were untestable.

10.40 a.m. *Jamie, aged four, arrives to see David Taylor, the consultant ophthalmologist, in the eye clinic. He has come all the way from Bangor in North Wales. Jamie has poor eyesight and is somewhat withdrawn. David Taylor tries to turn his eye-test into something of a game. He goes to the far side of the room and holds up a card bearing a letter: 'Now, Jamie, can you point to this letter on the card you have in front of you?' The game is played with both eyes and then each eye separately. 'It isn't too serious,' Mr Taylor tells the parents, 'but we need to patch the right eye to make the left eye do a little more work. He won't like it, I'm afraid, but he'll need to wear the patch for two hours a day.' Jamie's vision will be rechecked in three months' time and he may eventually need an operation to correct a squint.*

Jamie's sight was far from good, but there was enough to enable him to cope with reading, writing and other detailed work. Other patients this morning came after encountering difficulty focusing on school-work. Some, though, were more serious. One had a tumour close to the eye while Ying, a thirteen-year-old boy of *parents born in Hong Kong, had lost most of his sight over the years and had to be guided to a chair in the clinic. He'd had a series of operations for retina problems at Moorfields Eye Hospital and his parents had brought him to David Taylor for a second opinion. If they were looking for a miracle, sadly they were disappointed. After using some eye drops to dilate the pupils, David Taylor told Ying there was no way of making his eyesight better. He could see light and identify the direction it was coming from and this, said Mr Taylor, would help more than he might imagine in orientating himself. Ying appeared to anticipate the verdict, certainly he accepted it with astonishing good humour. His parents, though, were downcast. All David Taylor could offer them was a promise that he'd try to answer some of their questions about Ying's previous treatment; otherwise, they should go back to Moorfields since that was the place which specialized in retinal surgery. David Taylor himself specializes in (or has become known for) operations to remove cataracts in newborn babies. Most patients, though, are seen as outpatients and the thrice-weekly clinics see more than 2500 children a year. Three other doctors saw patients in addition to Mr Taylor plus opticians and specialists who conduct more elaborate and sophisticated tests of eyesight and the visual pathways between the eyes and the brain.*

10.45 a.m. *Mrs Ozal, wife of the Prime Minister of Turkey, begins an official visit to the hospital. Great Ormond Street is on the Government's hospitality office list as a possible place of interest for visiting heads of state, royalty, ministers and other VIPs. Mrs Ozal, accompanied by Turkish officials and more Turkish photographers than had been anticipated, toured a number of wards, inspected parents' accommodation and visited the play centre and out-patients department.*

10.50 a.m. *Kevin, aged fourteen, is examined by Dr Judith Chessells, the senior haematology consultant, in one of the twice-weekly leukaemia clinics. There are around fifty children on the list today and for their parents it is often a time of tension. They must wait while their child's blood (and sometimes bone marrow) is examined for the presence of leukaemia cells. The play centre is reserved for these children on clinic days to try and occupy them*

119

while they wait. The risk of recurrence is greatest in the first two years after stopping treatment; during this period patients are seen once a month. Kevin is coming to the end of those two years. He had acute lymphoblastic leukaemia but has been off treatment for twenty-one months; after four years off treatment he will go to a special long-term follow-up clinic no more than once a year – if he stays well.

In any one clinic there will be children like Kevin and others whose thin wispy hair betrays the fact that their chemotherapy treatment has only just ceased. The ages today varied from two to fifteen. Many of the younger children soon make themselves at home in Dr Chessells' room so that by eleven-thirty toys are scattered all over the floor. Judith Chessells explains the risks of infection or discusses aspects of 'shared care' with other hospitals, but she never forgets to talk directly to the children, however young they might be. She examines the children for any signs of an enlarged spleen or liver and checks the boys for testicular swelling. The parents know that these can be warning signs of a recurrence, but confirmation from the blood or other tests is nevertheless a shattering blow. Later this morning Sister Christa Muller, who works full-time for the haematology and oncology clinics, brings the results of a bone-marrow test: leukaemic cells have returned. It's a harrowing moment for the parents and little better for those who wait outside in the corridor, fearing that one day it might happen to them.

Polly

Eight children in every thousand are born with a heart defect, but most never need to worry. The abnormality will be so minor that their hearts function perfectly well, or it will correct itself as the child grows. But about two of the eight would die or deteriorate without treatment; for one of these two their defect will be so serious or complex that they will need open heart surgery, where the heart is stopped and a by-pass machine takes over its work and that of the lungs, so that the surgeon can repair the defective heart. Some of these children will not survive the operation or the crucial few days that follow; most will not only survive but grow up to lead a completely normal life.

Great Ormond Street has been performing by-pass surgery since 1961. Most children are from Britain but some come from Europe and beyond, even from Russia, for diagnosis and surgery so specialized and so skilled that it is not available in their own countries. Open heart surgery can be performed on very tiny premature babies of under 1.5 kg (barely 3 lb), but generally the cardiac team will wait, if possible, until the baby weighs at least 3 to 5 kg (5 to 11 lb). There are various kinds of heart problems: some children will need major surgery when they are small babies, others can get by, perhaps with the help of a minor, palliative operation, until they grow to a sturdier size and weight. Among them was Polly Logan-Banks who would face surgery for a complex condition including a hole in her heart; without open-heart surgery, she would die.

Polly's route to Great Ormond Street from her home in South London followed the normal process of referral from one hospital to another within the National Health Service. She was born on 29 March 1984, the first (and perhaps the only) child of Moira Banks and Ken Logan, an intellectual and individual couple who are nevertheless just as ruled by parental love and responsibility as the most conventional married pair.

Moira, blonde, elegant and articulate, was thirty-one when Polly was born. She had never thought of herself as at all maternal. 'I thought there was a possibility that I might never have children,' she says. 'But as I got to my late twenties, I realized I did want a child. It was an experience I wouldn't want to miss.' She considered going it alone and raising a child as a single parent, but then met Ken, a teacher at a school for children with emotional and behavioural difficulties in Camden, North London. They began living together. Marriage was not considered. Neither was religious and going through a civil ceremony seemed pointless; instead they had a party when Polly arrived. They are a settled couple, however, with a joint mortgage and a joint bank account (or, as Moira puts it, 'joint debts') and they have never found any disadvantages to being unmarried other than Moira's dislike of being called Mrs Banks. Though Ken feels his parents would initially have liked them to marry, she thinks her own are quite pleased they are not.

'My parents are very liberal. When I was growing up we always discussed everything and they never took the establishment or authority side,' says Moira. She earns her living as a freelance translator and proof-reader from French and runs a small business, with her mother, organizing bed and breakfast accommodation for American tourists. Work remains important to Moira even though the desire for a child was strong. Ken, thoughtful and analytical, agreed. 'There was a conscious decision to have a child. It seemed the right time – like our friends, they've had a solid ten years in a career and then think they'll have children before they are thirty-five when it becomes more difficult.' They conceived easily and the timing seemed auspicious. The pregnancy, though, was to change their lives.

When Moira's first ante-natal check-up produced the surprising news that she had a heart murmur, she didn't think too much of it. The doctors did not seem to suggest it was serious; she had never had any symptoms, although she recalls hating games at school and easily gets chilly. But four months pregnant, she passed out when shopping and her GP felt that the murmur should be investigated. She had tests at a local hospital. Moira – not an unquestioningly co-operative patient – found the tests had their ludicrous side. 'They gave me this box to wear on a great huge belt around my extended waist. I was supposed to wear it until I passed out again so that it could record what was happening. Needless to say I had it on for a week and never passed out. I thought I'm not going round for the rest of my pregnancy with this great box round me, so I just took it back with nothing on it.'

Nevertheless the murmur was diagnosed as an aortic stenosis, a narrowing of the aorta, the large artery rising out of the left ventricle of the heart which takes the oxygenated blood back into the body's circulation. Though the implications did not hit home at first, Moira may need surgery in the future, depending upon how the condition develops; this, plus the small chance that another child could have a cardiac problem, means that Polly will be their only child. The condition meant too that Moira felt ill throughout this pregnancy. 'I felt tremendously debilitated all through, flu-ish all the time. Then I developed high blood pressure and went into hospital, supposedly for a rest,' says Moira. 'The hospital was used to admitting mothers for a rest,' adds Ken. 'It may be right for older-style families with other children, but Moira got more rest at home because we share the shopping and cooking, like most of our friends do.'

Moira left hospital, which is not her favourite place, saying the idea of resting was a joke. Her strong personality probably helped her to absorb this blow and the uncomfortable pregnancy which followed. She is naturally forthright and combative and will not cave in easily, though events in the next three years were to cause her acute depression at times. She is also honest enough to admit that she is very glad she didn't proceed with the idea of having a child as a single parent – after what was to come. Yet although the pregnancy was miserable, neither her symptoms nor ante-natal scans ever suggested there was anything wrong with the baby. And subsequent discussions with doctors have indicated that the two heart conditions of mother and child are not related. Polly arrived at almost full term after a straightforward and, with the aid of an epidural, painless labour. Her parents were very happy and at

Polly's first examination immediately after birth, the doctors found nothing wrong.

The problems began that first night. Moira herself felt ill, very breathless and could hardly haul herself along to the bathroom, eventually collapsing; the night staff were unsympathetic, which hardly helped at such a vulnerable time. The following morning Polly was given another routine examination. The doctor listened to her heart with a stethoscope and said: 'Hello, there's a murmur here.'

'To begin with I wasn't tremendously worried,' remembers Moira, 'because I knew that there are lots of murmurs which don't mean very much. But the consultant came along and had a listen and he realized it was more than just a murmur. Then I began to wonder what was going on.' The doctors said Polly would have to go to a hospital which had an echocardiogram machine suitable for children; so late in the afternoon Polly was sent in an ambulance to Great Ormond Street, accompanied by her father. 'It was awful, it was pouring with rain and it was the rush hour, so we had flashing blue lights all the way because the traffic wasn't moving at all. It wasn't that much of an emergency, but I was very upset. I didn't know what was going on – I left Moira attached to a blood transfusion, not knowing at that stage if Polly would ever be coming back.'

Polly, less than a day old, immediately became the subject of further tests at Great Ormond Street to try to identify her heart problem and assess how serious it was. Already the doctors had listened to her heart with a stethoscope, the most basic diagnostic skill and one which has been available for centuries: the doctors can hear the sounds the heart makes as it beats and assess any murmurs (abnormal noises) which come from the way the blood flows through the heart. He or she would also see whether the baby was very breathless or blue and check her pulse or heart-rate and her blood pressure. At the maternity hospital Polly had also had an electrocardiogram (ECG) test. Electrodes are placed on the chest and limbs which record the electrical activity in the heart and a doctor can interpret the wavy patterns produced on the paper print-out, not only to see whether the heart's rhythm is normal but also to get an idea of which chambers may be enlarged. Later she would also have a chest X-ray to show the overall heart size and give a clue to the pattern of blood flow through the lungs.

The echocardiogram test for which Polly was transferred to Great Ormond Street is a form of ultra-sound scan using very high-pitched sound waves which partly pass through body tissues and partly are reflected back from the tissues. The reflected waves come back into the machine and can be analysed to produce a picture of the heart on a monitor. Because this test is non-invasive, carrying no risks and needing no anaesthetic, it is particularly valuable where children are already ill. It provides so much information that it has reduced the need to perform so many cardiac catheterizations, although in Polly's case this more involved and risky test would also be required before many months had passed.

But the pictures on the echocardiogram were sufficient to enable the Great Ormond Street cardiologists to come up with a diagnosis during that second evening of Polly's life. She had a defect known as Tetralogy of Fallot. It was an exotic sounding condition, but what it involved was explained to Ken; later that night he would get a consultant paediatrician to come with him to Moira to make sure she understood it too. Fallot was a nine-teenth-century French pathologist who correlated a group of four abnormal heart conditions which can occur together and identified them as an entity. The first of these four conditions was a Ventricular Septal Defect (VSD): a hole between the two ventricles which are the two lower, pumping, chambers of the heart (the upper chambers being the right atrium and left atrium in which the blood collects). The second aspect of the condition was the stenosed, or narrowed, pulmonary valve and arteries; these arteries, which carry blood from the right ventri-cle to the lungs ready for oxygenation and recirculation round the body, were in Polly's case small and narrowed. As a conse-quence this had induced the third problem: an obstruction caused by a muscle band which was impeding the flow of the right ventricle. The muscle tissue had become thickened as a response to having to push the blood through the stenosed valve and arteries. The fourth, and least serious, aspect of the condition is that the aorta, the great artery on the left side of the heart which supplies red blood to the body, is pushed slightly to the right.

Ken, having been a physical education teacher, knew some anatomy, but even so he had to have the condition explained to him twice, first by a cardiologist, then by a surgeon. The doctors drew diagrams for him to show the working of the heart. These showed the left side of the heart pumping out the oxygenated blood from the lungs round the system and the right side pumping the deoxygenated or blue blood which had come from the body into the lungs via – in Polly's case – narrow pulmonary arteries. They also showed the blockage in the right ventricle. This meant that the blood from the pumping part of the heart had difficulty in getting through the narrowed area to the lungs; some of the deoxygenated or blue blood was therefore passing through the hole between the two ventricles and going round the body. In simple terms, Polly would not be getting enough red or oxygenated blood. She was thus liable to become cyanotic or blue, cyanosis being the blueish appearance of the lips, tongue and nails caused by imperfect oxygenation.

It seemed to be clear, however, that Polly was not an emergency case. Some children with Fallot's Tetralogy will be so blue and distressed that they need a shunt, a palliative operation which will improve the blood supply to the lungs by connecting an artery that goes to the arm with the pulmonary artery. This relieves the condition, but does not cure it. Later their major surgery will close the VSD, the hole between the two ventricles, and tackle the problems of the stenosed valve and arteries and the obstruction to the ventricle. The condition has a range of severity; it is even possible for it to remain unsuspected for years, just as Moira's aortic stenosis remained unknown until the extra strain of pregnancy brought it to light. In terms of the range of severity, Polly was moderately ill. The hope was that she would be able to do without a shunt and gain weight until she could have her definitive repair.

It was about a quarter to eleven at night when Ken left Great Ormond Street. He found himself without any cash, but managed to find a cash dispenser so he could return to the maternity hospital in West London. He knew by this time that

Polly would be travelling back the following day. Moira had been hoping that they would come back together and when Polly arrived the next afternoon she went straight to the hospital's special care unit for observation. She remained in special care for two days, a depressing period for her parents, trying to come to terms with the revelations of the past twenty-four hours. Moira had post-natal blues and was still unwell herself.

'All the other Mums had their baby at the end of their beds but to get to Polly I had to stagger down the corridor and stairs with my blood transfusion. I'd get there to feed her and even though I had told them I was coming, they'd just have fed her. Things began to improve when she came back to the post-natal ward and I began to feel better.'

Both parents felt nervous when they brought Polly home. 'They offered us an apnoea mattress which rings an alarm if the baby stops breathing, but we thought in her case it was more likely that she'd breathe faster and faster than stop breathing. We thought we'd be forever jumping up and down with false alarms and drive ourselves into a terrible state. We decided to watch her very carefully, but try to make life as normal as possible,' says Moira.

'The worry the whole time was whether she would need a shunt or not,' says Ken. 'That was what I was told at the beginning, that first night. She would need to be ten kilos, the optimum weight for her surgery and if she didn't get to that and was getting distressed, then she would have a shunt which would help her through until she was big enough to have the main operation.' When Polly first went home, no one knew how serious the symptoms were going to be. 'It was nerve-racking not knowing whether she was going to go bluer and bluer at any time and it was only by having her home and living with her month after month that we got more reassured that she wasn't going to seize up,' says Moira.

Regular checks by the doctors became a feature of this period and when Polly was a month old she went back to Great Ormond Street to make sure she had not deteriorated. 'I had written out all the questions I wanted to ask and I had two sides of foolscap,' says Moira. 'The registrar we saw was extremely helpful and he went through every question and answered every single thing. We felt a lot more knowledgeable about it after that.'

But the first two and a half months were not easy. Moira had an infection on her stitches and for a while could not walk. Ken got up to fetch the baby for night feeds, but Moira's breast-feeding did not go smoothly. Because they are basically unwell, some babies with a heart defect may be irritable and poor feeders. Anxiety can also reduce milk production. Moira stuck at the breast-feeding but even though she sought the help of midwives and special feeding experts and she borrowed electric pumps, nothing worked. It would take an hour for a feed and then ten minutes later Polly would wake up hungry again. Her parents hardly slept. 'We got very intimate with the World Service,' recalls Ken about those long nights. 'But the day she went on boiled cows' milk at two and a half months, we never had another moment's bother with her feeding,' says Moira. It also helped that Polly seemed reasonably healthy. She was not distressed or going very blue at home, so her parents began to be hopeful that she could reach her target of 10 kg (22 lb); it helped to have something to aim for.

After the change of diet Polly slept normally and was a placid baby. She was a pretty child with blue eyes and red-gold hair. At about eleven months, though, she gave her parents a bad scare with a virus infection. 'She had a cold and an ear infection and we knew she was rotten. Then one evening she deteriorated quite quickly,' says Ken. They took her to their local hospital who gave her aspirin and oxygen. Fearing that she might have pneumonia, the hospital called in a consultant from home; but they were told to take Polly back to Great Ormond Street. 'By the time she got there she was a lot better and they must have thought what's all this fuss over an ear infection, though they kept her overnight,' says Moira. Like all parents they had various frights and they thought particularly hard about whooping cough vaccination which in normal circumstances they might have left alone. 'We were undecided but in the end came down on the side of vaccination because whooping cough could have seen her off. It would have been so much worse for her because of her heart,' says Ken.

Polly walked at thirteen months and her progress was very

normal. She had almost reached her target of ten kilos when her weight hit a plateau. Moira abandoned her earlier, preferred policy and began giving her biscuits as well as fresh fruit. A background strain lingered all the time as they watched for symptoms of blueness or exhaustion. At times, too, Moira was short of work which led to financial pressures and, as a freelance, she had to keep plugging away for more work. Devoted as she is to Polly, Moira has always wanted to work, to be a fulfilled and interesting person, for Polly's sake as well as her own. The strain was there, but it helped that Polly looked healthy and was doing things normally; she was an easy, even angelic child. The support of the hospital was also greatly valued. 'When you know that Great Ormond Street is there and you can ring them any time, then you know you have that back-up. With the slightest thing, they were always sympathetic and prepared to listen,' remembers Moira.

At the hospital itself Polly continued to have three-monthly check-ups where she was watched closely for signs of breath-lessness and deterioration. Doctors asked about her sleeping patterns: was she retaining the midday nap when other babies of her age would have been ready to do without it? Was she irritable and crotchety? Her condition is a progressive one and if she had been left completely alone, she would have been liable to cyanotic spells which can deprive the brain of oxygen. The body responds to lack of oxygen by producing more red blood cells and a very high red blood cell count can leave the patient vulnerable to strokes, cerebral abscesses and other problems including the possibility of lung damage. Ultimately a person with Tetralogy of Fallot will go into right-sided heart failure.

Polly, somewhere in the mid-range of severity, did make it through to her definitive surgery without a shunt. But at her clinic visits it was noted that she was becoming more cyanotic, more breathless; her parents, aware of the dangers and watch-ful as they were, tended to be less conscious of Polly's gradual deterioration. The doctors prefer to operate on this condition when the child is between 10 to 12 kg ((22-26 lb) so the timing of Polly's operation was a matter of delicate judgement. So, too, was the precise nature of the surgery, for Fallot's Tetralogy is a complex condition and there are various surgical options, depending on the exact status of the defective heart.

Polly would need one further test before these decisions could be made. She had already had many tests showing the range of diagnostic equipment which is available today, especially ultra-sound which has revolutionized the work of cardiac units everywhere in the 1980s. These diagnostic techniques are especially vital to paediatric cardiologists because they are dealing with congenital abnormalities which may be more varied and obscure (especially those which arrive at Great Ormond Street) than the degenerative problems of adults which tend to fall into similar patterns.

At this point the surgeons became involved in Polly's story, for one of the principal characteristics of Great Ormond Street's approach to cardiac problems is collective discussion and decision-making. 'This is one of the main strengths of our unit and in many ways it is unique,' says Czech-born Jaroslav Stark, who was to be Polly's consultant surgeon. He came to Great Ormond Street in 1965 for training and later settled in London with his family. 'In many hospitals you have the department of cardiology which is one entity and the department of surgery which is another – often in different buildings. The cardiologists investigate the child, make up their minds and more or less tell the surgeon what to do. Here we have what we call the Thoracic Unit and right from the beginning the surgeon and the cardiologist are involved together. The surgeon often suggests what details he has to know for that particular condition and the cardiologists can then adjust their investigation. We have joint conferences three times a week when we all look at the investigations; sometimes we may disagree on small details, but basically we all put our minds to it to jointly establish an accurate diagnosis and decide what is the optimal way to treat that individual child.'

'There is really no place today for what some surgeons still claim – "I open up and I look inside and then I fix it". It is occasionally possible but it's just surgical bravado, nothing else. If you want to do an operation safely a hundred times in a row, you can't rely on that. This is generally true of several branches of surgery but especially it applies to neonatal cardiac surgical work. In very complex congenital heart defects we have to assess very carefully the physiology and then decide whether we should repair all defects or whether it would actually be advantageous for the child to leave some of the defects unrepaired. This is important not only for the immediate survival of the child but also for the best possible long term results.'

Mr Stark is sure that the advantages of teamwork contribute to the good results of the unit which are among the best in the world. Yet physically, it is one of the least preposessing departments in the entire hospital. For years its staff have been waiting for the opening of a new seven-floor cardiac block which will increase ward space from twenty-nine to fifty-six beds and provide new investigation rooms, operating theatres, research facilities and parents' accommodation. There will also be better changing rooms and coffee rooms for the nurses, and proper storage facilities so that equipment does not have to be stacked in ward corridors as at present. The block was actually completed in 1980 at a cost of over £4 million but had to be evacuated just one week after it was handed over when a concrete beam collapsed. Six years later it was still being rebuilt, despite the outpouring already of an additional £13 million. Until the block is successfully re-opened the department is resigned to decrepit waiting rooms, small and inconvenient offices where consultants work amid stacks of files, and clinical facilities which lack space, although not 'state of the art' medical equipment. On first sight, the cramped conditions cause foreign doctors, especially those from the United States, to reel back in amazement. Yet the conditions do not stop many foreign doctors joining the unit for a year or two to gain experience.

About one in five of the patients are also from overseas, mainly private patients – some are from an EEC quota or government-sponsored. One unusual patient was eight-month-old Yuri Sobol who came from Russia in December 1985 under an Anglo-Soviet health agreement. He was born with a complex congenital heart defect for which treatment was not available in Russia. After long negotiations, Yuri was able to come to London for Jaroslav Stark to perform the first stage operation; if all goes well, Yuri will return to London for corrective surgery in about four years' time.

Mr Stark was to operate on Polly two months later. The diagnosis was already known from the echocardiogram: there was a hole in the heart and a severe narrowing of the pulmonary arteries that run from the heart to the lungs. The additional questions that needed clarification were where exactly was the narrowing, how long was the narrowing and how severe was it? These questions would be answered by the cardiologists who would perform the cardiac catheterization and angiography.

At sixteen months old Polly therefore returned to Great Ormond Street as an in-patient for her catheterization. This usually involves a three-day stay in hospital. Under a local anaesthetic and sedation, a fine plastic tube known as a catheter is passed through the femoral artery in the groin up into various parts of the heart, steered along with the circulation. The catheter is connected to a machine called a transducer which changes the pressure wave being picked up by the catheter into an electrical signal shown on a monitor. It can differentiate pressures in different parts of the heart and the great arteries; these are then compared against the normal pressures for healthy children. Small samples of blood are also taken from the various chambers in the heart and measured for their oxygen content. Finally, a radio opaque material which shows up on X-rays is injected, filling the appropriate chamber in the heart to show the structural abnormality; this part of the catheterization is known as the angiogram.

The catheter test showed that the narrowing of the arteries was very severe, more than the doctors had expected, and also indicated that the pulmonary valve was suspect. 'By this time they seemed into the realms of total technical detail and the catheter obviously told the doctors more than it told us,' says Moira. The catheterization was bad timing for her since she was recovering from peritonitis, following a burst appendix. Polly resisted sleep in hospital and Moira had to spend hours standing beside her cot trying to get her to sleep; she finally had to be given a sedative the night before catheterization. Ken and Moira had a foretaste of the tension in store for them when

Polly was away in the angiogram suite hours longer than expected; the delay was caused by problems, which do occur occasionally, in stopping the bleeding after the catheter is removed. When she returned Polly came round quickly and soon wanted to go back to the playroom, so her parents knew she was all right.

'We weren't really sure what they were going to say about her coming in for her operation,' says Moira. 'But at that point they said "We think she's ready."' Not an emergency, Polly went on to the waiting list which was about six months so her parents expected to receive a letter the following spring. Christmas was fun: Moira and Ken had friends to stay with a young baby of their own. Polly was well and she thoroughly enjoyed the two Christmas trees and their lights. 'It was ridiculous how many presents she had, although the boxes ended up being played with, of course,' says Moira.

But the summons for Polly's surgery came sooner than expected, one month after Christmas and two months short of Polly's second birthday. Because of cancellations, Polly's name had come to the top of the waiting list and out of the blue one Friday Moira took a phone call from the hospital asking her to bring Polly in on Monday, for surgery the following Thursday – just six days away. 'It was an awful shock,' says Moira, 'but really, in retrospect, it was the best way because we only had three days of anxiety before she went in instead of three weeks.' Moira immediately rang Ken's school, but he was visiting a museum with some of his students. He says: 'When I got back there was a message saying "Ring home" and there's never a message saying that. When I knew the reason, there was a mixture of shock and relief. First I wondered why are they doing it earlier, is there something they haven't told us? But we accepted that it was just a cancellation. Then we had a strong feeling of "Let's get on with it".'

Moira also felt Polly was at just the right age for her to have the operation: 'She was too young to be frightened or to be too aware of everything that was going on, too young to be conscious of anticipated pain. Yet she was old enough to have a firm grasp on life, not like the tiny babies that just waver away.' Ken was less certain. He wondered if the fact that she

133

was too young to understand what was happening or to talk about it would be more traumatic for her: could it leave her with a painful, subconscious memory?

The weekend before the operation was filled with making arrangements and both parents were fairly calm. Moira rang a couple of regular freelance clients to warn them that she would not be around for a couple of weeks. Ken decided to work normally from Monday to Wednesday, as Polly would then be having tests, but to arrange for time off after that. His school, where he had worked for nine years, was very understanding. Being busy made it easier for them; other parents preparing for the same experience find themselves hardly able to pack the child's things or to contemplate the child's room. Moira arranged for her mother to come up from Sussex and look after their house, s small but attractive Victorian terrace in Herne Hill, South London, and their large, vociferous dog, Pooter. 'She was ready to drop everything, she wanted to be here and my father was abroad on business, so that made it easier for her. We all thought "Right then folks, this is it" and got it all organized. Then off Polly went; we were obviously terrified, but felt that it had to come some time and that it was better that it came now.'

Moira took Polly into Great Ormond Street on that Monday and Ken joined them after school. The first few days went smoothly, except that Polly did not sleep and Moira had to ask a nurse for a sedative; she desperately wanted Polly not to be too tired by Thursday. Polly spent Tuesday and Wednesday having tests on ward 1D which is the less acute ward of the cardiac unit at the western end of the first floor. It is here that children are usually admitted before surgery and where they return a day or so later from 1A, the intensive care cardiac ward. That, at least, is the plan if all goes well.

Karen Eagles, 1D's playleader, went through the play preparations with Polly and Moira, using a Teddy who has all the tubes and drains that a child will have after cardiac surgery: he has a ventilator tube, a drip into his arm for liquid food, a medicine drip into his neck, two chest drains to clear up excess blood from the operation site and a catheter to drain urine so that it can be tested and measured – kidney output is an important indication of how well the newly-corrected heart is working. The Teddy also has an operation scar, pacemaker wires (these are inserted in case they are needed and taken out just before the child goes home), electrocardiogram stickers on his chest and a hospital name-band round his wrist. Karen emphasizes to the child that all the tubes and wires will gradually be removed as she gets better after the operation. To Karen Eagles, the play preparation is the most important part of her work. Children are also encouraged to ask questions and play out their fantasies with the hospital box, which contains equipment such as syringes, masks and a stethoscope. Polly was too young to grasp every detail, but she enjoyed going through a book of photographs compiled on the ward which followed the progress of other 1A children after heart operations.

What Moira also found particularly helpful was a talk with 1D Sister Jane Jacob. She went through the functions of all the post-operative tubes and warned Moira and Ken what to expect about Polly's moods: she would be dreadfully thirsty and would blame them because she couldn't have a drink, she would blame them for everything, in fact, and not smile for two or three days. 'It was very helpful to be prepared for that!' say the parents. The day of the operation and the few days following will be a great psychological ordeal, so the doctors try to prepare parents for it. Dr John Deanfield, one of the team of five cardiologists, advises them to pace themselves for a marathon rather than a sprint and to try to ensure that they don't have too many sleepless nights.

Dr Deanfield also understands the parents' feelings of helplessness: their child is at the greatest risk it has ever been and they have handed it over to other people. 'The most important thing is for parents to feel complete confidence in the medical and nursing staff,' he says. 'If they feel they have done everything they can, and the child is in the best place, that takes some of the tension away. If the child dies, one of the things I try to communicate is that it wasn't their fault, it wasn't the hospital's fault, sometimes problems can't be put right.' John Deanfield warns parents that in the post-operative period things happen fast and staff will be giving one hundred per cent attention to the child. He wishes the ward had a more adequate waiting room, but of course, it was designed long before this kind of surgery was envisaged and in the new cardiac block these needs will be met. 'When things are at their most tense, the facilities are least adequate,' says Dr Deanfield.

At least Moira and Ken would be resident for the two nights following the operation in 'The Home from Home', a house renovated by a charity, The Sick Children's Trust, where parents can stay while their children have treatment at either Great Ormond Street or St Bartholomew's Hospital. But at first they slept, or tried to sleep, at home. On 1D Polly kept little better hours, despite being given a sedative from Tuesday evening onwards: 'We would get there at six in the morning and she was always awake,' recalls Moira. On Wednesday, the really unbearable tension started. Moira coped with it by retreating; she just went silent.

Mr Stark, the senior cardiac surgeon, would be assisted during Polly's operation by his senior registrar, George Alexander, a tall and expansive American from North Carolina. It was Mr Alexander who, the night before Polly's operation, came to see Moira to discuss in detail what the operation would mean. 'Previously we had heard that there was a ninety to ninety-five per cent chance of her coming safely through the operation, but he put it a different way and said there was a five to ten per cent chance that she wouldn't survive the operation. It sounds much worse put that way round. He also raised the question of a number of bleak possibilities – even though they were very remote – that she could have a stroke, die on the operating table. Of course, I wanted to know every detail about the operation but the next day these thoughts kept coming back into my head,' says Moira.

On Thursday morning Moira again arrived at the hospital at six o'clock, later to be joined by her mother, Joy, and Ken. At one point Polly had been scheduled to be first on the operating list, but the day before she had been moved to second; this meant she would go to theatre at about one p.m. 'In some ways it was worse having to wait, but you suppress any tension for her sake,' says Moira. 'She had a bath and we spent the morning playing.' But inexorably the morning wore away.

Polly was given her pre-medication injection which made her cry; normally she never complained, even watched with interest when blood samples were being taken, but this was a fairly big injection and even a nurse will occasionally admit she doesn't like giving it. After the pre-med, Polly fell asleep on her mother's lap in the playroom. Then came one of the worst moments for any parent: handing over your child for her operation, so that she has passed right out of your hands, perhaps never to come back. Sister Jacob and an operating department assistant, already wearing a green surgical gown and a mask, came in for her; until then Polly had thought it was all play, she hadn't realized anything was going to happen to her. 'She was looking over the assistant's shoulder, shouting "Mummy, Mummy, come". Both my mother and myself burst into tears immediately – there's just no description of how you feel.'

There now stretched before them the long wait of at least four or five hours. They saw Dr Philip Rees, the consultant cardiologist looking after Polly. He was very sympathetic and said he knew what an unpleasant day it was for them, but it had to come. Some parents go right out of the hospital, perhaps to Hamleys to buy a toy for the child, Moira, Ken and Joy went to the parents' sitting room on the fifth floor. Here they spread themselves out on one of the sofas and prepared for the long wait. 'We were really grateful to Marks and Spencer for that sitting room*,' says Joy, Moira's mother. 'It was a relief to be there after the ward and have that bit of humanity, plants and comfort. When we got back to the ward and all the other anxious parents later we realized how much we had appreciated it.' Joy tried to knit, but couldn't; Moira stared at the floor and did her best to keep her mind a blank.

'I didn't want to sit there just remembering her, I didn't want there to be any question of it being a past thing. But your mind keeps coming back to thoughts of what could go wrong, the five to ten per cent chance that she could die. The second

---

*Marks and Spencer had recently refurbished the parents' sitting room, as explained and described in Kristie's story.

fear is that she might suffer brain damage. Of course you want to think positive, but it's such a huge thing that you are scared to be confident. You can't be blasé, you've got to do a certain amount of preparing your body for just in case, I think, so that your mind and your body would be a tiny bit prepared if the worst happened. Mostly I just sat and concentrated on a spot on the floor and tried to pass the time like that. Of course, it seemed like weeks.'

Ken kept making tea on the hour and going to fetch sandwiches for them all – anything to keep busy. 'He really didn't know what to do with himself,' says Joy. But for Ken the ordeal was not quite so bad as for Moira. 'I never really faced her death. I don't know if I was blocking it out,' he says. Ken's worst time had been his first visit to Great Ormond Street when Polly was diagnosed at a day old and he had been very distressed by his shock and concern for the two people with heart conditions — first Moira and now his daughter. By the time Polly had her operation he had developed confidence in the hospital and felt they had handed over Polly to a team of people who would ensure a positive outcome.

Polly had been wheeled to the first-floor operating suite and taken first to the anaesthetic room where, after she had gone to sleep, a catheter to collect urine and lines to monitor both venous and arterial blood pressure were inserted. Next door, in the theatre, technicians had already set up and tested pressure equipment and the ventilator which would be used during the operation. Fully anaesthetized, she was taken into theatre where a large team of people was already partly assembled. An operation such as this would require one theatre sister to be scrubbed and assist at the table, with a minimum of two nurses to fetch and hand things to her. George Alexander, the senior registrar, was scrubbed and ready to perform the first part of the operation with a houseman at his side; they would be joined later by Mr Stark. The two anaesthetists – a consultant and a registrar – took up their station at the head of the operating table. There would be two 'perfusionists' or pump technicians who would take charge of the heart-lung by-pass machine; one sits in front of the machine regulating the blood flow, the other acts as a back-up and performs regular blood checks. The blood is tested for its red cell count, acid base balance and the amounts of carbon dioxide and oxygen.

The perfusionists primed the by-pass machine, which stands near the anaesthetists, with blood matching that of Polly. The machine acts as the patient's heart and lungs while the surgeons are working inside the heart; it both pumps blood and exchanges gases, passing the deoxygenated blood through an oxygenator which is linked to an oxygen supply. After the blood is oxygenated, and excess carbon dioxide removed, it is passed back into the system via the patient's aorta, the vessel which transmits purified blood to the body. The by-pass machine also contains a unit which controls the temperature of the blood and this will be used to cool the blood right down from its normal thirty-seven degrees Celsius to twenty degrees. When cold the body's metabolic processes slow and need far less oxygen in the blood, so that the surgeon can work with a lower blood flow; in some children the flow of blood can be diminished or even stopped completely. A calculated amount of blood (based on body weight and height) is pumped round the body but the surgeon tells the perfusionist what temperature and what blood flow he requires to suit the surgical requirements. The perfusionist then regulates the blood flow and watches the patient's blood pressures; later, before the patient comes off the by-pass machine, he will increase the temperature of the blood.

Advances in the by-pass technique – the machine had to be miniaturized for babies and children along with other adjustments so that the child would be able to function properly afterwards – are not the only improvements in treatment which have made the success rate of this kind of surgery possible. Advances in diagnosis give the surgeons much more precise information beforehand so they know how to approach the heart, from the front or from the left or right chest. They have specialized micro-instruments which enable them to work on babies as small as 1 kg (2 lb). There is far better understanding of the physiology of cardiac defects: sometimes a small hole with which the heart is functioning well is better left alone. There is also much greater knowledge of how to protect the heart during the period when it is stopped. The heart is stopped – by placing a clamp on the aorta – because the surgeons can stitch (or suture) far more accurately when it is still. Generally the surgeons have about one hour when they can stop the heart without any consequence to the child.

The surgeons painted Polly's chest with antiseptic solution and then draped it with green surgical sheets. Then, at about one-thirty, George Alexander began the operation by opening Polly's chest, cutting through the breast-bone and exposing the heart. Mr Stark then joined the team. He put in the cannulas, or metal tubes, which would link Polly to the by-pass machine. When the flow from the machine was established, Polly was cooled. The aorta was then clamped and a special solution was injected into it to stop and protect the heart. Mr Stark first patched the VSD, or hole between the two ventricles, with dacron, a synthetic fabric, suturing it around the hole. Next he turned to the second stage of the operation which would open up the way from the heart to the lungs.

As expected from the angiogram taken during the catheter-ization – 'We get surprises in theatre about once or twice a year,' says Mr Stark – the narrowing was too extensive and severe merely, as can sometimes be done, to put a patch on the right ventricle. Mr Stark therefore removed the muscle obstruction within the right ventricle and also removed a thick-ened and very abnormal pulmonary valve. He then used a patch of pericardium, which is the outer membrane that encloses the heart, to enlarge both left, right and main pulmon-ary arteries. During this stage of the operation the aortic clamp was removed so that Polly's heart started to beat and she was completely rewarmed using the heat exchanger in the heart-lung machine.

When the temperature was normal, the by-pass was gradu-ally discontinued and Polly's heart was allowed to take over completely. At this point the pressure in all chambers of the heart were measured. The right ventricular pressure was still somewhat higher then the surgeons would have liked it. The line to measure right ventricular pressure was therefore left in place so that the pressure could be monitored continuously during the post-operative period; this was very helpful for the overall strategy of looking after a child such as Polly.

At about three-thirty Moira, Ken and Joy left the parents' sitting room and went down to 1A to wait in the playroom. Moira walked round to the sisters' desk, but the sister on duty (there are seven in this department) had heard nothing. Five minutes later, though, she came round to tell them that the main part of the operation was over and that everything was fine. 'I took this to mean that she was off the by-pass and they were tidying her up,' says Moira. 'The relief then was just totally enormous. She's come through, she's had her operation, she's alive. At least, it wasn't total relief because I didn't know what state she would be in when she came back but I knew I would see her again, that she would be coming back. My mother and I cried again.'

They all knew that Polly was not yet back in the recovery room so they could not go straight to see her. But at this point George Alexander came to explain how the operation had gone. Moira says: 'We knew that there were alternatives and that they wouldn't know for certain until they got to theatre. Mr Alexander explained about the large patch over the pulmonary arteries, the loss of the pulmonary valve and the raised pressure in the right ventricle. He said this did make recovery more rocky and that there was a risk of heart failure, so that dampened down the relief. I was thinking – 'Oh, God, is she likely to go at any minute?' There wasn't really any way they could tell whether there was a danger of it happening until symptoms actually started. He said that if she did well for the first seventy-two hours, that was a good indication that she would be all right.' Once again, George Alexander was warning them of what could go wrong, but Moira found her overwhelming need to see Polly swamped the worry. 'I knew that soon she'd be there and that was all I wanted to do – to see her back and OK.'

Half an later Polly came back to what the ward call the pump room, a three-bedded recovery room, extremely cramped for space, to which children return from theatre. She was ventilated and being given blood to replace the loss from chest drains. She was given sedation, ice packs and parace- tamol to reduce her temperature and a drug to strengthen the action of the heart. A nurse was assigned specially to her; she was to do the general observations of temperature, pulse, respiration and blood pressure and also to watch the ECG, arterial and venous blood pressure monitors. This nurse would be responsible for keeping the tubes open, measuring the urine output and administering drugs correctly as well as carrying out general nursing care such as keeping Polly's mouth clean and avoiding pressure sores; the nursing and surgical teams work very closely at this point. 'A good nurse,' says George Alexander, 'often makes the difference between whether a child does well or badly, sensing when a patient is in trouble, for instance, spotting that a child is cool even when the other signs are good. Peripheral temperature monitoring is another indication of how well the heart is performing – warm feet, the better the circulation. Spotting the first little hints can really make a difference.'

The nurse is also involved in the care of the parents. She must be ready to explain the child's progress to them, although at first parents are asked only to come into the room for ten minutes or so at a time. This is partly because the nurse has so much to do and partly because of the extremely cramped conditions caused by the plethora of equipment for each of the three beds and the frequent visits to the room from teams of doctors. Half an hour after Polly arrived in the pump room, Moira and Ken went to see her.

Many parents find seeing their child covered in tubes quite traumatic, but Moira and Ken were prepared for them and knew they were all normal and had their function. 'Straight away I noticed that she looked more pink – we'd never seen her lips that colour,' says Ken. Her face also looked good to Moira: 'It was a good colour and unmarked and that was reassuring. At about ten to eight in the evening, when we were there, she came to and said "Mummy" at me, so I was happy in my own mind that her brain was all right.'

After this crucial bit of relief, Moira began to collapse herself. 'At about eight p.m. I just felt terribly ill. We had eaten sandwiches but I'd had a migraine coming on, probably from the crying, and I had terrible heartburn from the pills I had taken. I had a feeling of total and absolute exhaustion and what worried me was because of my own heart condition I didn't want to push myself too far or I wouldn't be any good to her the following day when she needed me there. I hated to leave her but I knew I'd got to just collapse somewhere.'

Ken brought the car up the hospital driveway to the main door because Moira was shaking and incapable of walking even the short distance to the Sick Children's Trust house in Gray's Inn Road. Back at the house Moira got straight into bed with two duvets on top of her and went straight out. Ken had been very concerned about her and kept reminding her which extension to call if she needed any help, but she had urged him to go back to Great Ormond Street. 'It was important to me to know that Ken would be there while I wasn't,' she says. Ken slept in the 1A playroom, freezing cold; it was a bitter February night with snow on the ground.

The following morning, Moira woke up at about four-thirty feeling much better. Still exhausted, but not actually ill, she immediately got up and went to the hospital. Polly had had a good night. She was still being ventilated but the oxygen had been reduced from fifty per cent to forty per cent overnight. During the morning they gradually reduced the ventilation further and during the afternoon she was extubated – taken off the ventilator – and breathing oxygen through a face mask. 'That was great because that meant her face was back to normal and even by then we'd seen how pink she looked. Her face looked well, not harassed, or as if she had gone through something dreadful,' says Moira.

Jaroslav Stark, too, was pleased. That day he came to talk to Moira and Ken to explain the implications of the particular kind of surgery Polly had undergone. He says: 'The pulmonary valve had to be removed but fortunately in the majority of children it is not needed. But we will keep a good eye on her to watch the pressure in the right ventricle, to check that it can cope with the valveless system. For this reason we will probably re-catheterize in a year or two. We have no way of knowing in which child this ventricle will become tired, or the time scale, so we watch them in case they need a valve later. We could have put in a valve during this operation, but it's better to leave it and go back later as there is only a four to five per cent chance that Polly will need it.' Mr Stark managed to put over the information in a positive way so it was not alarming to Moira or Ken. By this time Polly's early and rapid progress – unlike some who may have a very difficult post-operative time – was already giving the surgeons reason to believe that the pressure in the right ventricle was coming down. Yet it remained important to know for certain which is why they would have to re-catheterize.

But Polly's good progress continued, although there were very minor delays: her chest drains were a little later coming out than expected, her urine output had to be encouraged with a diuretic drug and the first time they weaned her off the face mask, she couldn't quite manage and it had to go back on for a while. Although her parents were on edge, waiting for a set-back, these were small and temporary problems. 'Every time they told us about an X-ray or a blood gas test, it was good news. She started coughing early and this was a good sign. Although she was a bit chesty, she didn't seem to need as much suction as some of the other children,' remembers Moira. 'Our main problem was sleep. We just got exhausted being there. You didn't want to go away at all but it was a question of having to sleep. It would have been nice to have had the hospital accommodation a bit longer, until she was out of intensive care, but obviously there's such pressure on the house.' Over the weekend, when they returned home to Herne Hill to sleep, Moira's mother stayed there and cooked for them.

On Sunday Polly's chest drains, catheter and intravenous lines were removed. 'Suddenly she looked like a normal little girl again. There she was sitting up with a dress on,' recalls Moira. 'We had heard that her liver was in the right place which was one of the signs that they thought the pressures in her heart had dropped as they were supposed to. She was 'doing swell' as George Alexander put it. Ken adds: 'On the Monday evening she stood up and took a few steps holding on to our hands and on Tuesday she was off. Eating was never great, though she drank a lot once she was on free fluids from the following Wednesday. Although she was grumpy a lot of the time, she smiled earlier than they said. She never slept very well and it was "playroom, playroom" all the time, even when she was exhausted.'

Polly was showing a resilience typical of young children after major surgery when everything has been straightforward. It certainly impressed her parents. Ken: 'Polly always knew that we were around. It wasn't like a hospital with antiquated visiting hours. Even her language development, putting words together, continued while she was in hospital.' And Moira: 'She didn't have distress and pain in her eyes. She won't have the intensive care bit in her memory at all as she was so heavily drugged. She wasn't at all anxious to get out of the hospital; when the day came, and we said: "Shall we go home tomorrow?", she was shaking her head.'

'Children can bounce back even after a major operation,' says Adelaide Tunstill, clinical nursing officer of 1A. 'Seeing your child with all the tubes and drains can be worse for the parent than the child.' The nursing staff will do what they can to support the parents, but the parents also support each other. In the small waiting room on 1A, with its shabby furniture, always full of cigarette smoke and either too hot or too cold, there is always a group of parents talking. 'When there are people in there that you've got to know over the past week, you feel at home,' says Moira. 'They may be people you would never meet normally but everybody is interested in everyone else's story. Any heart story relates to your own and you want to get knowledgeable.'

Parents can help the new arrivals to get through the day of their operation. This is no place for anyone to be too euphoric about their own child's progress, but because they have been through it, this can be a help. Moira says: 'Whether it really is a support, as you'd like it to be, you don't know. They could be thinking – "Oh, it's all right for her, her little girl is doing fine". You can't go round saying: "Your child will be all right" because they might not. It's not the right thing to say.' Other parents had sadder stories than Polly's and were also apart from their husbands and worried about other children in Wales or Italy.

Polly, Moira and Ken left Great Ormond Street the following Saturday, just nine days after the operation. Moira and Ken, at least, were longing to get home and that evening they had a champagne dinner with her parents, her father having now returned from business abroad. They looked to a promising future although, as Mr Stark explained, Polly will have another catheterization eighteen months or so after the operation to check that the pressure in the right ventricle is not too high. It portends well that she has prospered since the operation, but the doctors will not know for certain until they do the catheterization.

'A child with a condition like Polly's,' says Mr Stark, 'we would expect in general to lead an entirely normal life, get married, do all the sports. There is the proviso as with any operation that there is always a small chance something will not go as it should; in some children you have a hundred per cent result, in some you have an eighty per cent result. It is our policy that children come for a check-up once a year because if something starts going wrong it's much better that we pick it up quickly. It's just common sense.'

'We'll wait for the catheter but a lot more hopefully,' says Moira. 'Before we had this great thing hanging over us and now we can be hopeful that we won't have it again. Polly certainly looks extremely well and is full of energy. She chats away to everyone and tells them that her scar is getting better. Everything looks positive, probably more positive than it has been since I was first pregnant. It has been a tough three years, but now the bad things seem to be receding and the good things turning up.' Moira has now got a lot more work coming through as a result of effort put in over the last two years, so financial pressures have eased as well. Her parents have offered to pay for a holiday: 'I'd like to be able to take her to a hotel which has a lot of catering for children, somewhere on a beach so that she can play with sand and see the sea for the first time.' Moira and Ken have never taken her anywhere beyond visiting both sets of grandparents; they were advised not to travel beyond a hundred-mile radius of London and certainly not abroad.

'We are thanking our lucky stars for the hospital – and for the NHS, such as it is these days,' says Moira. Like Moira, her mother Joy loathes hospitals but she, too, was very impressed with Great Ormond Street. 'The casualness appealed to me. Nobody pounced on us and said we couldn't do things. They let you make tea, they even let you borrow their tea and milk. The nurses are terribly overworked but relaxed. It is an inspiring place,' says Joy. 'There's an awful lot for other hospitals to learn from Great Ormond Street about the way people are treated and the way they are talked to,' agrees Ken. 'They do it because they know parents are anxious but adult patients are anxious, too, and I don't think in general hospitals it is done nearly as well. In an ordinary hospital they are under pressure because of staff shortages, they don't have time to deal with their patients properly and that's the political ballgame. At Great Ormond Street the limitations are those of the building.' Moira feels the staff experienced stress because of the cramped working conditions: 'But on the whole the nurses are very friendly and accommodating; you don't ask a nurse for something and she forgets.'

Nothing in their lives has ever matched this as an ordeal or for emotional intensity. 'Everything else you go through on your own account and you have a certain amount of control over it, but this is your child and you're helpless,' says Moira. Despite her closeness to Ken it was an ordeal which Moira felt she faced on her own. 'I felt isolated with it, inside myself with it, but physically and externally you help each other by just carrying on as per normal, always being around and knowing the other one is with Polly when you can't be there.'

Moira will always be there for Polly, who will always take precedence, even though work is important to her mother. She was an ambitious career girl who knew exactly where she was going until Polly came along. Perhaps it took her by surprise how intensely she would love her child and how those feelings would be tested when Polly's life was threatened. Just before Polly returned home from Great Ormond Street, Moira poured out her feelings of gratitude to the cardiac team in a letter to Jaroslav Stark.

Dear Mr Stark,

    I am sitting at home, late at night, knowing that my daughter, Polly, will be coming home from hospital within the next few days, fit, pink and full of health and life. Human language is totally inadequate to express what you have done for all of our lives. Ten or fifteen years ago Polly would undoubtedly have had a limited life expectation, and it is only due to people such as yourself that countless families have experienced hope where previously there was none, and life where only sadness and helplessness would otherwise have prevailed. I am not a religious person, and I do not thank a god for Polly's recovery, but please believe that I shall always, always, thank you. With inexpressibly grateful sentiments,

Thank you forever for the life of my child,

Moira Banks

Postscript: one year later
She is continuing to recover well from surgery. At three, Polly is a lively and forward child, already learning to read. Although there is the possibility of further corrective surgery, she is leading a totally normal life.

10.55 a.m. *Leanne, a sixteen-month-old girl, is seen by Meena Agrawal, a locum (or acting) consultant in the department of paediatric surgery. Leanne has a fatty lump on her back and X-ray changes in her spine which Miss Agrawal identifies as spina dysraphism. Eventually Leanne will need an operation, but as the lump is not interfering with her development, the surgeon would prefer to leave it for a while. 'She's at a very difficult age for post-operative care which could involve lying still for a few days,' Meena Agrawal tells Leanne's mother. She added that it was impossible to say what was underneath the lump; it could be cerebral spinal fluid or simply fatty tissue or both. Other children seen during the morning clinic do have spina bifida and related problems such as hydrocephalus which involves shunts to remove excessive fluid from the brain. Such patients tend to have bulging files of medical notes indicating a series of in-patient admissions as well as frequent out-patient appointments. There are also several children with various bowel problems. Ten-week-old Jake was born with what, for a mother, must be one of the most traumatic abnormalities – sections of the bowel lying outside the body. Yet once surgery has replaced the bowel inside the body Jake stands a good chance of leading a normal life. Other bowel problems may involve a lifetime of dietary restrictions to avoid potentially dangerous diarrhoea.*

11.00 a.m. *Jenny Collyer, secretary to the private patient wards, is on the telephone to Grenada where parents of a former patient are worried about how to obtain certain drugs. Life is only marginally more plush, but certainly more exotic on the seventh floor where the private wards are to be found. Multi-lingual notices give clues to the clientele with signs in Arabic, Greek, French, Italian and, more unexpectedly, Icelandic; children come here from Iceland for cardiac treatment. The mixture of nationalities is matched by a diversity of conditions. More than any other ward at Great Ormond Street, the private wards are general paediatric wards; with thirty-three consultants able to admit private patients to the wards, this is hardly surprising. Differing national traits and customs can pose problems for people such as Jenny Collyer and Sister Mo McAlea. Many Arab fathers are unused to being told what to do by women and will not allow their* *wives to sign consent forms. Occasionally a man will bring more than one wife with him to the hospital; one Arab father, hearing that his son had a congenital disorder, asked the doctor – 'Should I get a new wife?' There can also be problems of burial rites if a child dies. Preparing the bill for treatment if a child does die is Jenny Collyer's least favourite task. The cost is sufficiently high – in 1986 the charges set by the Government were between £241 and £265 a day – to bring in £1.7 million a year in the mid-1980s. And, as private health insurance schemes spread in Britain, the hospital is considering increasing the number of private beds to attract more British patients in order to boost the hospital's income – at present only one in twenty of the approximately 800 private patients a year. Ironically, many of the British children in the private wards come for one of the most routine operations performed in the hospital – the removal of tonsils and adenoids.*

11.05 a.m. *Christopher, aged three, arrives with his mother to see Dr Sarah Ledermann in a renal out-patient clinic. He is one of seventy-five long-term chronically sick children seen at the clinic, usually monthly, sometimes more frequently. A few will eventually need kidney transplants, but if they remain well, it is better to keep their own impaired kidneys than risk the complications of a transplant. Christopher was born with only one functioning kidney. There were other problems, too, notably three obstructions in the urinary tract. His treatment has involved two operations and several prolonged stays at Great Ormond Street. His kidney function fell as low as six to seven per cent of normal capacity, but is now around fifteen per cent. He is also eating better, after years of vomiting which were a nightmare for his mother. Not that life is particularly easy now. Five times a day he must take various drugs and his diet is still restricted in terms of protein such as dairy products.*

Dr Ledermann is pleased with Christopher. He looks well, is gaining weight and his renal problems were not affecting his bones. The blood and urine tests taken at the previous clinic visit were also fine; if they hadn't been she would have phoned his mother, with whom she is on first-name terms. Christopher, too, is at home in the doctor's office, going straight to the toy cupboard like the veteran visitor he is. So far he has not required any dialysis and he is not yet on the list of children awaiting transplants. The longer he can delay such a moment the better: he would be stronger to withstand the transplant and the chance of finding a suitable donor will be higher. Today, as Christopher scampers around the clinic, there appears to be little wrong with him. But his mother will never go far from home, never go on holiday to an area without a large hospital – just in case. She says: 'The doctors here have never had any doubts that he would make it, but you learn to enjoy him as he is now because there are going to be times again when he is deteriorating and when he is hard work and not so well. It's nice that he's got to the state that he is well enough to be a little bit naughty, like any other boy.'

11.10 a.m. *Catering staff begin to pack the children's lunches. On average the kitchens prepare meals for 200 children a day and in the next fifteen minutes all the meals must be packed in heated trolleys which are then wheeled off to the wards. The kitchens will also prepare more than 400 hot lunches and 150 salads which are sold each weekday in the staff cafeteria, seventy lunches in the outpatients' cafeteria, sixty snacks in a coffee lounge and 1000 rounds of sandwiches. Catering is a million-pound a year operation which has at least one outlet open for twenty-two hours a day, staff permitting. Getting staff to work at low NHS rates in central London is a perpetual headache for catering manager Anne Allen, as for other departmental heads. 'Hotels pay more for thirty-six hours than I can for fifty-six,' she says. Yet as a mass consumer she is able to exploit her power in the market place, driving hard bargains to keep down costs. Among items on her weekly shopping list: 550 lb of potatoes, 270 dozen eggs, 154 lb of flour, 30 lb of jelly powder, two sides of bacon (plus six gammons) and £150 on ice cream, £1000 on vegetables and salad, £500 on fruit and £700 on milk.*

11.25 a.m. *Naomi, nine years old, is examined by Dr Bob Dinwiddie in a chest clinic. She has frequently had trouble with her left lower lung and a sequence of X-ray photographs are displayed behind her. At one stage there was a worry that she might have cystic fibrosis, but a new analysis of sweat measure-*

ments developed by Professor Magnus Hjelm, head of the bio-chemistry department, demonstrated that this was not so. Naomi has been well throughout the winter – until yesterday when, to her mother's irritation, she developed a cough. Dr Dinwiddie prescribes some antibiotics to fight the infection and arranges for some sputum to be examined and for yet another X-ray to be taken. But he is more pleased by her good health throughout the winter than concerned about what appears to be a short-term problem. All in all it's a clinic where the children are doing well. Sometimes clinics are like that. One consultant said: 'You can have some clinics when everyone appears to be doing very well and you finish it on a great high. Other days there are nothing but problems or set-backs and your morale is shattered.'

11.45 a.m. *Penny Uprichard, the hospital's public relations officer, receives the first of several calls from the press about the condition of a child in intensive care. The child has been badly injured during a house fire the previous evening and is now on an artificial ventilation machine. Miss Uprichard goes to the ward to find out what is happening. Her days are rarely predictable. A Russian child flown to Great Ormond Street for open-heart surgery, a child with AIDS, or an emergency operation to separate Siamese twins will make national headlines, and there are always the more local stories for newspapers about children from their areas. In recent years television cameras have become regular visitors, recording everything from rare operations to* This is Your Life *about a long-serving sister. The weeks before Christmas are especially busy with a succession of pop singers, actors and sports stars visiting the hospital dispensing autographs and toys. Those are happier occasions than today's 'story': the child dies in mid-afternoon.*

12.10 p.m. *Susan arrives in the dental clinic for her biennial check-up. She is almost certainly the only patient today who will bring a fiancé to meet her consultant. At twenty-three she expects it to be the final appointment after treatment for a cleft lip and palate that has stretched over twenty-two years. She is a nurse herself nowadays – and an attractive one at that. Children are not normally treated at Great Ormond Street after their sixteenth birth-*

day, but cleft lip and palate patients tend to stay on a little longer because the final stages of their dental and plastic surgery treatment cannot always be tackled until they have stopped growing. Susan shows her fiancé the photographs of her mouth when she was a baby. If Dennis Plint, the senior dental consultant, beamed contentedly alongside he had every cause for satisfaction in a job well done.

The dental department is very largely an out-patient service, although it does have beds on ward 2C for patients requiring surgery. It also provides dental services for children admitted to the hospital for other reasons. Many of the children seen at today's clinic by Mr Plint, two senior registrars and a dental hygienist had rare congenital abnormalities such as a cleft lip and palate. Repair work here is often elaborate involving the construction of 'bridges' within the mouth or the use of bone grafts as well as complicated braces to realign the teeth. Young patients are rewarded with sticky badges proclaiming 'I don't cry' but fifteen-year-old Lillian had a more unusual souvenir: a plaster cast of her teeth as they used to be. She, too, is being signed off today after several years of treatment to straighten and realign her teeth.

12.25 p.m. *Elizabeth Smith, hospital number 490672, is taken to ward 6B by one of the voluntary workers who act as escorts for incoming patients. It is the orthopaedic ward and Elizabeth, who is thirteen, will be having an exploratory operation on her hip. She has been to Great Ormond Street before but not for five years and has only a hazy memory of where to find the bathroom. Her mother's memory is more vivid and she says the ward is brighter than when they were last there. Nor does she recall being offered a cup of tea so quickly after arrival as happened today. Elizabeth, like most patients, is a routine admission. On average there are between 9000 and 10,000 admissions a year with 1500 children on the waiting list. (Almost a third of the children on the waiting list come under the ear, nose and throat surgeons.) The children come from all parts of the country, although half come from the four Thames health regions. The average duration of stay varies from department to department with 2.7 days for ophthalmology being the shortest and 12.1 days for general surgery the longest. The statistics, though, are deceptive. Many children require treat-*

ment which involves a series of frequent admissions spread over many months. And a few children have been patients here for years.

12.30 p.m. *Lunchtime and, as the late shift of nurses arrive for the midday report, the hospital executive team meets over sandwiches and coffee in the office of Betty Beech, the director of nursing services. Among those present are representatives of the physicians, the surgeons and the medical advisory committee – plus the hospital administrator, Tim Walker. High on the agenda is the recurrent problem of restricting admissions to the hospital because they have too little money to employ enough nurses to keep all the beds open, particularly on the intensive care wards. The meeting is also a clearing house for items such as the ward cleaning programme and hears progress reports on building projects. Frequently it ends with administrator Tim Walker having a long list of items to follow up before next week's meeting. Otherwise he's very much at the beck-and-call of others. 'My role is to be the oil between the various cogs that go to make up a large teaching hospital such as this,' he says. 'The administrator is the one common factor throughout the hospital so I must make myself available as and when necessary to keep things running smoothly.'*

12.45 p.m. *Derren is seen by Dr Alison Leiper in the leukaemia clinic. It's going to spill over into the afternoon session. Dr Leiper, an associate specialist in the haematology department, is so accustomed to this that she now brings sandwiches to the clinic. She has been sharing the work-load with Dr Chessells ever since ninethirty and won't finish until nearly two-thirty. Derren is fourteen years old and had a bone marrow transplant nearly five years ago. He's doing extremely well, although he is also attending the growth clinic because he is not growing as well as he should. Possibly the pituitary gland, which produces growth hormone, was damaged by radiation treatment. But growth hormone deficiency along with cataracts in the eyes is one of the prices many children pay for a successful bone marrow transplant.*

Robert

'Robert should never have got as far as being born. I had a threatened miscarriage at twelve weeks, I was in bed for a month, then bleeding for the rest of my pregnancy. I suppose it was nature's way of saying this one isn't really to be. But because I had such good medical care, it went on. As it ended up with Robert having so many things wrong with him, I did wonder in the beginning whether it wouldn't have been better if I had lost him,' says Helen Payne, Robert's mother.

'I don't feel that now. He's Robert, he's so much a personality. But, at first, although we were fighting for him and hoping to goodness that nothing would happen, there was a little part of me that wondered. For a few days, I don't think anybody thought he was going to get very far. But the older he got, the more the doctors and nurses willed him to make it. The hospital has always been so positive.'

Helen Payne and her husband, Charles, have also learned to be positive, but it hasn't been easy. Robert, their first child, spent virtually all of the first thirty months of his life in hospital. Every day usually both parents would visit him so that they spent almost as much time at Great Ormond Street as they did at their home near Heathrow airport. Robert was born with so many problems that he needed all the surgical and intensive nursing skills of the hospital to survive at all.

Helen and Charles – he is always called Charlie by his family – had been married for five years when Robert came along. They had met when Charlie was still in the sixth form and Helen was at a teacher's training college; she later left and worked for the local office of the Department of Health and Social Security. In their mid to late twenties, they both come from stable, happy family backgrounds – each is one of five children – and they both wanted children of their own. They had been trying to conceive for four years and, in the ironic way it often happens, Helen had just attended her first appointment for infertility investigations when she discovered she was pregnant. Even the day of discovery was not entirely joyous: she started bleeding and had to leave her job.

Though she then went to bed for a month, the bleeding continued for the rest of her pregnancy, warning Helen that something was wrong. The difficulties acted on Helen's natural tendency to expect the worst; honest and self-deprecating, she admits that she has always taken a fatalistic view of life. 'I'm always in trouble for being a pessimist. I used to think – "It'll be me. All my friends are having nice little babies but I'll have the handicapped one". I was carrying a lot of fluid, but nobody told me until later that this was an indication that there could be a problem with the baby. I just thought in the back of my mind that there was something wrong.' But if Helen admits to being one of nature's pessimists, Charlie, large, relaxed and athletic-looking, takes a cheerful view of life. It never crossed his mind that there would be anything wrong with their baby.

Thirty-four weeks into her troubled pregnancy, Helen was at home resting when her waters broke. She went into Queen Charlotte's Maternity Hospital in West London. The doctors hoped they could delay Helen's labour, but said that she would have to stay in hospital until the baby was born; they expected that this would be in two weeks' time. Helen settled herself into the ante-natal ward, but only twenty-four hours later the placenta ruptured and she had to undergo an emergency Caesarean delivery.

Robert William Payne was born at ten seconds to midnight on 31 August 1983. He was six weeks premature and weighed just under 1.92 kg (just under 4 lb 4 oz). Charlie was present in the operating theatre; in the heat of the moment, a doctor said he could stay if he wanted, though this was not normal. 'I just thought it would be quite an experience. This was our first baby, even though Helen was unconscious and I couldn't offer moral support,' remembers Charlie. Afterwards, Charlie went to relax in a waiting room, thinking, having been in on the birth, that everything was all right. 'Then I overheard a nurse say "Pity about the baby's hand". I was hoping to God it wasn't ours,' he says. But then, during the night, doctors came to see him and broke first one bit of bad news about his baby's condition, then another.

Calm, equable Charlie Payne was suddenly in the middle of a nightmare. 'They came and told me that the baby's left thumb was missing and the forearm foreshortened. They had also had a problem getting a catheter down, which they didn't explain at that point. A bit later they came and told me that he had an imperforate anus – the normal opening from his bowels was missing.' All this happened in the small hours of the night. Charlie was on his own at the hospital and Helen was still unconscious. 'You worry about things like Down's Syndrome and spina bifida, but these were bizarre things I'd never heard of. I thought about ringing my parents, but it seemed pointless getting them up at three o'clock in the morning. I phoned them about six. At first, they got hold of the wrong end of the stick and thought the baby was dead. I think I started crying or something, I was in a bit of a state. My parents were even less able to grasp what had happened than I was.'

Queen Charlotte's is one of the most famous maternity hospitals in Britain, but it does not do any major paediatric surgery. If its doctors diagnose a surgical problem, they trans- fer a baby as soon as his condition is stable. They explained to Charlie Payne that Robert would have to go to either the nearby Hammersmith Hospital or the Hospital for Sick Chil- dren at Great Ormond Street. At first, Charlie hoped it would be Hammersmith; it was nearer, their side of London. Great Ormond Street was just a name; Charlie didn't even know where the hospital was. But Great Ormond Street had room for Robert and so, on the first full day of his life, Robert Payne went to the place that was destined to become, in effect, his home. Charlie had to decide whether to go with him in the ambulance or to stay with Helen. 'I didn't know what to do. I knew they would be operating and so I stayed. I felt I could be more use with Helen than with him.'

Robert travelled in an incubator in the ambulance for the seven-mile journey across London from Chiswick to Blooms- bury. An incubator is a small cot on a stand covered by a perspex lid which provides a warm, controlled environment for a sick baby; it allows clear observation and, if necessary, oxygen can be given. This, though, was not enough for Robert. He was already attached to a ventilator which controlled his breathing via a tube inserted down his throat and windpipe. Another tiny tube was inserted into a vein and through this there flowed a dextrose-saline solution which would keep his body fluids stable and prevent dehydration. Thus he arrived at Great Ormond Street at ten minutes past two in the afternoon of 1 September. He was still less than one day old.

Robert was received as an emergency admission and transferred quickly to ward 6A, the neonatal surgical intensive care ward for premature or very young babies on the sixth floor of the hospital. The ward, like much of Great Ormond Street, has come to specialize in rare conditions and so the 6A staff were not surprised by the complexity of Robert's problems. Robert was examined and slotted into that day's theatre list, for it was clear that he needed surgery urgently. In charge would be Lewis Spitz, the hospital's senior general paediatric surgeon. He had been appointed Professor of Paediatric Surgery* in 1979 after a career spanning hospitals in his native South Africa, Liverpool and Sheffield. In the months to come Helen and Charlie Payne would hold many discussions with him, but the first contact they had was on the following day when Charlie overheard Professor Spitz telling his entourage of junior doctors that this baby had 'Vater's Syndrome'; the Professor told them to go away and look it up in the medical journals.

This is what the junior doctors would have found. Vater's Syndrome is a cluster of associated congenital defects, 'Vater' being merely an acronym formed from the different elements. 'V' stands for vertebral anomalies – and Robert had scoliosis, a malformation of the spine. 'V' also stands for ventricular septal defect, a heart problem which in fact Robert did not have; fortunately, cardiac checks showed that his heart was virtually normal. 'A' stands for anal abnormality – the absence of a normal opening to the bowels about which Charlie Payne had

---

*The title of Professor reflects his role in the adjoining Institute of Child Health, a centre for paediatric research and postgraduate teaching, with which the hospital is closely linked.

been told in those bewildering hours at the maternity hospital. 'T' and 'E' stand for tracheal and (o)esophageal abnormality† – not only the failure of the oesophagus or foodpipe to reach the stomach, but also a link between the oesophagus and the windpipe so that food and fluids spill into the lungs. Robert had this, too, as he did the radial and renal problems associated with the letter 'R'. A shortened left arm and missing left thumb – Robert's only visible defect – immediately illustrated the former, but more serious were the renal defects discovered during the first operation: his left kidney didn't work at all while the right kidney did not work at full efficiency.

It was a forbidding list. Yet all the abnormalities were surgically correctible. The process would begin that evening, as soon as possible, like much of 6A's surgery, out of regular hours. 'All the consultants here are not reluctant to come out at weekends or at night, because we know that the first operation is the baby's best chance,' says Professor Spitz.

Robert's reconstructive surgery thus began at eight p.m. when he was barely twenty hours old. This first stage consisted of a series of basic repairs which would correct the life-threatening anomalies he had been born with; once completed, these would enable Robert to grow and to put on weight ready for more surgery. First, the tube connecting the oesophagus or foodpipe to the trachea or windpipe was sealed off. But the oesophagus still didn't reach the stomach, rendering feeding impossible. A gastrostomy was performed – this involves making an opening into the stomach through which milk (or other liquified food) can be pumped via a tube. Even though Robert could not feed normally, he could still produce saliva in his mouth which – because of the abnormal oesophagus – could spill over into his lungs causing infections or potentially fatal breathing problems. So the end of the oesophagus was brought to the surface in the neck to form a surgical opening known as an oesophagostomy; this would allow saliva to drain freely and later be the escape route for milk when Robert was enjoying feeds by mouth – 'sham feeding'. This left, of the

---

†'E' originates from the US spelling of esophagus; the usual UK spelling is oesophagus. See also Stacey's story.

immediate problems, the question of what to do with his waste matter as he lacked a normal anus. A colostomy was therefore performed so that his bowel movements were discharged via a surgically created opening on the abdomen over which plastic colostomy bags are placed to collect waste. It was noted that the appearance of the kidneys was abnormal but operation number one, the first of many, was over.

At ten-thirty p.m., Robert was wheeled back from the sixth floor operating suite to 6A. Keith Holmes, then Professor Spitz's senior registrar, phoned Charlie Payne to tell him how the operation had gone while 6A's night shift took charge of the baby. Robert's temperature, pulse and blood pressure were monitored frequently through the night. Around two a.m. his temperature and pulse began to rise, but by morning his condition was once again fair. He remained dependent upon the ventilator in order to breathe. The machine was set to give Robert thirty breaths a minute with air that contained forty per cent oxygen. As he gained strength, doctors would reduce the number of machine breaths and lower the amount of oxygen closer to the twenty per cent in normal air. The hope was that he would gradually be able to breathe on his own.

Artificial ventilation is potentially hazardous in very young babies, particularly premature babies such as Robert: inserting tubes down narrow windpipes can cause the trachea to become ulcerated or permanently narrowed. This is more likely to happen where hospitals are unaccustomed to ventilating babies, and is one reason why babies are referred to specialist units such as Great Ormond Street's ward 6A. At such units today there is far greater expertise in the use of ventilation on tiny babies. Yet these facts may only gradually comfort distraught parents; at first it is bound to be frightening that such a basic function as breathing has been seconded to a machine, and that the baby's face is almost covered with tubes and tapes. Thus Robert appeared on the morning after his operation when Charlie Payne visited him for the first time in Great Ormond Street. It was not a sight Charlie will ever forget.

'People get choked when they walk into Great Ormond Street for the first time. Later you become more hardened to the sight of very sick children. He looked like such a wreck. He was lying there, he looked pathetic, strung out like a little frog with so many wires. I couldn't believe anybody could have so many wires and tubes. I had never even seen a baby in hospital before.'

The shock is all the more harrowing because parents such as Robert's father, days or even hours ago, may have been expecting their baby's birth to be a normal, happy event. Instead they have to adjust to the sight of a very sick baby amid bewildering technology and cope with their fears about whether the baby is going to live. The ward sisters on 6A, or a staff nurse if she is in charge, watch out for the arrival of new parents, making sure that they talk to them before they see their baby and explain what the surgery will achieve. The most common problems are forms of intestinal obstruction, oesophageal atresia, defects of the abdominal wall, diaphragmatic hernia and spina bifida. Even though 6A sees these conditions all the time, they remain rare in the population at large; multiple problems such as Vater's Syndrome are even more obscure. The specialization, while good for the children, is recognized as a potential problem for student nurses who don't see enough of the commoner, less serious problems when it comes to taking exams. (The problem is resolved by the nurse training also at the Queen Elizabeth Hospital for Sick Children in Hackney – see *Casualty* section of this book.)

Neonatology has expanded rapidly in the last twenty years. More premature infants with more serious problems can now be saved; among them are babies born as much as three months premature, occasionally even earlier. 6A, one of the hospital's three intensive care wards, was established as a neonatal unit in 1974. 'Our results on this ward,' says Professor Spitz, 'are as good as anywhere in the world. We hardly ever lose a patient because of an unexplained event. Either the child is extremely premature or had such a combination of abnormalities that he or she didn't stand a chance.' Many technical factors have contributed to this dramatic progress. Ventilation is much better understood, anaesthesia has improved and intravenous feeding is available, which it was not two decades ago. 'There's not a whole lot new in surgery, but there have been major advances in intensive care and nursing,' says Professor Spitz. 'It's the one to one nurse-patient relationship when children are very ill that gives this tremendous level of care. The fact that the children are being so closely monitored means that events are anticipated before they occur, so that problems can be prevented. The reasons are partly the technical advances, but it's more the nursing expertise. I would rather have a good nurse next to the patient than a good monitor.'

The skill of the surgeons has increased too and this is one of the areas where Great Ormond Street is unique. '6A is probably the biggest unit of its kind in the world and, although we are under-staffed, the surgeons here build up expertise. The experienced general surgeon, inexperienced in paediatrics, who deals with one case of a certain condition in a year is not going to get such good results as someone who is treating that kind of case all the time. Here we are devoted to these problems and we are always looking for new and improved ways of doing things. If we just followed the textbooks all the time, we would just be standing still,' says Professor Spitz.

Two ward sisters, Mary Wallis, in her forties, and Hilary Graves, in her thirties, head the 6A nursing team. Their full complement of trained staff (State Registered Nurse or State Enrolled Nurse) is twenty-one including the sisters. At 'Report', the conference which is the handover to the next shift coming on duty, the sister or staff nurse in charge will go through the list of patients, detailing their condition and care, and nurses will be allocated to each, with the student nurses going to the least ill children. The sisters work closely with four consultant surgeons and other regular visitors would be the senior surgical registrars and housemen, as the senior house officers are known. A physiotherapist attends the ward frequently, often many times a day. A dietitian is also in daily contact with ward staff, as finding the best feed for these often highly premature, ill babies requires delicate skill. (On average one in three patients in the hospital as a whole is bottle fed and such is the range of dietary problems that there are thirty-five varieties of milk feeds.)

The ward is brightly lit – night and day – for better observation of the babies and the nurses wear all-white intensive care dresses rather than the pink and white stripes of the general wards. But alongside the technology endure the comforting, traditional babycare rituals. The nurses might be feeding or cuddling a baby on their lap; the white walls, uniforms and hard surfaces are softened by toys sitting beside even a very ill baby and by mobiles hanging over the cots. Colourful, hand-made crochet blankets are used instead of factory products.

The focus of all this activity are the patients, tiny and vulnerable in their immaturity and in the defects which fate has dealt out to them. So tiny and so vulnerable, in fact, that first-time visitors can scarcely comprehend how they can exist, let alone how surgeons can operate on them. The minutest babies might be no more than 0.9 kg (2 lb) in weight and 38 centimetres (15 inches) long.

Communicating with parents ranks very high on the ward's priorities. The sisters have become experts in assessing the kind of people the parents are and in explaining the technology simply. 'Parents learn technical terms very quickly and even parents with very low educational skills can cotton on to the vital things,' says Mary Wallis, the senior of the two ward sisters. The doctors talk to parents, too, but can sometimes be over-technical without knowing it. Mary Wallis and Hilary Graves will therefore repeat explanations patiently and as many times as necessary, often resorting to simple diagrams because most people's knowledge of anatomy is sketchy. Strange new words are in any case harder to understand when a parent is in a state of shock, scarcely adjusted to having a child in hospital at all. Not surprisingly, the sisters quickly become reassuring props for the parents who are going through this awful experience.

For Sister Wallis, her basic motivation in caring for babies and their families is her Christian faith. She has a serenity which typifies the calm and happy atmosphere of this ward where the nurses seem a particularly united team. 'I think you sort of fall in love with the nurses,' says Charlie Payne. 'Sister Wallis is a kind of mother figure. She explains things but won't give people a load of bull. She has years of experience and knows how to handle people. She has seen a lot of babies who haven't made it up there, she's been through all the traumas. Robert would be going through several crises, but the nurses would always come up and say – "Don't worry, there is something they can do".'

Charlie got to know ward 6A first; it often is the father rather than the mother, for the babies' mothers are initially among the least frequent visitors. Many will be recovering in the post-natal wards of other hospitals, often from Caesarean deliveries which will take longer to get over. At first, all they will have is a Polaroid picture of their baby, taken by nurses at the time of the child's admission. (Great Ormond Street is a hospital where children are nursed, not where they are born; ideally, there should be a post-natal ward so that mothers and babies could be transferred together.)

Five days therefore passed before Helen Payne saw Robert. The news was broken to her of his many problems as she was slowly recovering from anaesthesia. 'They did tell me that various things were wrong with him but at first it was washing over me. It only began to sink in over the next few days so it wasn't such a horrendous shock as it might have been. By the time I was fully aware I did know and I tried to accept it.' To her this seems less painful than the shock her husband suffered, but 6A staff remember her first visit and knew she was absolutely shattered.

You cannot see much of a baby's face when he is being ventilated, as adhesive tapes hold the breathing tube in place. They took Robert off his ventilator, using a hand-held oxygen bag so that Helen could hold her baby for a few moments, but she was too apprehensive to enjoy the experience: 'I was petrified and nervous. I wanted to put him back.' At first Helen could hardly realize that Robert was her baby; the bonding attachment grew later when she was able to cuddle and care for him.

And so began what became a way of life for Helen and Charlie Payne. Each day Helen would travel on the tube from their semi-detached home at Heston, near Heathrow, to visit Robert in one corner of ward 6A. Charlie went back to work; he is an assistant to a general manager at an international bank in the City. He began his habit of calling in at the hospital every evening on his way home. Sister Wallis remembers him as a faithful visitor, always with his briefcase. Work at least offered Charlie a distraction from thinking about Robert's problems.

Robert did not do too badly in the days immediately after his first operation. Helen was encouraged to express breast milk – the hospital regards breast milk as the best feed in most circumstances, if the mother can provide it, and Helen did well to provide it for as long as she did. The expressed breast milk was fed to Robert via the gastrostomy tube into his stomach – at first just five millilitres at a time. Tiny babies require frequent, tiny volumes of feeds; drugs, too, have to be controlled with great precision which is why intravenous fluids and drugs are controlled by machines rather than the gravity 'drips' normally acceptable for use with adults. Sometimes Robert could not tolerate even these minute feeds. Milk volumes are calculated on body weights and general signs of well-being or tolerance. The sisters know how to upgrade the feeds almost instinctively, though they always calculate as well.

Getting the strength and frequency of Robert's feeds right was just one of many problems in his first weeks of life. Like many neonates and premature babies especially, he became jaundiced and received photo-therapy treatment due to high levels of bilirubin in his blood. Bilirubin is the end-product of the natural process of the breakdown of red blood cells. This 'light treatment' helps to break down the potentially toxic bilirubin in the blood so that it can be excreted. If bilirubin levels become too high, brain damage can occur. He also required frequent suction to prevent secretions causing infections in his windpipe and lungs. He was seen by the hospital's cardiologists to check his heart and one of his rare pieces of good luck was that his heart was virtually normal. But the main task facing the doctors was to wean Robert off the ventilator: the longer any child is on artificial ventilation, the greater is the risk of long-term damage to his windpipe and his lungs.

The process is a gradual one performed under close observation to see how the baby copes on his or her own. The checks include blood gas monitoring to check the blood's oxygen and carbon dioxide content. The first step, when Robert was three days old, was to reduce the number of artificial breaths from thirty to twenty a minute. Although the rate had to be increased for a while, two days later he had made it down to fifteen breaths a minute. He was again examined by an anaesthetist and switched to something called CPAP, pronounced 'See-pap' and standing for Continuous Positive Airways Pressure. What it means is that the machine supplies gentle pressure to keep the airway open, but the actual breathing is done by the patient, not the machine: it is the penultimate stage of artificial ventilation. Robert had several tries at CPAP, but the machine had to be switched back to full ventilation when he began to have difficulties breathing. Once, when he was nine days old, he appeared to be doing sufficiently well for the breathing tube to be removed from his throat and windpipe. But again his condition deteriorated and the tube had to be re-inserted.

The last stages of the artificial ventilation involved the use of a shorter tube or prong inserted into his nose instead of the tube being down his throat. This seemed to work quite well and by the time Robert was fifteen days old the nasal prong could also be removed. He was now being nursed in a 'head-box', a clear, perspex box fitting round the baby's head which was supplied with a mixture of air and additional oxygen. One week later he had made the progression to breathing 'normal' air, although he was still in an incubator.

At this point everyone was pleased with Robert's progress: he was coping well in ordinary air, he was tolerating his feeds, now thirty-five millilitres of expressed breast milk every two hours, his colour was good and he was showing no signs of respiratory or heart-rate problems. Even at one month old, he was still two weeks short of what would have been a full-term, forty-week pregnancy. Nurses noted that he enjoyed being cuddled by Dad and, increasingly, Helen and Charlie could do things for their baby – they could change the nappies, assist with the gastrostomy feeding and help to keep him clean. Nurses encourage parents to become involved with their children's care. The signs promised well for transferring Robert to ward 4AB where he could continue to gain weight ready for the next stage of his 'reconstruction'.

First, though, he had to begin 'sham feeding'. This is an

important stage in the care of babies such as Robert born with oesophageal atresia. The initial phase of their surgery is to create an opening in the stomach so that they can be fed through the gastrostomy tube. Babies depend upon this until the next stage of the surgery reconnects the oesophagus with the stomach thus enabling normal oral feeding. Such an operation usually has to wait until the child is a few months old, but by then the child may have lost irrevocably the instinct to feed normally. Therefore the process of learning to feed by mouth, called 'sham feeding', is started as soon as the baby is up to it; otherwise the sucking reflex will be lost or sucking will not be associated with feeding. Sham feeding consists of giving a bottle feed in the normal way at the same time as a gastrostomy feed is given. In this way the baby learns to suck and also associates an oral feed with a full stomach. But of course the feed taken orally never reaches the stomach; it drains through the oesophagostomy opening made in the neck, initially to remove saliva. Robert was a little surprised by his first sham feed and became a little breathless. Nevertheless he took twenty millilitres of SMA, a commercial baby milk.

When Robert was twenty-five days old, he left 6A to go down two floors to ward 4AB. Two hours later he was back, once again seriously ill. 'I was holding him and we thought he was just going off to sleep,' says Helen. 'Then we realized he was going bluish and then bluer, and we called a nurse. At the time we didn't know enough to be worried, then later we realized, My God, he might have died. But the staff nurse grabbed him and threw him in a cot and got the oxygen going and called a doctor – she knew just by looking at him how bad he was.' Some of his sham feed had gone into his lungs, probably because he had not co-ordinated his swallowing reflex properly. He was taken back to 6A and put back onto full ventilation. All feeds were stopped – gastrostomy as well as sham feeding – and he was fed intravenously. A chest X-ray was done which showed that part of the right lung had collapsed and become infected. An antibiotic called Gentamicin was given to fight the infection caused by the milk feed which had spilt over into the lungs. But why had the problem occurred?

The first operation had sealed off the tube connecting the oesophagus or foodpipe to the windpipe. Occasionally, this link re-forms and so a barium X-ray was performed – barium is a radio-opaque dye which shows the progress of fluids through the body. Yet this had not happened with Robert. He now had everyone worried. He remained on full ventilation and ten days later a second chest X-ray showed that he still had fluid in the right side of his chest which suggested that it was leaking from the lower oesophagus. A needle was inserted into his chest and through this nearly seventy millilitres of milk were removed, but the leak needed to be sealed. He went to the hospital's sixth floor operating theatres the same day, again for an emergency operation. The date was 6 October. Robert was just six weeks old.

This time the lower end of the oesophagus was excised and closed to make a more effective seal to the stomach. An X-ray after the operation showed some improvement, but four days later Robert again got into breathing difficulties. Yet another chest X-ray showed that there was still fluid around his right lung. A drain was now inserted into the right side of his chest and this removed no less than a hundred millilitres of fluid. After this he improved steadily, although he remained on intra-venous feeding and ventilation. Four days later he was back on gastrostomy feeds which were increased steadily, and in four more days he was off the ventilator and in a head-box with oxygen and coping well. Eleven days later Robert resumed sham feeding and was well enough for Helen to give him a bath. By the end of the month Robert was doing well and, now two months old, was ready once again to leave the familiar surroundings of 6A for ward 4AB.

By this time the Paynes had bonded thoroughly with the environment of 6A and were surprised and reluctant at the prospect of moving. 'I was absolutely horrified at first,' says Charlie. 'It hadn't occurred to us that Robert would be moved to another ward as he got older – 6A was 6A, we'd started off there and we didn't want to go anywhere else. Moving to another ward was like changing jobs; we had to get to know everybody, start all over again.'

On descending the two floors to 4AB the Payne family

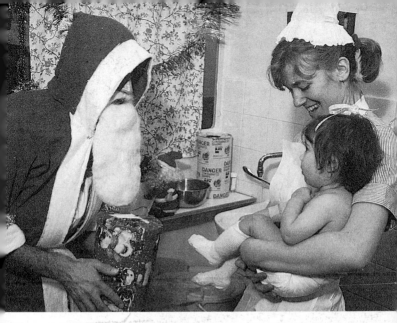

The magic of Christmas: for some, illnesses are temporarily forgotten

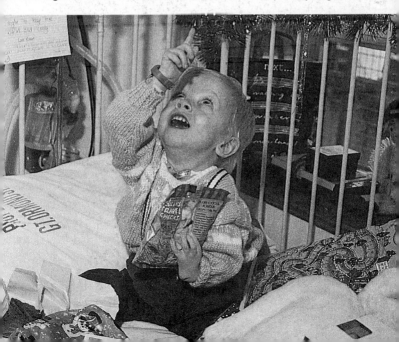

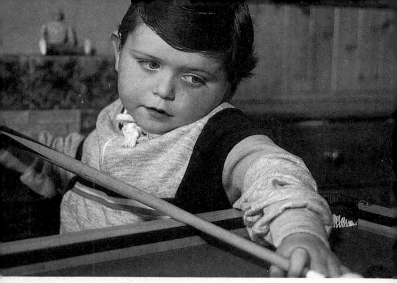

Declan Carroll: his mother worried that he wasn't growing, but she worried more when they discovered he had a brain tumour

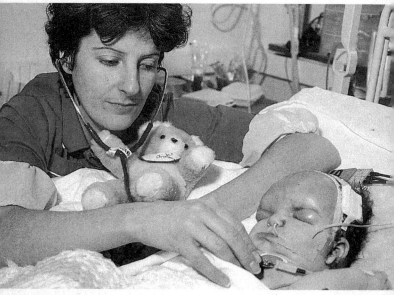

Sister Lindy May nurses another child on the neurosurgery ward who, like Declan, has just had brain surgery

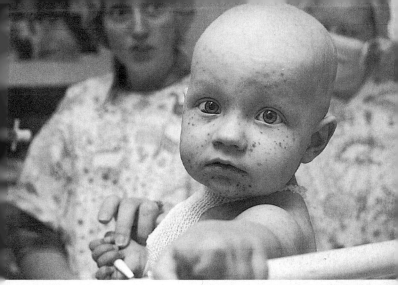

Anna Wells (with mother, Janet, in background without mask): tiny and short-lived spots called petechiae didn't bother Anna, but they were a warning of trouble to come

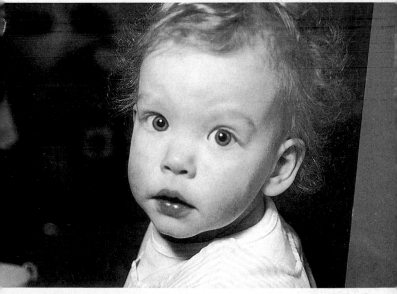

Polly Logan Banks, who faced major heart surgery before her second birthday

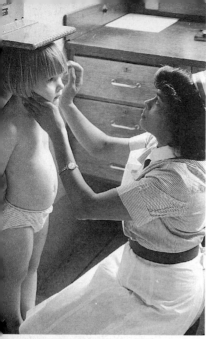

Measuring up:
preparing for an out-patients' clinic

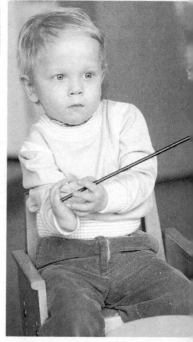

Robert Payne,
engrossed in a music play session

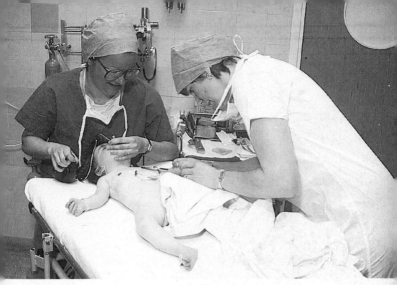

In theatre: anaesthetists prepare a patient

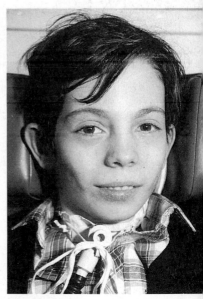

Gus Grieco,
paralysed from the neck down

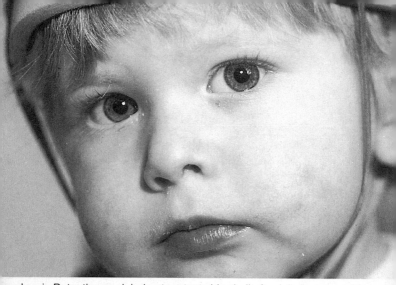

Lewis Pate: the crash helmet protects his skull after injuries caused by a car crash, but that wasn't what brought him to Great Ormond Street

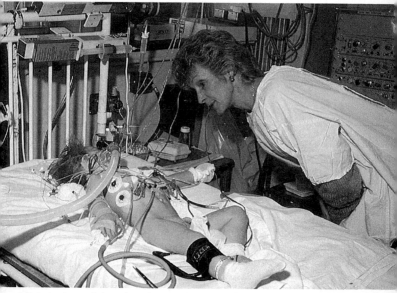

High-tech medicine: the wires and machinery of intensive care all but obliterate the tiny patient

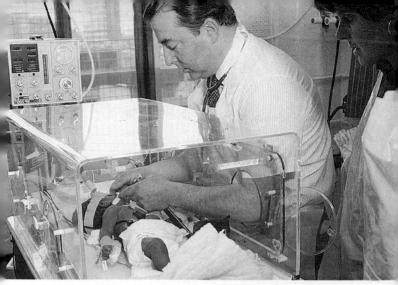

Consultant Dr Bob Dinwiddie examines a child being nursed in the optimum environment of an incubator

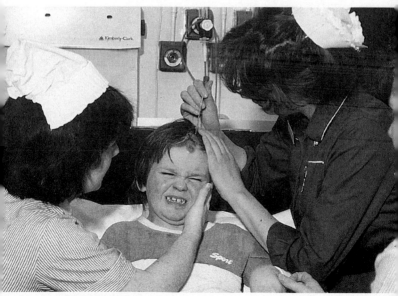

Casualty: twenty-five thousand children a year are examined, patched, stitched and treated by the Casualty staff of the Queen Elizabeth Hospital for Sick Children

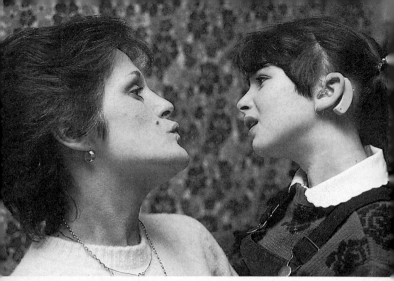

Stacey Tyrrill: after twenty-eight operations and almost seven years, she was well enough to live permanently at home. Now deaf, she communicates with her mother Pauline by sign language and lip-reading

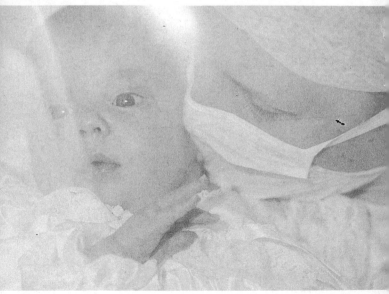

Kristie McWilliam and her father Steve, inside the plastic bubble

passed into the charge of Hannah Wright, the senior of two ward sisters, an attractive but sometimes formidable girl then in her late twenties. She lacked the gentleness of the 6A sisters, but made up for this in her indomitable energy and efficiency and the bracing emotional support she gave to parents. Not one for sitting in her office while the nurses do all the nursing care, Hannah loves the drama of surgery: the fact that, if all goes well, she will see the children recover, often surprisingly quickly, and walk out of the hospital with their problems solved or substantially reduced. Supervising their recovery is a vital role, because even the most brilliantly innovative surgeon depends on a nursing team to ensure that a child survives after leaving theatre. Being in the confidence of the surgeons is one of the most rewarding aspects of the job to Hannah Wright. 'The sisters can criticize as much as they like and make helpful comments, which they do,' says Professor Spitz. A luckless houseman was once put in his place by the Professor for failing to listen to Sister Wright; she knew, he said, more about paediatric surgery than the houseman perhaps ever would.

Hannah Wright was also demanding of herself. 'A sister is always responsible. If something goes wrong in the middle of the night when you are not there, it's still your fault because you should have trained your nurses properly,' she says. Training her nurses meant more than just practising procedures, for paediatric nursing requires special skills. Ginnie Colwell, sister of ward 4CD at the less acute end of this surgical floor, puts it this way. 'You have to be more observant because the patient will tell you less than an adult would. And babies and small children can change into a critical state much more quickly than adults because their blood volume is smaller. Sometimes ordinary observations [the basic pulse, blood pressure and temperature checks which are performed at varying intervals, depending on how ill the patient is] may tell you very little, but a nurse will be able to see that there is something wrong, some kind of obstruction, for instance. It becomes almost intuitive.'

Although the consultants may retain a touch of grandeur, most are on first-name terms with the sisters. On the whole, like paediatricians in general, they are also more skilled in communicating with parents and more likely to recognize the claims of parents to information than many doctors in general medicine would be with their patients. 'They are absolutely straight with you here,' is a remark frequently heard in the parents' sitting room at Great Ormond Street, from people who value what they have not found to be the case elsewhere. It is not so very unusual for parents here, because of their intimate involvement, to know more about the specific condition of their child than their GP or the local hospital which they may attend later as out-patients.

Professor Spitz and the Paynes were to reach a good understanding. But by being around much more, and having the daily care of the children, the sisters form the closest relationship between the parents and the hospital. The other sister on 4AB, Val Green, a softer personality than Hannah Wright, was also to become a firm family friend of the Paynes and continued to visit Robert long after she had stopped working at the hospital. Helen and Charlie Payne soon learnt to appreciate the way the ward was run. 'Sister Wright inspires confidence in you when it's needed,' says Charlie. 'She knows the hospital inside out, she knows the kids inside out, she gets things done, knows how to buttonhole doctors and doctors' secretaries.' Charlie and she developed a relationship outwardly full of banter but concealing enormous mutual respect underneath.

The Paynes also adjusted to the freer, less clinical atmosphere of 4AB. Like most of the hospital it is rather antiquated-looking, yet scrupulously clean and with plenty of visible high-tech equipment. Parents chat and make coffee in the kitchen, toys spill out from the playroom and children toddle up and down the corridor, trailing their drip stands behind them. Not far away there is often tension with seriously ill children, perhaps being ventilated. But the children here are mostly old enough to be mobile and when they feel well, and have had their parents with them, they bounce back, lively and happy; the resilience of children, who mostly do not understand what has happened to them and therefore do not worry, ensures that they are less depressed and subdued than adult patients would be.

One ward sister, recalling her tour of American children's hospitals, felt she had seen huge, beautiful modern buildings, palaces in comparison with Great Ormond Street, but she was surprised to find so little play on the wards. On her ward, she said, you could hardly walk without falling over a couple of tricycles. (In the United States a different philosophy sometimes applies, where the playroom is regarded as a sanctuary for the children and medical staff are not allowed in.)

Robert was just over two months old when he arrived on ward 4AB and encouraging him to take sham feeds was still a priority. Sometimes he took them well, but once or twice he would become breathless, sometimes severely, so that the feeding would have to be stopped for a while. For more than a year Robert was nursed in a cubicle, rather than the open section of the ward, because he had a persistent urine infection which was resistant to Gentamicin. Since Gentamicin is a commonly used antibiotic in the hospital, the spread of resistant organisms was a serious risk, and Robert had to be isolated from other children. Once he was well, the second phase of his surgical reconstruction could go ahead. This meant an operation on his kidneys: his right kidney would be repaired while, eventually, his useless left kidney would be removed.

Robert's renal problems had been identified almost as soon as he arrived at Great Ormond Street. On his first examination his left kidney was palpable, or able to be felt, which indicated that it was swollen. This was a hint that something was wrong and during his first operation, on that day of admission, the left kidney was found to be in a dilated condition known as hydronephrotic. What it meant was that urine did not drain away from the kidney as it should. A few days later there were further tests, including an ultra-sound scan and a DTPA scan in which a radio-isotope is injected and shows up DTPA, a chemical excreted by the kidney. Both the scans revealed that the left kidney was not functioning at all and, even worse, that there was an obstruction affecting the right kidney as well. The obstruction would have to be surgically investigated and removed as a matter of urgency.

'This was one of our most worrying times because we knew he'd only got the one functioning kidney,' says Charlie Payne. So when he was eleven weeks old Robert went back to the operating theatre for an operation known as a pyeloplasty which would remove the obstruction on the right kidney. The urological surgeons found blood vessels compressing the pelvi-ureteric junction, the point where the kidney drains into the ureter, the tube which carries urine to the bladder. First, the blood vessels were divided; then, a 'nephrostomy' tube was inserted to drain urine directly from the kidney, thus temporarily by-passing the site of the surgery. But all did not go smoothly. After the operation the nephrostomy tube did not work correctly and began to leak urine.

Three weeks after his first kidney operation Robert returned to theatre for more investigations. These were inconclusive and the nephrostomy tube was left in place. Ten days later another X-ray with contrast showed that there was now good drainage into the right ureter and the bladder. Now the nephrostomy tube could be clamped, which was just as well since a couple of days later Robert pulled it out altogether. Luckily, by then he was passing urine quite well in the normal way. This was a great relief to his parents and Helen was there to spot the first flow since the operation. 'I just happened to be changing his nappy and there it was,' remembers Helen. 'That was exciting.'

It was a happy omen for Robert's first Christmas. He was in such good form on Christmas Eve, happy and smiling, that he was allowed home. He was a little under four months old and it was the first time he had been home. Robert slept most of the time, but his parents did not. 'We were up every half minute looking at his cot to see if he was still breathing,' says Helen. On New Year's Eve Robert was home again and they took him to a party at Helen's sister's. On the way home he suffered a breathing attack and they had to rush him to a local hospital; here, he soon recovered and by the time the paediatrician arrived, he was smiling. But Helen and Charlie were relieved to get back to Great Ormond Street.

In the New Year Robert's feeding progressed well until, in February, he became first very chesty and then turned grey-blue and had to be nursed in humidified oxygen for a few days. He got over this scare, but more worrying were a series of urine infections. Could there be something still wrong with his one functioning kidney? A second DTPA scan confirmed the presence of a further obstruction. A blood test showed that the level of creatinine – a chemical which should be excreted by the kidneys – had crept up a little, also suggesting a continuing renal problem. Professor Spitz, who had not performed any of the kidney surgery, decided to bring in the hospital's senior urology surgeon, Philip Ransley.

Mr Ransley, a very experienced paediatric urologist, reviewed the case and operated the next month. Finding that the pelvi-ureteric junction had become blocked again, he removed the obstruction and used a different technique to ensure that the ureter healed correctly. This time, although Robert would still need long-term antibiotic cover to guard against urine infections which could seep back up the ureter and endanger the functioning kidney, he progressed very well after the operation. 'Robert was a different person after that operation,' says Helen. 'When he got over his first set of operations, he seemed to be a really happy little child, then he started getting really grumpy. We thought we were just going to have a grumpy baby, one of those that always happened to cry all afternoon. But eventually they found he needed that kidney operation re-doing. After that he was a changed character.'

Yet, as for any child with serious renal problems, anxiety over the future of his sole surviving kidney will always be there, says Charlie. 'It would be so easy for the one kidney to suddenly pack up. There's no reason why it should, but having had problems with it, you half expect them to recur.' The right kidney undergoes periodic scans to check that it does not need further surgery and the doctors say it has enough function to keep Robert healthy. 'Robert's kidneys are a very weak point in his armour,' says Charlie, 'what little armour he's got.'

Nevertheless, the Paynes were relieved that at least one phase of Robert's surgery was over. In April, as the weather turned brighter, Robert was well enough to be taken out of the hospital for a walk. 'Mum and I, accompanied by a staff nurse, wheeled him in a pram round Queen Square, round the corner from the hospital. The wind was blowing and he kept gasping and gulping. I was a bit worried because that was what had started off his breathing attacks,' says Helen. His gastrostomy feeds were also going well. Only the sham feeding presented difficulties, causing him occasionally to turn blue and breathless. It was decided to enlist the aid of a speech therapist.

Feeding was a relatively new area for speech therapists, when, as in Robert's case, there was no obvious physical reason why the child could not suck effectively. But the movements required for sucking are clearly related to those required for speech, and in Debbie Sell the hospital had a progressive specialist who had recently returned from observing pioneering feeding therapy in the United States. Tips from her coupled with the hard work of the nurses were eventually to turn Robert into a champion sham feeder. 'Robert was the best sham feeder we've ever had,' says Professor Spitz. Months later, Debbie Sell would also push forward his language development.

Robert sucked well on a dummy, but was apt to panic when given a bottle. Debbie Sell tried putting him in different positions, using an eye-dropper to give tiny quantities and touching or stimulating the mouth. None of these ploys succeeded in getting Robert to suck well on a teat: it was a basic babyhood skill that he had never really acquired. Helen said sadly: 'All I want is a baby that can suck so that I can feed him.'

However, when they later introduced puréed feeds, he took to this quickly; the thicker consistencies seemed to reduce his panic. 'It was such a thrill when Robert did eventually start feeding, even though it was sham feeding,' says Helen wistfully. 'At first it was a real fight, an hour's struggle to get three teaspoons of food into him, then one day he ate a whole tin of Heinz Turkey Dinner.' Later he began to enjoy other tastes and textures such as cereals, fruits and vegetables. It was a messy procedure because the puréed food still came out through the oesophagostomy drain in his neck. Charlie sometimes found it frustrating. 'Later on, when he was really eating well, he would demolish a banana in two minutes and it seemed such a pity that it wasn't doing him any good. Also it was hard to explain to other people; I was convinced that lots of visitors to the ward just thought he was a messy eater.' Nonetheless it was an achievement which pleased everybody.

The spring weather was fine and Robert was able to be put

on the balcony of 4AB in a pram. Thoughts began to turn to going home. He went home for an afternoon in mid-April; it was a trial run, particularly for Helen. She had earlier expressed misgivings about how she would cope with Robert at home. It was therefore always part of the nursing plan to build up her confidence by encouraging her to care for Robert on her visits; the colostomy care, gastrostomy and sham feeding would mean far more responsibility for her than ordinary babycare. So, when Robert began to tolerate his sham feeds so well and was gaining weight and his urine was free from infection, the doctors decided it was time for him to go home. Not indefinitely, because there was more surgery to come, but for the first time 'home' was where he would sleep rather than a place for an occasional day visit. The date was 28 April and Robert was just under eight months old.

Helen and Charlie were now responsible for all their son's care. Charlie rigged up a stand from a dowelling rod on which to clip the syringe in order to give the gastrostomy feeds. Helen had been given detailed advice from the dietitian about how to prepare Robert's feeds; these were by no means straightforward. The gastrostomy feeds were of *Chix*, a complex feed of finely minced chicken with five or six additional ingredients calculated for the individual's needs. The sham feeds were ordinary SMA, but even this had to be thickened with cooked cornflour to help Robert cope with it. Helen was grateful that her mother came and helped for there was hardly a spare minute in the day when something didn't need to be done for Robert; but generally everything went well.

Then, one day in late May, Helen took Robert for an appointment with the local health visitor for a routine hearing test. Her mother gave them a lift to the health centre. On the way home in the car Helen noticed him watching the sunlight and shadows of the trees flashing past the car. Suddenly he was twitching and jumping as if something had frightened him. 'Mum turned the car straight round and we rushed back to the health centre. By the time the doctor came he had stopped and then he went off into a deep sleep, as they said he would,' recalls Helen. But Helen's GP said she should telephone Great Ormond Street to tell them that Robert seemed to have had a fit. The hospital said they should bring him in the following day.

Although Robert was seen initially in an out-patient clinic, he was readmitted to ward 4AB so that his apparent fit could be investigated and his other problems reviewed. Among the tests would be a CT scan of his brain for which he would have to be sedated. Initially the drug which Robert was given as a sedative or relaxant before the scan seemed to have no adverse effect. He had gone quietly to sleep after the scan when, at about two o'clock in the afternoon, he had what the medical staff call a respiratory arrest. Or, in more simple terms, he stopped breathing.

Over Robert's life, and his innumerable ups and downs, Helen and Charlie Payne have had several phone calls first thing in the morning to tell them – in the code which doctors and nurses use to break bad news – that Robert hasn't had a very good night. This afternoon was one occasion when Charlie was abruptly summoned from his desk in the City. '"Can you come? Robert isn't very well," they said. I thought for them to phone me at work, it must be quite bad. I just leapt into a taxi. It was only about ten to fifteen minutes away, but it was an awful ride,' says Charlie. Helen was already on her way to the hospital when the arrest occurred and the staff were in control by the time both parents had arrived. Robert was resuscitated with oxygen via a face mask and suction via a tube passed down the nose to the back of his throat. He responded quickly, although his breathing remained laboured. As evening came he grew more settled, but he was still nursed in a head-box with fifty per cent oxygen.

Robert was watched closely overnight, with hourly observations. But the next morning his condition was satisfactory and the oxygen was gradually reduced. He was sufficiently stable by the afternoon for a gastrostomy feed, half the normal amount, to be given. After a good night's sleep, he was cheerful and seemed well the next day. But the ward took no chances: for three more days he slept on a special mattress which sounds an alarm if it detects that a child has stopped breathing. The alarm did not sound and six days after the arrest, he was well enough to go out for the afternoon with his mum and dad.

After recovering from this drama, Robert's luck, for once, was in. The neurological investigations of the apparent fit which he had suffered at home – an EEG test* to measure brain waves and a CT scan to assess brain function – both proved normal. The fit remained an isolated incident. His parents' nerves were slower to recover. 'If the phone rings, I automatically think it must be the hospital,' says Charlie. 'It gets me every time. You get so used to it that I get the same feeling even on the odd occasion when Robert has been at home, then I think, oh ... he's here.'

Robert did make it home for another month, from mid-June to mid-July, but although there were some good times for his parents, he was never an easy or restful baby to care for. He had to be re-admitted in July with a high temperature, chesty cough and yet another urine infection. In any case, the next stage of his reconstructive surgery was only two weeks away.

Professor Spitz then performed what is known as a 'pull-through' operation. The rectum, the lower end of the bowel, is pulled through and connected to a new anus. This was also the right time to remove the useless left kidney; had it been left, it could have been responsible for more infections.

The day after the operation Robert was noted by the doctors to be 'looking good' and his recovery was, for him, unusually smooth. He went briefly home again, then later had another operation to tidy up the new anus. All in all, the weeks around Robert's first birthday were a good phase in his life. While he was home the Paynes celebrated the birthday with a quiet family day. 'Some of his cousins popped round during the day and in the evening we had a barbecue for the adults,' recalls Helen. A slight squint, which came and went, had been detected, but the ophthalmologists did not think any action was necessary. More good news came with the X-rays to check the pull-through repair undertaken by Professor Spitz. This appeared to be perfectly satisfactory and so, in mid-October, Robert's colostomy was closed. Another stage of his surgery was over; he was now reconstructed from the stomach to the anus and could excrete bodily wastes in the normal manner.

---

*See pages 230-1 for more about EEG tests.

Robert was a little miserable and grumpy after the operation which closed the colostomy, but he began to pass proper stools satisfactorily. 'It was quite incredible when he passed his first stool,' recalls Charlie. 'Sounds funny, but that was quite a landmark.' People felt a general sense of achievement, as the nurses monitored the progress of Robert's new system, but Helen's sardonic view that one problem solved usually led to another was soon to be endorsed. Robert entered a long phase of chronic diarrhoea which resisted the attempts of several doctors and dietitians to cure it.

Robert's diarrhoea began in October 1984 and continued right through until he had his major operation to reconnect his oesophagus and stomach in August 1985. It was a frustrating period when different diets and drugs were tried but the diarrhoea persisted. It meant Robert was not gaining weight because he was not absorbing food properly, and the doctors wanted to sort out this problem before contemplating the big operation. He needed meticulous nursing care. His gastrostomy feeds had to be maintained as it was essential for him to gain weight and strength, ready for future surgery. His sham feeds had to be continued in preparation for the day when his neck drain and gastrostomy would be closed. Maintaining a good fluid balance was essential because of his renal problems. The diarrhoea meant frequent nappy changes and bottom care. Robert was home for his second Christmas, but had to be re-admitted at the end of the next month with severe diarrhoea – not surprisingly, he had also lost weight. The diarrhoea made his bottom so horrendously sore that Helen felt he needed hospital care.

Yet in spite of this problem, which meant he was often unwell, Robert was to develop faster in the next few months than ever before and to fulfil some of his potential as an intelligent and responsive little boy. The nurses had already noted that his development was a little delayed so he had been encouraged to roll, sit, crawl and walk in the baby walker. Play with the ward playleader was important, as were the occasional outings with Helen and Charlie to discover the real world outside the hospital. At the end of a long list of nursing care tasks, the nurses noted: 'Give parents support and help for the day when Robert goes home.' And once again, they enlisted the aid of Debbie Sell, the speech therapist who had coaxed him into sham feeding on solids. This time, she was more concerned with his language development.

In January, when Robert was about sixteen months old, Debbie Sell noted that his language development was delayed. He wasn't responding to the names of common objects and was making no attempt to talk. She knew that Robert was a little boy of normal potential, but a hospital is a poor environment for learning language. Nurses come and go on different shifts and the environment is narrow and routine, lacking most of the stimulation and the need to develop language that a child enjoys in his own home. Debbie aimed to open up some new territory for Robert while involving Robert's mother as much as possible. She says: 'Mrs Payne is a bright lady, but she needed a few guidelines, a few ideas for positive play. I showed her how she could use play to stimulate language, for example taking turns with common objects like brushes, shoes, socks and toy telephones, continually stressing their names. Paddington Bear, with his hat, coat and wellingtons, is a useful toy, even though these were not so meaningful in terms of Robert's little life.'

The next stage was to encourage listening skills by using rattles and squeaky toys, making the right noises when looking at pictures of cars, dogs and cows, then progressing to understanding a few simple phrases like 'All gone' and 'Down and up'. Nurses – once chided by Debbie Sell for using babytalk to Robert – are mostly too busy to hold intense conversations with a child. Robert, though, loved this kind of play.

'Robert is a delightful, sociable little boy who seems to be in a rapid stage of development ... excellent prognosis for developing language,' noted Debbie Sell in her case records. He was so responsive that she made a training video of him, playing and talking to Paddington and the toy telephone, recognizing objects in picture books and imitating simple words. Debbie would come and see Robert in his cubicle where he was also visited by Janet Corderoy, then the ward physiotherapist. She, too, was concerned with Robert's development.

There was nothing physically wrong with Robert's legs, and

the physiotherapist was determined to get him walking. But a successful programme of physical therapy depends upon having a stable child and Robert's intermittent diarrhoea, and resulting low state, hindered his progress. Janet Corderoy says: 'Robert was always up and down like a yoyo and if children don't feel well, they don't want to explore the environment. Until they want to move, there's not a lot you can do. It was also very limiting being in the cubicle – no other children to interact with and fewer toys to make things interesting. You can't keep taking things in and out because of the infectious precautions, so you just have to improvise with the chairs and the rails of the cot.'

Janet also aimed to work with Helen to give her ideas. One of the first was to get Robert sitting on a mat and putting things just out of his reach to entice him to move on his bottom. The next stage was kneeling and pulling up, although Robert did not like being made to stand. 'It must be scary to be shifted into standing when your legs are weak from lack of use and sensation. Moving from one position to another needs a lot of balance and muscle work,' says Janet.

Some days were not so good – 'Bottom sore, feeling a little grizzly' Janet wrote in her case notes – but it was largely a matter of perseverance. And Janet could be tough with him. Once he was happy taking weight on his feet, she would get him to maintain the position while he played with toys. Robert was also helped by attending sessions at the hospital's Paul Sandifer Day Centre, where physiotherapists, speech therapists and a teacher, among others, operate what in effect is a specialist nursery school. Janet noted that, at seventeen months, Robert could walk, holding on, along the length of two chairs, 'which is lovely'. He progressed to walking with a trolley and then grew in confidence to cruising around the room holding on to the chairs. By mid-April, at nineteen months, he was 'taking six or eight steps unaided now'.

Like everything else, walking had been harder than normal for Robert. But this was one conspicuous achievement he had made. One consequence of Janet's persistence was that, although she had grown fond of the whole family, she herself was not Robert's favourite person. 'I had to put him in positions he didn't like and persevere. If I hadn't, progress would have been much more slow. Originally he didn't have the motivation to do anything, but you can't explain to a child why you are doing what you are doing. In an ideal world I'd like him to run to me when he sees me, but I understand why he doesn't. But it was very satisfying seeing him walk, and also because his Mum was so pleased.'

Janet Corderoy and Debbie Sell used their expertise to push Robert's development forward, often co-ordinating with each other; Debbie, for instance, gave the physio department a list of hints on how to play with Robert and how to talk to him during this period. The common element for each of them was play, also fulfilled in Robert's sessions at the Paul Sandifer Day Centre. Here Sue Hammond, the indefatigable teacher, often understaffed but helped by a nursery nurse and volunteers, oversees the developmental play of a group of mentally and physically handicapped children, both out-patients and in-patients, sometimes accompanied by their mothers. Robert continued to attend the Centre through 1985 and 1986. It offered him much-needed socialization; at first, he could only stand and stare at the other children. Sue Hammond, feeling he needed to be bombarded with sounds and stimulation, pressed for him to spend longer periods at the Centre. For Helen it was good to see him start to do normal things, and to get away from the ward. It also did her good to see that other children have problems.

Robert was observed to love cleaning: his favourite toy was a mop and for a year or more he kept his own special mop in the corner behind his cot. He was frequently seen trundling round the ward behind Leonie, the cleaner. He also loved Sue Hammond's singing sessions and playing musical games round the piano. Charlie Payne was quite moved the first time he went to watch. 'Seeing him get up when they called out his name, going to the front, joining in and taking turns – they were such normal things. It was great seeing him in a different environment.'

Meanwhile, on the ward, efforts continued to find a diet which would stop Robert's diarrhoea. His sham feeding was going well, but the dietitian, who already had a heavy file on

Robert, sought vainly to find the right gastrostomy feed. He had already dropped milk feeds and gone on to Chix, the complex feed based on comminuted chicken. He was seen by the hospital's gastro-enterology team who suggested diminishing the amount of Chix to minimum strength, then gradually increasing it until the point where Robert once more developed symptoms, so that the right amount would be established. Jeanette Ellis, one of the hospital's dietitians, spent four months changing the recipe almost daily, but Robert did not improve.

Finally in May the gastro-enterologists reluctantly had to suggest that Robert be put on Total Parenteral Nutrition (TPN), a course of intravenous feeding which would go straight into the blood stream, by-passing the stomach altogether. And so Robert went to theatre to have a Broviac catheter inserted into the right atrium of the heart through a neck vein so that he could be fed a complete diet of nutrients – fats, proteins, carbohydrates, sodium, potassium, minerals and vitamins – through this in-dwelling, long-term catheter. Though Robert later developed infections from the catheter and had to be treated with antibiotics, the TPN did achieve its objective and he began to put on weight.

Robert had also been seen by the orthopaedic team to assess his scoliosis – curvature of the spine – but it was felt that at this point he did not need any treatment. The slight squint detected some months earlier looked a little more noticeable, however, and for a while he wore a patch on his good eye; surgical registrar Keith Holmes nicknamed him 'Patch' and the name stuck. Sister Hannah Wright was by now so pleased with Robert's developmental progress that she pleaded with Sue MacQueen, the senior nurse responsible for infection control, to reconsider his 'infectious precautions' status. He had been put in a cubicle because of his liability to Gentamicin-resistant germs, but Hannah Wright wanted him out in the more stimulating environment of the open ward. Her argument was helped by the fact that Robert had tampered with his Broviac line and more than once bled profusely. He needed the more continuous surveillance of the ward where at least one nurse is always present, she argued. Sue MacQueen agreed, provided that the nurses kept up some extra precautions, such as additional hand-washing and wearing disposable gloves when changing nappies. So, when Robert was twenty-one months old, he was moved to a corner of the open area.

Although they knew that this would be far better for him, at first his parents missed the privacy of the cubicle. Helen and Charlie had set up home in there with their own chairs and all Robert's things. The ward, designed in an age when there was far less equipment and far fewer visiting parents around than today, quickly becomes overcrowded when all six beds have a patient. Robert, as a long-stay patient, amassed more toys than the other children and they were always getting lost.

But in the hurly-burly of the ward the nurses got to know Helen Payne much better. They had thought of her as rather shy and reticent; they admired the way she stayed contentedly in the cubicle with Robert and his books, and made few demands of the staff. Also, within a matter of weeks, Robert's walking, talking and general sociability had come on amazingly. It might be thought that all his experiences would have made him withdrawn, sad and indifferent to life, but he is not. When he is well, he is very quick to smile, respond and talk to people, and he draws visitors to him. Sometimes it seems that everybody in the hospital knows Robert.

'Everybody remembers him,' says Helen. 'I'm forever meeting nurses in the lift; they ask me how Robert is and I hardly remember them, so many nurses have passed through the ward.' 'Robert is so easy to love,' says Linda Davies, a staff nurse who joined 4AB when Robert was nine months old. 'When you have done something for him, he will always smile and talk to you. He's so sweet to look at and he knows how to tease the nurses.' Much later when Linda left Great Ormond Street to take up a new post in Manchester, she found she missed Robert more than anything. Julie Chapman, the ward clerk, who has worked there for eight years, is one of Robert's best girlfriends. As long-stay patients, the Paynes got to know all the staff, including dietitians and physiotherapist, much better than ordinary parents would.

Inside the hospital Helen and Charlie built up a close relationship with the sisters on the ward which would stand them in good stead in the times that lay ahead. They felt unstinting admiration for all the nurses. 'I always feel guilty about how little they earn,' says Charlie. 'I'm just pushing paper around and getting well paid for it, but they are spending long hours on their feet and they're very devoted; every minute of the day, when they're not on an official break, they're doing something. And when you see them on a one-to-one when Robert has had an operation, you see how skilled they are. They work so hard for such pitiful money. Yet still they do it. Obviously they get a lot out of the job, but they've still got to live like everyone else.'*

There was a new second sister on the ward now, Brìd (pronounced Breeje) Carr, younger and less extrovert than Hannah Wright, but equally dependable and with a gentler way with parents and junior doctors. Brìd is often seen working in the sisters' office, hours past her official off-duty time, even though she is in a minority of nurses at the hospital who are married. Charlie Payne may have been struck by the nurses' poor pay, but there are other disadvantages to the profession. The anti-social hours are one reason why extremely attractive nurses often stay unmarried; boyfriends sometimes just cannot understand why they can't change shifts and nurses tend not to join clubs and activities where they would meet men because work is so exhausting – and fulfilling. (The fact that Great Ormond Street does not teach medical students might also be considered by some nurses to be a disadvantage.)

Once Helen and Charlie Payne had got used to the rigours of the open ward, that spring was a happy period. The TPN line, though not a permanent solution to Robert's eating problems, had made him put on weight and he was often stable enough to be taken for walks. 'We'd lock off the TPN for a couple of hours and we would take him to Coram's Fields,† a

---

*See Appendix for examples of pay rates for nurses and other hospital staff.

---

†Coram's Fields are on the site of a foundling hospital established by Captain Thomas Coram in the eighteenth century. It remains an area, like Great Ormond Street, where children come first. At the entrance is a sign: "Adults only admitted if accompanied by a child."

lovely old park with a children's playground round the corner from Great Ormond Street. We'd go shuffling off round there and get out of the hospital,' remembers Charlie. Then the doctors started talking about doing the gastric interposition, the big operation which would reconnect Robert's oesophagus and stomach so that he could begin to eat normally. And what really pushed them into it was Helen's pregnancy.

In March of that year, when Robert was eighteen months old, Helen had told Charlie, in her quiet way: 'I think I'm pregnant.' It was a surprise because the Paynes did not consider themselves a very fertile couple. 'We never actually set out to have another baby. Robert had taken four years to produce and I was thinking, maybe we could try in a year or so when Robert would be at home and all fixed up,' says Helen. Initially Charlie, who had always vaguely imagined himself with a large family, was more pleased than she was; Helen had had a very uncomfortable first pregnancy. Then there was the underlying doubt.

Because the baby was unplanned, they had not sought advice from the hospital's genetic counselling clinics, as they would have done had Helen's tentative schedule for another baby worked out. There was, in fact, a very small chance of a recurrent problem, but easy confidence in the future had left them both. 'Having been exposed to Great Ormond Street and the million and one things that can go wrong with babies, you worry,' says Charlie. 'Even though you are aware that they are a very small percentage and that thousands and thousands of very healthy babies are born.'

Helen felt very sick during the first months of this pregnancy, but there was no bleeding and everything seemed to be fine. Yet concern for her and the new baby very much entered into the doctors' planning for Robert's operation. The form of the surgery was clear. The basic objective was to fill in the gap between the oesophagus and the stomach. The 'luckier' children with oesophageal atresia have such a relatively small gap that the two ends can be joined directly; if they are well enough, this can be done straight after the birth when the condition is discovered. This, in fact, is what happens to most babies born with oesophageal atresia. But in Robert's case, the gap had been too big and he had been too tiny and ill for anything but the time-gaining procedures of gastrostomy feeding and the oesophagostomy neck 'drain'. Ways of closing the gap included transplanting a piece of the colon or bowel (as in Stacey's story) but for five years at Great Ormond Street all the oesophageal replacements had been gastric interpositions: the stomach, which normally lies horizontally in the abdomen, is moved up towards the neck and joined to the stump of the oesophagus.

This form of operation had succeeded colon transplants at Great Ormond Street because of the far greater complication rate of the latter. Follow-up and assessment are vital to the surgeons' decisions. 'We are looking at our results all the time and we watch what's happening elsewhere. And of the children who had had gastric interpositions, most had done incredibly well,' says Professor Spitz. 'We have got over twenty children who are running around, eating everything, developing normally and obviously we keep a close watch on them. So that was the procedure we would follow for Robert.'

The unresolved question was when to do the operation. Robert's intestine was not absorbing food, as the diarrhoea showed; maybe reconnection would help. His renal surgery and then his prolonged diarrhoea, which they had hoped to sort out first, had already delayed the time at which the gastric inter-position might have been considered. Professor Spitz says: 'Normally we do this operation at about seven or eight months but because of all his other problems we said we must wait. But the question is how long do you wait. Sometimes you have to make a decision, because you just can't leave them as they are. The other thing that swayed us was Mrs Payne's pregnancy. She was going to have another child and if we could have Robert in one piece by then it would be so much nicer.'

Not only nicer, but safer; if Robert died after an operation towards the end of Helen's pregnancy, the shock might send her into premature labour and harm the new baby. But was Robert up to it? The diarrhoea had been nutritionally devastating, even though the TPN had now made him gain a little weight. This would be a major operation for Robert: was he really strong enough? There was a good case to be made for leaving it, too. Intense deliberations continued among the doctors until, finally, Professor Spitz said that he had been loitering about the ward for too long: he set the date for 31 July.

'In July Robert was so well and happy,' remembers Hannah Wright. But the prospect of the operation hung over the otherwise happy month. Robert himself could not be told, even though by now he had had so many operations and investigations that he knew when he was going to theatre. 'You can see it on his little face – he doesn't want to go where he is going. If he has got one of those little gowns on and the trolley comes, he knows there's trouble ahead,' says Helen. She and Charlie knew that this was a major op. and Professor Spitz had told them of the risks. Helen says: 'It was a long while since he'd had an operation and he hadn't been on a ventilator since he was a couple of months old. We knew he would be coming back absolutely flat out and ventilated. It wasn't much fun.'

The night before the operation Robert was on his best form. His parents took photographs and let him stay up late. He was running cheekily round the sisters' desk, making everyone laugh. Charlie and Helen said their goodbyes and went home. To the nurses' consternation, a short time later Robert, who had been so well, suddenly 'spiked' a temperature of thirty-nine degrees ('spiked' is the nurses' term for a sudden rise in temperature, coming from the pattern it makes on a patient's chart). Half an hour after the Paynes arrived home, there was a phone call to say that because of the temperature Robert had been taken off the next day's operating list. 'We just sat there, we were absolutely numb. The phone was going all next day as people rang up to see how he was and we had to keep explaining the operation had been postponed.'

Somehow Helen and Charlie went through the same routine again, for Robert's temperature proved short-lived and the operation was rearranged for one week later, on 7 August, barely three weeks short of his second birthday. As long-term residents on this surgical ward they had watched many parents break down as their children went off to theatre and had time to work out what their own coping mechanisms would be. They planned to arrive at the hospital when Robert was

187

already there and wait on the ward for the next couple of hours. But the actual operation was very straightforward and took less than the usual three or so hours. Professor Spitz was very pleased with the way it went; the stomach did not leak, in fact it didn't do anything unexpected.

Helen and Charlie were sitting in the playroom of ward 4AB, expecting to be there for another couple of hours, when the operation was over. Charlie says: 'First of all, the Prof. breezed in and said, "Very good. All done. They're just sewing him up now". Two staff nurses had been up to watch the operation and they came down to tell us all about it, quite elated. They were so full of admiration for the Professor, so delicate and gentle the way he manipulated the stomach into position.'

Robert was wheeled back to 4A and Hannah Wright said, in a deliberately flip, offhand way to his parents: 'All right, you can come and see him now.' Helen, who has only once broken down into tears on the ward and prefers to do her crying at home, was glad she had made a joke of it: 'If anyone had come up and put their arm around me, I would have collapsed.' Robert was on a ventilator, heavily sedated. He was being 'specialled' which meant a nurse was with him all the time. A replogle tube had been passed down his nose and was used to drain the contents of his stomach; this enabled the wound to heal and also ensured maximum expansion of the lungs. He had a catheter inserted to collect urine and a line into the femoral artery in his thigh so that blood could be collected easily. His gastrostomy and oesophagostomy had been closed, but there was a new opening into the jejunum or small intestine. This was to provide for feeding directly into the small bowel until the reconnected oesophagus functioned effectively.

His parents were not the only people to feel tense. Brid Carr, who was off duty that day, could hardly bear waiting to find out what had happened. Hannah Wright phoned her at home to give her the news, which at first was good. Robert had an excellent first post-operative night and for the first couple of days he did very well. 'Everyone was a bit amazed and said "This isn't Robert"', recalls Helen. Professor Spitz and Dr Ted Sumner, the consultant anaesthetist, visited him and were very buoyant. On the day after the operation the Professor suggested removing the arterial line, but he bowed to Sister Wright who felt they ought to keep it in for a few more days. The ventilation was reduced a little and everyone remarked on how well he was doing. The Paynes, cautious and with their characteristic, self-defensive note of pessimism, would reply darkly, 'Yes, he is at the moment,' or 'It's early days and you know what Robert's like.'

On the fourth night Robert proved his parents right. Earlier that day the physio had thought his chest slightly worse and during the evening he became more and more restless. At one-thirty a.m. his breathing rate, heart-beat and blood pressure had gone up so high that the night staff called the duty registrar and the anaesthetist. The registrar thought his lungs had too much fluid on them and Robert was given a diuretic to stimulate urine output and reduce the fluid. He was also put back on full ventilation with sixty per cent oxygen. By morning he was fair, but the next few days brought several episodes of breathing distress. He had frequent visits from the physios to help remove secretions from his chest. One week post-operation he was still on full ventilation.

Once more, just as had happened during his period of ventilation when he was a tiny baby on 6A, Robert was proving difficult to wean off the ventilator. Prolonged ventilation, although life-saving, may carry complications such as tracheal or lung damage and the medical team will always be working towards reducing it. If Robert seemed well, the doctor or anaesthetist would say it could be turned down; either by reducing the amount of oxygen, the number of breaths or the pressure exerted by the machine. When the ventilation was reduced, the nurses would monitor the child carefully, watching for signs of breathing difficulties and sending blood samples to check for oxygen and carbon dioxide content. After a major operation such as a gastric interposition, Robert might have been expected to be ventilated for a week, but no more. However, he ran into respiratory problems which no one had anticipated and the Paynes, with Helen now more than six months pregnant, were forced to live through a nightmare of setbacks for the two months after the operation. For a month they stayed near the hospital at the Sick Children's Trust house in Bloomsbury in order to save Helen the long daily tube journey.

The ventilation went up and down. Parents and visitors would come into the ward to see Robert and immediately ask about the figures on the ventilator: how much oxygen, how many breaths? About two weeks after the operation Robert seemed to pick up a little, with more settled and comfortable nights when he hardly woke. He seemed cheerful during the day and the physiotherapist said his chest was clear. The doctors therefore decided to switch him to the less intensive form of ventilation known as CPAP – Continous Positive Airways Pressure – where the patient has to do the breathing.

At first Robert appeared to be coping, but the following morning his breathing deteriorated so badly that he had to go back on full ventilation. Towards the end of August there were two more attempts to establish him on CPAP, but with the same unsuccessful result. In this uncertain, unstable state Robert Payne approached his second birthday on 31 August. It was a mixed day; there were lots of cards, presents and visitors from inside the hospital, but he was still on full ventilation and miserable because of the discomfort caused when his breathing tube tapes were changed. A few days later there was another attempt to switch him to CPAP, but with no more success than before; at first he coped well and then once more became unstable.

One month after the gastric interposition, everyone was profoundly worried. Professor Spitz called in the ear, nose and throat surgeons and in early September they took Robert back to theatre to look down his trachea via an instrument called a bronchoscope. But the trachea looked all right. Professor Spitz saw Robert's increasingly anxious parents to explain the situation. In mid-September he did another bronchoscopy and found that the trachea or windpipe was soft; there was tracheomalacia, or collapse of the trachea, which should be a rigid tube. Professor Spitz decided to do an aortopexy, a procedure in which the aorta, the large artery rising out of the heart, is pulled forward and stitched to the sternum or breastbone, which in turn pulls forward the trachea and prevents its collapse.

But the aortopexy did not sort out Robert's airway problems. Towards the end of September he had been ventilated for more than seven weeks since the gastric interposition. He was at the limit for ventilation so the ENT surgeons and the anaesthetists urged a tracheostomy, the insertion of a small tube directly into the trachea just below the Adam's apple.* The damage which could be done to airways by prolonged ventilation made the tracheostomy inevitable, to the dismay of the Paynes who had desperately wanted Robert to avoid it. The tracheostomy was performed on 27 September so that the ventilator now pumped air into his lungs via the trachy rather than through a tube in his nose. It was an enormously stressful period for the doctors and nurses involved. 'We felt we had been destructive because in the summer he had been feeding and walking so well,' says Hannah Wright.

It had been even more desperate for Robert's parents. At the beginning of October, nearly two months after the gastric interposition, Helen began to have regular contractions. She was only thirty-two weeks pregnant and, in view of the outcome of her first pregnancy, her doctors could not take any chances. She went straight into Queen Charlotte's maternity hospital for a few days. Here the doctors were able to give her a drug which would inhibit labour. (Although she did have to spend a further two weeks in hospital later, she then came home again for a further fortnight and managed to make it to her booked Caesarean delivery.)

'I was very upset because I had just disappeared from Robert's life and he wouldn't know why,' says Helen. Feeling that he was just too little to understand, they didn't try to explain to Robert but Charlie kept up his routine of always being there to put Robert to bed, then dashing off in mid-evening to Queen Charlotte's where the ante-natal ward gave him permission to visit after regular visiting hours. Charlie was anxious about the new baby as well as Helen and Robert. 'We had asked for a second scan and that time the scan operator

---

*See Stacey's story for detailed description of tracheostomies.

took ages. I was convinced she'd found something and even when she said it was all right, I still didn't believe her.'

At this point everything could have fallen apart for the Paynes; this had been the worst period they have ever lived through. For most of Robert's stay on 4AB they had been visibly coping: Charlie cheerful, witty and quick to see a joke, Helen calm and controlled. On the ward everyone felt for them. Valerie Sheldon is the ward social worker and had got to know them during that year. She looked for ways to offer support even though these were not obviously apparent. 'The Paynes may be feeling dreadful but they are not a family who would normally seek a social worker's help,' she says. 'When parents have marital or financial problems, a social worker has something tangible to focus on. But the Paynes are not in this category. With many couples going through a situation like this the cracks would open up very quickly.'

Nonetheless Val Sheldon, a sensitive judge of a situation, knew how bad this one was. She wanted to get involved if there was anything she could do. Openings for practical help might be limited in the Paynes' case, but she offered emotional support, too. 'When people are going through this situation of having a child desperately ill for a long time, their emotional reserves are used up very quickly and they can dry up without support and encouragement. You try to offer support but in a different way from family or friends.'

'In a chronic situation a feeling of helplessness sets in for the staff – a sense of "There's nothing we can do". When Robert was slow coming off his ventilator I would go and see the Paynes, and we would often end up joking – a reaction to the desperate situation we were all in. I realized that the Paynes have found their own way of coping and I didn't want to change that in any way, but to remain alert to needs that were not being met.'

During the day, in the absence of Robert's mum, Sue Osborn, 4AB's playleader, spent a lot of time with him. Most of her day is spent organizing play for the older and less sick children, but she already knew Robert well. Robert, if fit enough, would be in the playroom painting, sticking or glueing. The playroom, says Sue Osborn, ought to be like a little home;

there is a television and the children have their meals there. But playleaders also become emotionally attached to many children: they are not associated with painful procedures in the children's minds, although there will be hospital play to help prepare children for unpleasant tests or minor operations such as the insertion of a Hickman Catheter. Playleaders are also a continuous weekday presence in the ward where student nurses change every eight weeks and staff nurses rotate between different shifts. Robert would therefore go to Sue Osborn and ask for her more than the nurses.

'It's part of my job to offer comfort and reassurance if Mum is not there,' she says. 'But Robert loves his Mum and Dad which is very important. I don't want to try and take their place. The Paynes are lovely parents; they were always here. Dad came every day and so did Robert's mum except when she had to spend time in hospital. But if he needed reassurance, if he had had physio, or tubes changed, or was coming back from theatre, I would try to look out for him and be there.'

It was a great deprivation for Helen to be parted from Robert, but at least when she went into the maternity hospital in early October, he began to improve. His nights became more settled and on 2 October Robert was well enough to be on CPAP once again. He was able to get out of his cot and sit, painting, on a playmat. He went for a short walk. After twenty-four hours alternating between CPAP and an oxygen mask, he was finally extubated – taken off the ventilator – on 3 October.

During October he continued to be fed via his jejunostomy tube into the small intestine, but as soon as he was well enough he was given ordinary meals in the hope that his newly-connected oesophagus and stomach would work. Everyone was optimistic because he had been such a good sham feeder and when he ate two morsels of his dinner on 7 October the fact was triumphantly recorded in the nursing notes. He was tempted with jelly or chips and received lots of encouragement from his parents, nurses and Sue, the playleader. At one point his jejunostomy feeds were stopped, in the hope of stimulating his appetite, but his oral intake was poor and they had to be restarted.

On 5 November Helen Payne gave birth to her second child. It was a straightforward Caesarean delivery: a perfect baby boy whom they called Simon. 'Everyone was so pleased that something had gone right for us,' says Helen. Charlie found it hard to believe that the baby was healthy, even after the doctors had examined him and one had showed Charlie the baby's bottom. 'I didn't really believe he was all right until I'd seen him eat something,' he says. He joked with Hannah Wright that he had been right round the baby ten times, checking that everything was there.

Sister Wright took Robert by taxi to Queen Charlotte's to visit Helen and Simon. Even though Simon's arrival had not been planned, now that he was safely here he was cause for rejoicing. 'Simon will be good for Robert in the long term,' said his father. 'If he's going to be small and weak, he may run into problems with other kids. Now he has somebody who might look after him.'

Robert, though, had undergone a tremendous ordeal and was nowhere near back to being the child he was in the summer. He remained lethargic and miserable and his eating was disappointing. At the end of October speech therapist Debbie Sell saw him again. The idea was discussed with the doctors that they put a little valve into the opening of the tracheostomy tube. This valve opened for air to be breathed in and shut as the air was expelled, allowing air to be breathed out through the vocal cords so that Robert was able to make an audible sound. She did not want his language to slip back; if the 'speaking tube' did not result in Robert beginning to talk, they would consider teaching him Makaton, a simple sign language, and Sue, the ward playleader, went on a Makaton study course in preparation. But fortunately Robert tolerated the redesigned tube and did begin to talk.

Robert was not well enough to go home for Christmas, so for the first time he experienced the organized jollity of a hospital Christmas. In the New Year the ward said goodbye to Hannah Wright. She was off to Oman for a year to help run a paediatric surgical unit at a hospital there which has links with Great Ormond Street. Bríd Carr would now be in charge, so the ward was still in capable and reassuring hands. Later another sister, Katie Lewis, joined the team.

On 21 January Robert clocked up one full year of continuous hospital residence, depressing confirmation of how slow his progress had been since the gastric interposition. His parents remained outwardly cheerful, but little seemed to be happening clinically. Robert had a series of chest infections and a replogle tube was inserted to keep his stomach drained. Though there were other children with complicated conditions being nursed on the ward, most recovered after their surgery and went home; their parents expected events and developments on a daily basis. However, the Paynes were now resigned to a much slower time scale. Maybe in March Robert's tracheostomy would be reviewed; but nobody was talking about coming home.

For the foreseeable future, ward 4A was Robert's home. 'He's got no concept of families and houses,' says his father. His mother wonders what he thinks about 'home'. 'He hears the phrase "going home" all the time. I said to him the other day "Would you like to come home?" He said "Yes, I would," but I don't know what he thinks about it,' says Helen. Charlie adds: 'He just equates it with people not being at Great Ormond Street. If he's playing up and I threaten that I'll go home, he clutches my hand and he normally settles down.' Robert has been to another hospital, visiting Queen Charlotte's after Simon was born. 'He might have thought that was home,' mused Helen. 'Perhaps he thinks that everybody lives in these big buildings with lots of beds in them. It would be lovely to get into his mind – because he must have such a narrow view of life.'

After Simon was born Helen had to combine looking after a new baby with visiting the hospital. She had always been meaning to learn to drive, but never got round to it. Val Sheldon, the social worker, asked herself: 'What can we do to help Mrs Payne while her life is virtually split in two?' She saw it as part of her role to help keep Helen Payne visiting and was able to arrange funding for drivers to bring Helen and Simon to the hospital during the week. Charlie continued his habit of calling at the hospital every day after work. Hannah Wright used to tease him with jokes about having abandoned his child if he ever failed to turn up, but in fact he has only missed the odd day since Robert arrived on the ward.

At teatime, Robert will start looking out for Charlie. He seems to know what time it is and sometimes walks to the lift to meet him. In his office, two or three miles away across London, his father is getting ready to leave for the hospital, where he will give Robert a bath and play with him until he goes to sleep. 'Sometimes, especially if it's been a hard day at work and I'm tired and if he's been horrible the two or three nights leading up to it, I sometimes think – Oh, God. But when it comes round to a quarter to five I nearly always find I'm looking forward to seeing him. I never get fed up with going to see him, it's part of our routine now. And I know he waits for me. I couldn't come home and think of him sitting there.' On Sundays Robert will often go to sleep clutching the Sunday colour supplements. 'Charlie brings them into the hospital to read and Robert plays with them all day, then hugs them as he goes to sleep,' says a nurse, 'because they are Daddy's.'

The Paynes have paid a price for their fidelity as parents. They enjoy little normal social life. Charlie, a keen footballer throughout his teens and early twenties, hung up his boots the week Robert was born. Nor have they had a holiday together since then. 'We did go away for one weekend to York when Robert was about six months old and we both felt so mean leaving him,' says Helen. 'Now it would be impossible to leave him because he would miss us more.' They cannot move house, as Helen would like; they cannot afford to move further into London, while further out, where property is cheaper, would make visiting the hospital too difficult. Charlie Payne does not believe the situation has affected his performance at work, but it may have affected his objectives in life. 'Your materialistic ambitions just go out of the window when something like Robert. He becomes the be-all and end-all of your existence. Even some of our friends found our situation brought things into perspective for them; people are so wrapped up in their jobs, they forget the most important thing is the health of their family.'

Great Ormond Street is not a place for long-term conditions, but an acute-stay hospital, and inevitably when a patient like

Robert becomes a chronic case, the environment is not all that it might be. In an ideal world there would be a special unit within the hospital for the small group of long-stay children with staff based there for much longer periods. A life confined to hospital may have caused Robert's serious feeding problems: no one is really sure how much of this stems from behavioural origins, caused by the lack of normal stimulation, and how much is a physical problem.

But many people at Great Ormond Street maintain that Robert will one day live at home – and they are sure that he is not institutionalized. Although affectionate, he is selective in his response to people; he will not hug a stranger, as some institutionalized children will in their hunger for contact. He has always been well aware of who his parents are and the hospital has done everything it can to strengthen this bond. Robert is also not spoilt. 'He is not a typical hospitalized child,' says Hannah Wright. 'We've managed to keep the discipline going and Helen has been so good in this way. Robert gives so much – there's no resentment about what's happened to him.'

Where have the Paynes found the strength to carry on? 'They are outstanding parents,' says Professor Spitz. 'Many people would have cracked, their marriage would have broken up, they would have abandoned the child. The stresses are worse now that they have a normal child. They will realize Robert's limitations, even though he's an intelligent kid; he doesn't seem to be mentally affected at all, even though he's been through absolute hell and back.' Brid Carr, who also knows them very well, agrees the Paynes have a staying power not many people have. 'They are deeply religious and there is a family network behind them; it's not overpowering, but the support is there. But basically, they wanted a child very badly and they are just very giving.'

Helen is not sure if religion helps you to cope, because she knows that plenty of people without religion also cope. But she and Charlie do value the fact that many people pray for Robert. 'Sometimes I wonder, with all these people praying for him, why he isn't better. But my mother says perhaps he would have done even worse without them.' Helen's mother always cooks a meal for Helen and Charlie on Sundays which frees them to spend the day at the hospital. And, says Helen, she is always there if needed.

Though grateful for their family's help, and realistic about Robert's chances, Helen and Charlie always clung to the hope that one day they would lead a normal life and spend a day, even a complete weekend in their own house. So when could Robert go home? His reconstructive surgery had now been achieved: his imperforate anus had been sorted out, his remaining kidney, though it would always need scanning and antibiotic cover, had been repaired. His oesophagus and stomach had been connected, though had yet to prove that they worked effectively. His lesser problems, like his scoliosis and his deformed arm, would be reviewed as he grew older. For Robert to go home, he would need to be eating well and gaining weight, free of chest infections. And his trachy would have to be closed, since Helen was reluctant to look after him at home with a tracheostomy, given his complicated history.

In February, seven months after the gastric interposition, Robert suddenly seemed a great deal better. Professor Spitz examined his stomach in theatre with an instrument called a gastroscope and it looked normal; then a barium meal, X-rays taken after Robert swallowed a radio-opaque dye, showed that his stomach was emptying normally. He began to eat a little and all his old sparkle came back. He suddenly had a lot more energy and would try to hop and jump, play hide and seek and football with the older children on the ward. He was taken to the nursery school at the Paul Sandifer Centre for the first time for months and ran in to the Wendy house, so delighted to be back. He put on a little weight and Sue Osborn, the play-leader, began potty-training. Robert was talking much more and putting sentences together. He was taken to the entrance hall to meet his parents and ran to meet them. Everyone was so pleased; could Robert have turned the corner?

Robert certainly deserves some luck. He was born with an appalling collection of defects, but they were such that doctors believed they could set them right; then he ran into problems which no one anticipated. He has had to bear more than anyone ought to have to bear, let alone a two-year-old boy. Yet he has still had more good days than bad, says his father, and when he is well, he has a happy life.

More than anybody else his parents have given him the will to survive. For them, as for others, the hospital experience has proved that parental love can bring forth incredible strength and devotion. Their son's ups and downs have been so many that the image of Robert going home alternately fades and clears; but until they can all walk out together, Helen and Charlie Payne will go on walking into Great Ormond Street hospital to be with Robert. 'We will never let him down,' vows his father.

Postscript: one year later

He went home for Christmas 1986. Although he had to return for minor surgery the following month, he returned home again and has since done remarkably well. Robert is eating well and beginning to thrive; doctors hope to remove his tracheostomy during the summer and plans are beginning to be made for his education at a special school. For now, though, he just loves being at home.

1.15 p.m. *A group of student nurses meet in the canteen to compare notes as they come off duty after their first real shift on the wards. During their initial eight-week period of theoretical training the students are given two trial shifts, but all admit nonetheless to having been petrified before their first stint of duty on a ward. Afterwards there is a universal feeling of fatigue; they are exhausted by being on their feet virtually the whole time, although this is something they will have to get used to. One or two have been bored by not having enough to do because they cannot, of course, take care of the really sick children. Others have been on wards which were short-staffed or had a rush of admissions and so were expected to do a great deal. All wear pink caps to mark them out as novice students but they say that some doctors, as well as the parents, don't understand the significance of the caps. So one or two were annoyed that doctors expected them to know more than they possibly could have done. All felt insecure because they were constantly asked to fetch things without knowing where things were kept. But there were the satisfactions of their debuts on the wards. One 'pink hatter' described how she had bathed a baby for the first time. The baby had a Hickman Catheter in her chest and the nurse had to avoid getting the catheter or the area around it wet; afterwards the child ('a nice little Indian baby') looked really lovely, she said.*

One in three paediatric nurses in Britain are trained by the Charles West School of Nursing which comes under the Great Ormond Street umbrella. The increasingly specialized nursing at Great Ormond Street has got to be balanced by more general paediatric training at the sister hospital in the group, the Queen Elizabeth Hospital for Children in Hackney. But what the students will learn at both hospitals is that children are different; they're not just smaller versions of adults but individuals whose metabolism, physiology and pathology will vary at different ages in ways absolutely crucial to their health. 'They develop at different rates with different needs at different stages of development. This quality of development offers the potential for improvement but also makes them susceptible to damage. It is the potential for improvement which makes children so special. We have to train our students to look after the emotional and social needs of children as well as coping with their clinical condition,' says Betty

Barchard, who, as chief nursing officer, is in overall charge of the nursing school as well as the two hospitals.

1.30 p.m. *Afternoon school sessions begin. These are optional, unlike the morning sessions which for older children can involve work for GCE examinations (see the story of Gus and Lewis). But many children come to join in music or painting sesssions. There is also a music session beginning at the Paul Sandifer Centre for handicapped children and the play centre is opening its doors for the afternoon session. Play is an integral part of hospital life. Each ward has (or should have) a playleader and others are based, along with volunteers, in the play centre situated off the out-patient department. For children in hospital, play has a thera-peutic value. It promotes normal development and helps children cope with the stresses of hospital life. There is also 'hospital play' through which children can become familiar with medical equip-ment and be prepared for hospital procedures. But play is also fun. It helps the children to relax and be happy while in hospital and, by doing so, gives the hospital its fundamentally cheerful and buoyant atmosphere.*

1.35 p.m. *Dr Mike Dillon, the renal consultant, is coming to the end of his 'morning' clinic. He had seen eleven patients with varying forms of kidney problems, asking how they've been doing, checking blood pressures and taking blood samples for analysis. In a week he and his colleagues will see around 150 out-patients. For some, like four-month-old Stephen, renal problems are part of more general ailments; for others, such as Jonty, the kidneys were the prime cause of their difficulties. Jonty is now seventeen and came unaccompanied by parents, a sporty student who was the first patient of the day to be taller than his doctor. Nine years earlier he had been critically ill with a condition called polyarteritis nodosa. This involves widespread inflammation of the arteries which causes severe kidney disease. Not too long ago it carried a hundred per cent mortality rate and even with intensive drug treatment one in five victims still die.*

Jonty came through his ordeal and arrives for his penultimate appointment at Great Ormond Street. At seventeen he should be transferred to adult hospitals, but his parents have asked if this

201

could be deferred until after he has completed his A Levels in the summer. He also asks whether it would be safe to have the injections necessary for a visit to India. Other mature patients also asked questions about the safety of drugs: 'Would it be okay for me to go on the pill?' queried a sixteen-year-old girl. Five minutes earlier Dr Dillion had been grappling with the problem of a baby whose cancer treatment had caused renal problems resulting in a dozen or so wet nappies a night. Dr Dillon believes that out-patient work is sometimes undervalued. 'You have to make decisions on the spot without any back-up system. On the ward there is group of doctors and you have some time to think about problems. Out-patient work is very exacting if done properly. It's too easy to say "Come back in two weeks" and not make a decision.' Nor does the work end when the final patient has been seen. Doctors usually have at least an hour's paperwork ahead of them, dictating letters to GPs or other hospitals about their patient's condition. Dr Dilln arrived at the hospital this morning at eight-twenty, having only left at eleven-fifteen the previous evening after two ward rounds, two clinics and hours of subsequent dictation.

2.00 p.m. *Frank Bruno, boxing champion, arrives accompanied by Disney characters from Smart's Amusement Park to distribute Easter eggs to the children. So many eggs are given to the hospital that three large boxes full are sent to Queen Elizabeth Hospital for Children in Hackney. This sister hospital receives fewer gifts and fewer visits so presents are often shared. Even the stars of the BBC's 'East Enders' visited Great Ormond Street rather than the children's hospital in the East End!*

2.10 p.m. *The afternoon out-patient clinics are beginning. First to be called in to the neurology clinic is Sarah, a fourteen-year-old girl who is suffering from progressive muscular failure. She is in a wheel-chair, but is reluctant to use it at school – and that's what is worrying her mother. She fears Sarah is trying to do too much and perhaps overstraining her heart; there have been frequent giddy feelings, she tells Dr John Wilson, the neurology consultant, and once Sarah passed out. Dr Wilson examines Sarah tenderly. He asks her to squeeze his fingers and then tests her co-ordination. He* *looks in her ears, eyes and mouth and whispers instructions in a simple test of hearing. He listens to her heart but can find nothing wrong. However, to try and reassure Sarah's mother he arranges for her to have a special test known as an echocardiogram as well as a standard chest X-ray. Throughout the examination he talks not only to the mother but also to Sarah, as he did to patients throughout the afternoon. 'Is there anything you want to tell me or to complain about?' 'Can I look at your back?' 'I'd just like to do a few things, but none of them will hurt you.'*

His kindly, courteous manner does much to put patients and parents at their ease. One or two mothers are anxious, but many seem remarkably cheerful and resilient in the face of conditions which foreshadow depressing and debilitating futures. Failures of the nervous system produce not merely mental handicap but muscular and psychological problems. Those which come to Great Ormond Street tend to be the problems which are not susceptible to quick or easy 'cures'. Dr Wilson says it is a question of following the old medical truism: 'cure sometimes, relief often, comfort always'. Not that this should imply a passive acceptance of neurological conditions. 'Twenty years ago people often made a diagnosis and didn't try to prevent the complications which developed. Now we are much more aggressive in trying to keep problems at bay,' says Dr Wilson.

2.15 p.m. Dr Richard Lansdown, chief psychologist of the Department of Psychological Medicine, sees Claire (not her real name), a nine-year-old girl who suffers from eczema. He will try to help her through hypnosis; it won't cure Claire's skin problem, but it may help her to control the irritation. He asks her if there are times when the itching seems particularly mild; is it in cold, dry, hot or wet weather, for instance? Each child is different and Claire said she liked cool conditions; Dr Lansdown then induced a trance. 'In your mind I would like you to go through a magic door into a room and in that room you can go anywhere,' he said. 'So you can go to a pine forest, full of Christmas trees with snow on the branches. You touch the tree and put snow on your hands and the part of your skin that is itching.'

Dr Lansdown has been using hypnosis for a couple of years but only recently to try and help patients with skin problems, in

*conjunction with dermatology consultant, Dr David Atherton.
Usually it takes four or five sessions lasting around twenty minutes
to teach children how to induce a pain-relieving trance themselves.
So far, he says, the results are encouraging. The Department of
Psychological Medicine is one of the largest departments in the
hospital. It only has one ten-bedded ward for in-patients since the
thrust of the department's work is through family-oriented out-
patient services which include a day centre which parents attend
with their children. Consultations can take up to two hours and
involve psychologists, psychiatrists and specialist social workers.
The range of problems encountered is notably diverse, ranging
from learning difficulties and bedwetting to child sexual abuse and
anorexia. There is also a heavy commitment to research, often
conducted jointly with doctors from the hospital or the Institute of
Child Health.*

2.25 p.m. *John Fixsen, the consultant orthopaedic surgeon, sees
the second patient of his afternoon clinic – ten-year-old Giles, who
is accompanied by his father. Giles' feet turn noticeably outwards,
a very unusual condition which is known as femoral retroversion.
The deputy head at his school has suggested that they seek a second
opinion. Mr Fixsen asks if Giles has had any problems with his
legs but Giles, a bright and cheerful boy, replies that he has none,
other than not being able to run very fast. His father adds that he
gets some ragging at school, but is in no pain and does not seem
unduly worried. John Fixsen remarks that Charlie Chaplin probably had femoral retroversion – which accounted for his distinctive walk – and says that it is a cosmetic, not a functional problem;
he would very rarely consider operating in order to relieve the
condition. Giles and his father are happy to accept this verdict,
stressing that they have come just to make sure nothing is being
overlooked. An X-ray was taken to ensure there is no other source
for the problem and they go home quite happily.*

*Mr Fixsen sees many patients, like Giles, whom he assesses but
does not refer for surgery. Giles' father was positive and sensible
about the condition but later in the afternoon another parent very
much wanted surgery to correct what appeared to be a relatively
insignificant abnormality. 'Parents don't like accepting that a
child appears to differ,' says Mr Fixsen. 'They have a blueprint in*

their minds and no conception of the normal range.' Other patients this afternoon illustrate other problems commonly seen in the orthopaedic clinics: parents in search of a miracle cure for a handicapped boy who is slow to walk and children who have been operated on elsewhere with less than perfect results. Much of John Fixsen's work consists of providing second opinions, perhaps on rare conditions or to judge a clash of opinions. As ever, the conditions seen at Great Ormond Street are very complicated and Mr Fixsen frequently discusses cases with his registrar (who is also seeing patients in the same room) and two visiting foreign doctors. With his visitors, he explores differing attitudes such as the greater willingness of doctors in Mediterranean countries to operate on essentially cosmetic problems (such as unequal leg length) than in Britain. But amid the bustle, he never forgets the parents and his courtesy plus an obvious zest for the job makes the atmosphere constructive and relaxed, at least for most of the parents. Even when there is no miracle cure, reconstructive surgery can be very worthwhile. In cerebral palsy patients, for instance, spines can be straightened so that they can sit in a chair or use a communicator, something for which the children will be very grateful. Today there is a much better understanding of normal child development which may make surgery and splintage unnecessary, says Mr Fixsen. If surgery is planned, he adds, it must take account of the child's future growth and it is this which makes paediatric orthopaedics fundamentally different to that of adults.

Gus and Lewis

'Welcome to ward 5A where the people are crazy but nice,' says the poster outside the intensive care ward. It was painted by Augusto Grieco, or Gus to his friends. It's a colourful poster with a style uncramped by the fact that Gus painted the poster with a brush held in his mouth. He has lost, among other things, the ability to paint by hand, yet if it had not been for 5A he would have lost his life. On average one child in every five admitted to the ward does die. But children are only admitted to intensive care if they are in danger of dying, so it would be fairer to say that four in every five live. 'We're the end of the line,' says Bob Dinwiddie, one of the unit's three consultants. 'There's nowhere else to go.'

Gus was referred to 5A by ward 1C, the neurology ward at Great Ormond Street, when his condition deteriorated twenty-four hours after arriving from a hospital in Watford. Most children on 5A have been referred there directly by other hospitals. Among them was Lewis Pate, his ambulance's path cleared through the rush-hour traffic by a police escort which reminded his mother of something out of TV's *The Sweeney*. Minutes, even seconds, can count when a child is critically ill. They certainly did in the case of Lewis: he was virtually dead by the time he reached 5A. Even if he lived, his parents were told, he would probably lose his hands and his legs might have to be amputated at the knees. Gus's parents, too would have to adjust to a 'different' child – if, that is, he pulled through the crisis which in forty-eight hours transformed him from a football-playing teenager to one fighting for his life.

Gus and Lewis were two of around 250 children who, on average, are admitted to 5A each year.* It is not the only ward

---

*Children rarely stay on 5A for long so two stories are better than one to show what can happen to patients in intensive care; the contrasting fates of Gus and Lewis also posed different problems, not only for 5A, but other members of the Great Ormond Street staff.

with intensive care facilities in the hospital; there are also 1A, the acute cardiac ward, and 6A, the neonatal surgical ward. Other wards, such as the neurosurgical 1B, also have children on ventilators from time to time. The fact that intensive care nursing is so spread around the hospital is a matter of regret to many medical and nursing staff and there are plans to concentrate all intensive care, except cardiac, in one unit in a future stage of hospital rebuilding. Until then 5A will remain the only general paediatric intensive care unit at Great Ormond Street – and one of only two for the London area as a whole.

Nowhere are the pressures greater at Great Ormond Street than 5A. The whole hospital deals with seriously ill children, some of them with incurable conditions. Many wards have to cope with grief and bereavement, but none more so than 5A where the staff are confronted weekly, sometimes daily, with decisions about whether or not to turn off life-support machines. The ethical dilemmas are intense, not only in determining whether or not a child lives at all but also in contemplating what quality of life the child might enjoy if treatment is continued. It is little wonder that senior nursing staff talk about a 'burn-out syndrome' affecting nurses on 5A. And yet it is a happy and cohesive team. 'There is always a sense of failure if a child dies,' says charge nurse Kevin Purvis. 'But it is very rewarding to have helped support a child and you have the knowledge that you've done everything possible to keep them alive.'

Keeping them alive is the first priority. Often the staff will not know the cause of the illness which has brought a child to 5A; while investigations continue, the patient must be helped to weather the crisis. So it was with Gus. He arrived on 5A at eleven o'clock at night from 1C, the neurology ward, complaining of severe pain in his neck and legs; he was also having increasing difficulty in moving his arms and legs. He was classified by the 5A staff as grade 4 severity, the worst of their four admission grades: 'unstable patient needing intensive nursing and frequent adjustment of their treatment.' Gus was thirteen years old and only the day before he had been at school near Watford. Now his anxious mother feared he was going to die.

Augusto Grieco is the only son of Italian parents who met and married in England. His mother, Filippina, was then in her early forties and his father, Rocco, in his mid-fifties. In the best Italian tradition Filippina, a short, intense and dark-haired woman, was the dominant voice in running the home and bringing up the family. She had arrived in England from Sicily in 1957 in search of work and found it, among other places, at a hairdresser's in Finchley and a shop at the American air-base in Ruislip. After she married Rocco, an assembly-line worker, they settled in Watford which is where Augusto was born on 3 September 1971. Three months later he was back at Watford General Hospital because of 'failure to thrive'. The problem was diagnosed as thalassaemia major, an abnormal form of haemoglobin in the blood which causes severe anaemia. Both parents were found to be carriers of the disease – which is quite common in Mediterranean countries, especially Italy and Greece – so they decided to have no more children. For Gus, it meant blood transfusions and check-ups throughout his life.

Two days before his first birthday Gus was in hospital again, this time with a fever which turned out to be caused by meningitis, inflammation of the membranes of the brain or spinal cord. It is a serious condition, often causing severe neck pain, and the Watford Hospital referred him to Great Ormond Street. Penicillin treatment eventually caused the fever to subside and Gus suffered no recurrence of this illness. He would not be so lucky when he returned to Great Ormond Street almost thirteen years later. Until then, despite worries about his thalassaemia, he lived a normal life, doing respectably well at school and enjoying playing games such as football with his friends, although by secondary school he was finding this very tiring. He was slightly short for his age, and somewhat anaemic, but beyond that there was nothing to make him appear different to anyone else at school. When the problems began, they did so with startling suddenness.

'One day he woke up in the morning and said he had got pain in his back,' says Filippina Grieco. 'I thought perhaps he had slept in a funny way or something but anyway he went to school as usual. At ten o'clock the telephone rang and he said "Mummy, come and fetch me because I don't feel well". I took a taxi because we do not have a car and brought him home. But he said the pain was getting worse and so I called the local hospital. They sent a nurse with a car because the pain made it difficult for him to walk. By now he was saying the pain was terrible and then he said "I can't feel anything in my leg". He went to Watford General Hospital and they did some tests and then he was transferred that evening to Great Ormond Street.'

Gus was admitted initially to ward 1C, because at that stage he had no difficulty in breathing. The neurology team, headed by consultant Dr John Wilson, sought to establish whether a problem with the nervous system was causing the loss of movement and sensation in the limbs. Within two hours of arriving at the hospital he was taken to the operating theatre for a myelogram, an X-ray done under anaesthetic which can show damage to the spinal cord. At one point it appeared to be inflamed. During the next day his condition worsened. His pulse rate and temperature were high and he was often writhing in pain. He was losing sensation in his legs, unable to tell which one was being touched and finding it increasingly difficult to sit up or move. His hands were also becoming numb so the doctors began to worry about something they called 'ascending paralysis'. Other tests had been done, including a CT scan, but no condition had been diagnosed. Yet it was clearly sufficiently serious to warrant intensive nursing and so, at eleven p.m., one day after his arrival at Great Ormond Street, Augusto Grieco was transferred to 5A.

Roughly one-third of 5A admissions come from elsewhere in the hospital. They may be children from the oncology ward or children experiencing difficulties after surgery. They may be patients in acute renal failure or, like Gus, suffering from neurological problems. Dr Wilson, the neurology consultant, would continue to be involved in Gus's care, just as other consultants retain a role when their patients are transferred to 5A; at least one other medical team is involved in four out of every five cases handled by 5A. But the prime responsibility now rested with Dr Duncan Matthew, Dr Bob Dinwiddie and Dr Peter Helms, the three consultants in charge of the intensive care unit.

The unit was established in 1977, thanks to the generosity of the Variety Club which funded most of the building alterations necessary to house the high-tech equipment required for intensive care nursing. Britain lags behind the United States and several other European countries in providing such paediatric intensive care facilities and there are times when children have to be refused admission: the ward's nine beds may all be occupied or, as is more often the case, there may be too little money to employ sufficient nurses with paediatric intensive care training to provide the one-to-one, round-the-clock nursing which is an essential feature of intensive care. In such cases, children have to be sent to adult intensive care units where staff will lack paediatric knowledge. This matters because, as people at Great Ormond Street constantly stress, children are different. Their metabolism, physiology and pathology all differ from those of adults. 'All the things which make children different become all the more crucial the more critically ill a child is,' says Duncan Matthew, the unit's senior consultant. 'The different fluid requirement for a one-year-old, five-year-old and twenty-year-old, for instance, will be vital in intensive care. And the diseases which children get are different.'

Nobody knew what disease was afflicting Gus when he arrived at 5A; what they did know was that it was getting worse. As the paralysis ascended it was becoming increasingly difficult for him to breathe or to cough. 'The priorities were to manage the breathing until we found out what was causing the problems and to protect the chest from infections and inhaled secretions,' says Dr Bob Dinwiddie. Thus, one hour after arriving at 5A, Gus was attached to a ventilator. Only a proportion of 5A patients have something wrong with their lungs, but because they tend to have difficulty in breathing as a result of their other problems, virtually all the patients are put on ventilators. Getting them off the machines is often trickier.

Outwardly, Lewis Pate had had an even more turbulent life before he, like Gus, arrived at 5A and found himself attached to a ventilator. He was then one day short of his second birthday. Yet he had already been in and out of hospital several times, including the intensive care ward of an adult hospital. His troubles began with a road traffic accident when he was four months old. He had been flung out of his carry-cot, severely injuring his head. The injury did not heal as well as expected and it was not helped when he fell out of a hospital cot a year later when his head injury was receiving further treatment. This left Lewis with a thin and fragmented skull on the right side of the head. He had to wear a safety helmet to protect his head from further injury and a device known as a 'shunt' was inserted to drain excess fluid from his brain. More ambitious surgery would attempt to repair the skull when Lewis was older, but meanwhile there was one little operation to remove a cyst called a hydrocele from the scrotum. It should have been routine. Yet it started the process which first brought Lewis Pate to Great Ormond Street.

Ironically, the operation could have been done at Great Ormond Street, but to avoid delays it was done elsewhere. His mother, Jackie, says Lewis had a slightly high temperature before the operation and afterwards he remained feverish with some vomiting and diarrhoea. This was put down to gastro-enteritis which Jackie Pate says she was told could be treated just as well at home with standard medicines. When she got home, she called a local GP because Lewis's temperature was now over 40 degrees Celsius (or 104 degrees Fahrenheit). Again gastro-enteritis was diagnosed and Lewis spent the best part of two days living naked in the living room with his mother setting an alarm so she could check his temperature every hour.

Jackie Pate was not an inexperienced or immature mother. She was then in her mid-thirties with a fourteen-year-old daughter, Debbie, from a previous marriage. She lived with her husband, Malcolm, in a council house in Staines, west of London. They all escaped serious injury in the car accident which first put Lewis in hospital; since then his various scrapes with hospitals had left them wary of believing that everything would automatically turn out all right in the end. So when Lewis's temperature did not subside she called out another GP. 'Lewis was getting very restless and he couldn't settle or even fall asleep. His temperature was still over forty but his arms and legs were absolutely frozen. By late afternoon on the second day his arms and legs were going blue. He was thirsty but couldn't seem to drink anything. I had to syringe drinks into his mouth. The other GP said it was probably gastroenteritis but to play safe we'll take him to our local hospital at Ashford.'

Lewis was kept in hospital for observation which by four-thirty the next morning had become anything but routine. His breathing was becoming laboured and his skin was a mottled red colour; although his temperature remained over forty degrees, his limbs were getting colder.

Doctors were summoned and quickly recognized the symptoms as those of collapse and shock. He was transfused with blood plasma while the Ashford doctors contacted Great Ormond Street: Lewis was to be an emergency admission to 5A. Jackie Pate, who had stayed with Lewis at Ashford, had already phoned her husband to tell him that something was wrong. Only when she began the road journey through the morning rush hour traffic to London did Jackie begin to realize the seriousness of her son's condition.

'They got a police escort for us and I've never been so frightened in my life as by that drive. The way they were driving, I never thought we'd get there. It was like something out of *The Sweeney*. A lady doctor and a nurse came with us. Lewis was lying there and every now and again he'd open his eyes and he didn't look too bad. They hadn't told me what was wrong with him and I was assuming that perhaps it was something to do with his head. Because we had a police escort I thought perhaps he's a bit more ill than I thought, but I still didn't think he was near to death's door. Seriously ill and nearly dying, to me, are two different things so I never thought that we might not make Great Ormond Street. But when we got to the hospital there was a nurse standing on the steps actually waiting for us. Before I knew where we were, Lewis was in a lift and being wheeled straight through a door saying intensive care.'

Jackie Pate found herself, like Filippina and Rocco Grieco a few months earlier, ushered into a tiny, smoke-filled waiting room to be given a cup of tea and asked to wait. Normally parents are encouraged to spend as much time as possible with their children – in 5A as in every ward of the hospital. But when children are first admitted to intensive care it is a time of great activity in a very small space. As many as three doctors and two nurses will be crowded around a tiny cot, setting up lines to infuse drugs or blood – or both. And in Lewis Pate's hour of crisis, there was no time to lose. 'He reached us just alive,' said one doctor. 'He was virtually dead.' In his case, unlike that of Gus, the doctors had a fair suspicion of what the illness was – a rare condition called toxic shock syndrome. Duncan Matthew was one of the authors of an article about toxic shock which had recently appeared in a medical journal, but he had never seen anyone so acutely ill from this condition as Lewis was and as he became.

Whatever 'shock' may mean to a layman, to a physician it is a precise, clinical condition, as Dr Matthew explains: 'In a shocked state the circulation of blood is inadequate for one reason or another. The heart rate is also high as the heart tries to compensate for the system not working well. If the circulation is not working well, this may show itself in the blood pressure being very low or by only having reasonable circulation to the body's most vital areas. The system maintains circulation to these areas by shutting down the blood supply to peripheral areas with the heart and brain being the last to be shut down.'

Toxic shock has only been recognized as a distinct syndrome in the 1980s. It occurs when a particular infection has produced not only the features of shock described by Dr Matthew but also skin rashes, conjunctivitis and ulceration of the mouth. The shock is often severe enough to damage other organs such as the kidneys or the brain. It seems likely that Lewis got toxic shock after he developed a wound infection following his minor operation on the scrotum just four days before his admission to Great Ormond Street. This infection released toxins (or poisons) into the blood which produced severe side-effects and caused him to collapse. The shock, the blotchy skin, the poor circulation and the immediate medical history immediately made the 5A doctors suspect that Lewis was suffering from toxic shock; it would only have been their sixth such case but this is more than any other children's hospital in Britain. 'When Lewis arrived here he was very cold and very shocked. He was conscious but drowsy and miserable, a consequence of low blood pressure because the brain is deprived of blood. We had to try to stabilize the situation and resuscitate him,' says Dr Matthew.

The first forty-eight hours would be crucial – for Lewis, for Gus, for almost every child admitted to 5A. One-third of children only stay on the ward for forty-eight hours but of these one in three die. This high mortality rate increases the pressures on doctors and nursing staff because there is little time to establish a relationship with distraught parents which may help to support them through a bereavement. Often parents find it hard to accept that their child is critically ill at all, especially if the collapse has been sudden and unexpected.

In these first hours the differences between children's illnesses do not always affect the course of treatment, even if the doctors have a working diagnosis as they did with Lewis. For in the most acute stages of illness, many different diseases share what is sometimes known as a 'final common pathway'; there are many ways of being ill, but a more limited number of ways to die. Whatever the original cause of an illness, or its symptoms, its final stages are likely to produce one or more of a handful of conditions. Of these the most common are failures of breathing, kidneys, heart, metabolism and blood circulation.

'What we have to do is to take over as much of the body's functioning as possible to try to prevent any further collapse and to revive the system that is failing,' says Dr Matthew. How the intensive care unit shores up the system will depend upon the precise form of the collapse, but there are certain similarities, as Gus and Lewis found. Or, rather, as their parents found since the patients most at risk are invariably heavily sedated to relieve pain and anxiety and often given paralysing drugs to facilitate artificial ventilation. When the Griecos and Pates were summoned from the waiting room to see their sons something of a shock awaited them, even after all that they had been told to expect by the staff: both boys were attached to ventilators with wires and tubes leading from their bodies to a battery of monitors.

Gus and Lewis were nursed in cubicles approximately fifteen feet long by eight feet wide. Although there were significant differences in what the machines were doing, these would not have been immediately apparent to anyone without medical knowledge. Malcolm Pate and the Griecos were among the parents who did not want to know what the various machines were doing; Jackie Pate, in time, would ask what the flickering needles, fluctuating figures and oscillating green graphs all meant. But at first it all seemed too overwhelming, too baffling and too unreal to grasp. The apparent impersonality of intensive care was heightened by the featureless all-white uniforms worn by most of the staff. These uniforms (or the surgical greens worn in operating theatres) are changed daily to minimize the risk of infection with only red or blue epaulettes to signify respectively a staff nurse or sister. Few nurses wear name badges and although nurses always introduce themselves to parents, it inevitably takes time to get to know the individuals. And time is what parents in intensive care do not always have.

Gus faced his crisis five months before Lewis. The fact that it was the middle of the night made little difference: 5A has the same number of nurses by night as by day and the duty doctors get little sleep. 'The priorities were to manage his breathing until we found out what was causing the problem and to protect his chest against secretions,' says Dr Bob Dinwiddie. The increasing inability to cough meant there was a danger of saliva and secretions from the mouth causing chest infections. Stomach secretions may also regurgitate and cause problems; a tube was therefore passed through Gus's nose into the stomach so the nurses could suck out any secretions. Later that day another tube would be passed down his nose into his small intestine through which he could be fed. With plasters holding these in place, and the ventilator tube, there wasn't much you could see of his face.

The ventilator could be adjusted to vary the proportion of oxygen, the number of breaths and the pressure of air delivered into the lungs. Dials on the ventilator showed these figures while another machine registered the oxygen and carbon dioxide in the blood stream. The accuracy of these readings was checked regularly by analysing blood taken via a line into an artery of the right wrist. This arterial line, kept open by a gentle flush of an anti-coagulant solution suspended on a drip stand, also measured blood pressure. Another intravenous line enabled Gus to receive regular blood transfusions for his thalassaemia. There was a third 'peripheral' line which would be used to infuse drugs, intravenous nutrition or blood. Finally, a catheter was inserted to allow the collection of his urine and electrodes placed on his chest to give a reading of his heart-rate. It is a daunting list, yet Lewis Pate was to have an even greater array of lines.

There was always a nurse with Gus. Although the high-tech equipment is often the dominant impression of intensive care, one-to-one nursing – known as 'specialling' – is another characteristic. So, too, is a greater preponderance of senior nursing staff. There are five sisters including one charge nurse, the male equivalent of a sister; they are headed by Kay Blacker, the senior sister, and at least one is always on duty. The extra training required for paediatric intensive care work tends to mean that staff nurses may be slightly more mature than many on other wards. Finding sufficient numbers of appropriately trained staff is a perpetual problem for the hospital; intensive care work requires (and evokes) great commitment, but the pressure also produces a regular high turnover among nursing staff.

The atmosphere is invariably tense as parents react nervously to every bleep of the machines. So much activity, yet so little noise beyond the hum of machinery. There might be a television in the open ward and a nurse may play a radio for background music, but you rarely hear a child cry, let alone see one moving about, because most are sedated and intubated. There is no clatter of plates as meals are served because most patients are too ill for anything but intravenous feeding. More than most hospital wards, intensive care becomes a world apart where, day and night, staff wage ceaseless battles to keep life going.

The machinery dominates first impressions of intensive care. The staff try to soften its impact by covering walls and ceilings with drawings of animals, rainbows or cartoon characters. They also use hand-made crochet blankets to provide some individuality to each tiny bed or cot. Visually these small gestures symbolize a more important fact: that no amount of high-tech equipment can take away the need for skilled and sensitive nursing. Many patients are sedated and paralysed by drugs so the nurse cannot expect any verbal indications of distress; it is up to her (or *him* – 5A attracts more male nurses than any other ward at Great Ormond Street) to observe and anticipate the patient's needs. For instance, children have faster heart and breathing rates yet lower blood pressure than adults: nurses need to watch for changes which may be small statistically but significant medically.

'An intensive care nurse must be able to respond to things that are going wrong with their patient more quickly than an ordinary nurse on a general ward,' says Duncan Matthew. 'They are trained to understand a child's condition and to anticipate the problems which are likely to occur.' To nurses like Kay Blacker and Kevin Purvis this is part of the attraction of 5A. 'People like it because they work more closely with the patient and because they have to work more on their own initiative. You need a thorough knowledge of basic physiology and anatomy, but personality matters a lot. You have got to be an adrenalin freak,' says Kevin Purvis.

Certainly a nurse does more, much more, than sit and watch the machines. Detailed observations of temperature, pulse and breathing must be made or recorded, usually every half-hour; there is suction to be done, drugs to be changed, food to be syringed into tubes, urine to be checked. Paralysing patients helps to keep them stable but immobility can cause bed sores so nurses often have to move patients to different positions every hour or so; the mouth and eyes also need regular care to avoid sores or infection. Many patients require neurological observations which involve seeing how (or whether) the eyes react to light or the limbs to various stimuli. This was particularly important with Gus as he began his first full day on 5A. One other problem for the staff was that Gus, at thirteen, was old enough to appreciate the seriousness of his condition; they had to cope with his fears as well as those of his parents.

Once on the ventilator his breathing soon stabilized, but the paralysis seemed worse. He could not shrug his shoulders and was unable to move his legs or arms. A physiotherapist flexed his limbs regularly, partly in the hope of restoring movement but also to ensure that they did not get stuck in awkward positions. What should have been painful jabs on the feet now produced no reaction from Gus at all. Yet despite pain-killing drugs, he still experienced some discomfort in his legs and back. Three days after being admitted to 5A his pulse rate dropped to below fifty, occasionally as low as forty-five. This alarmed his parents who feared that one day he might not recover. The doctors were also concerned about where the paralysis might stop; if it rose above his neck and into the brain stem, he would die.

The myelogram – a special X-ray of the spine – performed shortly after he had arrived from Watford showed inflammation of the spinal cord. A week later a Nuclear Magnetic Resonance scan (a computerized non-radiation body scan performed at the National Hospital next door*) also showed an enlarged cord. So what was causing the inflammation? One possibility was that an antibody had created an immunological disturbance. Another 5A patient recently presented similar symptoms and had responded to prolonged treatment recovering the use of all his limbs. Such treatment would involve the use of steroid drugs and plasma exchange, but it would not be quick. During this time Gus would continue to need ventilation and so, it was decided, he should have a tracheostomy – an opening directly into the trachea or windpipe which could be connected to the ventilator. This would avoid the damage which can be caused by the prolonged insertion of a tube in the trachea; it would also enable Gus to move his head more freely and talk more easily. The tracheostomy would only be done when his condition was stable; his breathing remained fine, but the incidence of low pulse rate – bradycardia – was getting worse.

One week after admission, his pulse rate dropped twice during the night; on each occasion he appeared to become unconscious. The first time he recovered spontaneously, but after observing the second episode at two a.m. a doctor pre-

---

*At that time Great Ormond Street did not have its own NMR scanner. One was later acquired thanks to a private donation of £1.5 million to the hospital from overseas.

scribed a drug to aid the recovery. It happened again at seven-thirty and, although this time Gus remained conscious, his parents were now extremely frightened and needed constant reassurance about his condition. The first two incidents occurred after a nurse had sucked secretions from his tracheal tube and for the time being the nurses decided to ask his parents to leave the cubicle while this was being done. The staff tried a number of ploys to reduce the risk of a recurrence; a drug was infused during suction, his breathing was done by hand and the suction itself was speeded up. These prevented any further loss of consciousness, but the episodes continued on and off for another week. What finally appeared to solve the problem was the decision to switch the ventilator to one hundred per cent oxygen immediately prior to suction. With his breathing and heart-rate stabilized the way lay clear for the tracheostomy.

Two weeks had passed since Gus arrived on 5A. He remained dependent upon the ventilator but at least the tracheostomy would enable him to eat normally and so lead to the removal of the line into his foot. After the 'trachy' was inserted, a nurse noted: 'Gus has been very alert. He has been smiling and cheerful, looking forward to a cup of tea and tomato soup tomorrow, if possible.' His parents were also relieved that the bradycardia seemed to be under control. The first phase of 5A's care for Gus was over: they had kept him alive and the paralysis had halted at the neck. Five months later Lewis Pate presented a more difficult short-term challenge.

Lewis had many of the same lines into his body as Gus, although it always looks worse to see so many leading from such a small child. There was an arterial line in his right arm to indicate blood pressure and from which blood could be taken; a peripheral line through which blood or drugs could be infused; a line into his neck to give a constant reading of central venous pressure; a catheter for his urine; a rectal thermometer to give central bodily temperature; a naso-gastric tube through which secretions can be removed from the stomach; electrodes on the chest to register heart-rate; and a heated electrode on the skin which measured blood oxygen levels.

Lewis was extremely ill. His central temperature was over forty degrees, yet the peripheral temperature of limbs ranged from 28.4 to 34.1 Celsius – a difference of two or three degrees would be normal. But you needed neither a thermometer nor a medical training to know that something was seriously wrong. The tips of his fingers and toes were extremely blue and felt cold. So did his ears. The blood circulation was clearly very poor, a fact confirmed by low blood pressure. His heart, trying to compensate for the low pressure by pumping extra hard, was beating more than 200 times a minute – for a child of Lewis's age ninety to 140 would have been normal. He was also drowsy, his eyes reacting only slowly to light. And in addition to these symptoms of shock, there were the peculiar features associated with toxic shock: blotchy, red or purple skin on his chest, arms and legs. A battery of tests was instigated – twelve were listed in the first day's nursing notes – but none of these delayed the commencement of treatment. With Lewis's condition, there was no time to lose.

'The other hospital had quite correctly started his resuscitation by giving him blood plasma,' says Dr Duncan Matthew. 'In a state of hypovolaemic shock you are unable to keep up the blood pressure and so we had to restore the blood volume by giving either blood or plasma. Usually you give plasma because it doesn't need cross-matching. Lewis had very poor circulation and bleeding into the skin had produced a purpuric rash. We had to try and stabilize this situation and continue the resuscitation. We started to do this by replacing fluids on a massive scale and by taking over the ventilation to make sure he was getting enough oxygen. You need your circulation to be adequate to take the oxygen around the body.'

The plasma was infused into a vein on the left side of his neck. In the twenty-four hours Lewis received 1400 millilitres (2.5 pints), roughly ten times the normal dose based on body weight. Between plasma transfusions, the same line infused drugs which would dilate or open up the blood vessels in the peripheral areas of the body. Dr Matthew explains: 'By restoring blood volume we allow the heart to work more efficiently at a slower rate. By opening up the arterial blood vessels we help the heart because it is not pumping against narrow vessels.' Dr Matthew was anxious to do more than simply take the strain off the heart, vital though that was; he had to restore circulation to the cold extremities for without blood they would die.

At first Lewis got worse, not better. Not only was his heart-rate staying above 200, often with an irregular racing beat, but his breathing was becoming more laboured. The toxins in his system had reduced blood volume but increased the passage of fluid into his bowels. Ultimately this would be excreted as watery diarrhoea but meanwhile the abdomen was swollen, causing it to push against the diaphragm muscle and making it difficult to breathe, even with the ventilator. The oxygen was increased to seventy per cent and the breathing rate from twenty-four to thirty per minute. At the end of his first night his condition was deteriorating and there were unmistakable signs of gangrene on his fingers and toes. As the morning progressed, the oxygen was increased to ninety per cent. It was 26 October, his second birthday, but nobody was celebrating.

During that morning Malcom Pate asked Kevin Purvis, the charge nurse, if Lewis was stable enough for him to go home to collect a change of clothing; it had been such a rush yesterday, they'd come without anything and had slept in their day clothes on camp beds in the waiting room. 'Kevin said "No, that's not a good idea. In fact, if any close relatives wish to see Lewis, they should do so as soon as possible",' says Malcolm. He put his head in his hands and broke down.

They had been prepared for the worst since talking to Dr Matthew the night before, but now it seemed appallingly imminent; it would only have taken Malcolm four hours to go home and return to the hospital, yet the charge nurse thought that might be too long! Dr Matthew had said that Lewis's life was on a knife-edge. He and Kevin Purvis talked to both parents again. 'It was then that we realized that our child could die and that he might die at any second,' says Jackie. 'Dr Matthew said they would do all they could, but there might come a time when they could do no more and they might then have to make a joint decision with us about the ventilator being turned off. A lot of what happened would be up to Lewis himself.'

It is ward policy to prepare parents for the possibility of their child's death: if it happens, they should be better able to cope with their grief and if the child survives, the progress will seem all the more welcome. 'Parents have a right to know the truth and we have no right to withhold it,' says Dr Matthew. 'One of our major concerns is preparing parents, when appropriate, for the possibility of death. It is particularly difficult to establish adequate communication with parents to support them and to help them cope with a bereavement should it occur in the first forty-eight hours which is when most deaths occur. It is often very difficult for parents whose child may have been romping around perfectly normally twenty-four hours ago and who then find themselves in an intensive care unit with a doctor saying that their child is dying. It is very hard to explain and very hard for them to accept.'

The initial news is broken by one of the consultants or occasionally by a senior registrar. But they are supported by the senior nursing staff who aim to offer comfort, explanations and a willingness to listen. 'There is nothing passive about listening,' says Derek Bacon, the hospital's Anglican chaplain who says he spends more time on 5A than any other ward at Great Ormond Street. 'To be with people who are sitting waiting while the world caves in around them can be important, if only to stare down the helplessness or accept the anger. It is very delicate. The base line is ordinary human support, presence, attention. There may be other things to do with the chaplain's representative role or a family's expectations, but it depends on them. My job is to help them find that they can meet whatever is bearing down on them, and meet it in the way that is true to them.'

Derek Bacon believes that the 5A staff respond sensitively to human needs, summoning him via his bleep not only when a death is imminent or in response to requests but also when they think he might help people simply by being available to talk or listen. He also attends regularly the 'psycho-social' ward round when staff voice any worries about how families are coping with their children's illnesses. A social worker and psychologist join this weekly discussion and the social worker in particular will frequently spend considerable time with parents. But death is most likely to occur within forty-eight hours of an admission and is confined neither to weekdays nor office hours. This means that nursing and medical staff, supported by the chaplain, bear the brunt of the emotional strain imposed by preparing parents for the death of a child. Nor does the strain end there. If a child does die, the doctors may have to ask parents about a post-mortem and nursing staff, sometimes helped by the parents, will have to prepare the body for transfer to the mortuary. If the death has been anticipated, parents will have been invited to be with their child at the moment of death. Sometimes they cannot face such an ordeal. In these cases, a nurse will hold and cuddle the child: no child is allowed to die alone.

On Lewis Pate's second birthday, the nursing staff were bracing themselves for the trauma of a death on the ward. Jackie and Malcolm had called their parents and other relatives. A chaplain – not Derek Bacon, who was on holiday – came to christen Lewis. Neither Jackie nor Malcolm regard themselves as particularly religious, but Jackie particularly wanted Lewis christened, just in case he didn't make it. 'It was all I could think of, he's got to be christened. My mind went blank, I remember being very upset and I think I did some screaming. Somebody came along, some mother from 5B I think, and practically dragged me down to the chapel and I sat in there for a while. It didn't seem like reality. It didn't seem as though it was happening to my child,' says Jackie.

'I spent as much time as I could with Lewis but I didn't want to get in anyone's way. The most important thing was I wanted them to look after Lewis; I couldn't do anything there at that stage. I was also scared to be in there, to be honest. I was scared that he was going to die in front of me. I don't think I could have taken that. But then I'm not sure whether it was worse sitting in the waiting room and every time you heard the door open, you thought it was someone coming to see us and to tell us. So I used to just pop along and have a look through to make sure that the heart monitors were still going.'

Yet, towards the end of this bleakest of birthdays, he seemed a little better; for the first time the doctors began to think he was as likely to live as to die. But the battle was by no means over. 'We were very concerned that the demarcation lines between healthy tissue and damaged tissue were about mid-forearm and mid-shin. He might lose the whole of his hands and feet,' says Dr Matthew.

Nevertheless Lewis, like Gus, had overcome the first hurdle of admission to 5A. He was still alive and now the ward staff could turn their attentions to tackling the underlying condition. Lewis had taken two days to reach this point, Gus two weeks. Both sets of parents had put aside some of their worries about their sons' long-term outlook by fastening their immediate attention on survival. 'Just let him live,' thought Jackie Pate to herself as Dr Matthew outlined the problems which still awaited Lewis. Like the doctors, the parents tried to deal with one problem at a time. Once the initial crisis was past, they tried to adjust to lives which now revolved around the hospital.

Filippina Grieco had stayed in the hospital ever since Gus had arrived from Watford. So did husband Rocco at first, but then he began to commute there from home each day. He had retired from work and Filippina naturally abandoned her part-time job to be with her son.

For several weeks one of Filippina's sisters, Rena, came to join her in the hospital. They rarely left the ward, arriving before breakfast and rarely leaving before midnight. It was a dogged vigil and the combination of family protectiveness and Latin closeness caused some tension as Gus's stay lengthened. 5A is a ward for acutely-ill children from where most patients depart within a week; the cubicles are too cramped, too claustrophobic and too full of equipment for comfort. The waiting room is also small and, given the nature of 5A, frequently occupied by grieving families – the lack of space and therefore privacy which afflicts the hospital as a whole is rarely more acute than here. Nor was a ward where, on average, one child died each week the best of places for a mentally-alert boy, especially once Gus was stable enough to be moved from a cubicle into the open ward.

Awareness of his surroundings intensified a depression caused by the apparent failure to improve his condition. One month after his admission another myelogram showed that the swelling of the spinal cord had subsided but the cord itself now appeared damaged. Dr John Wilson, the neurology consultant, thought there was still a chance that it could be the reversible 'Guillain-Barre Syndrome' caused by an antibody. As much in hope as expectation, the doctors started Gus on a course of immuno-suppressive drugs and called in the renal team to begin a process called plasma-pharesis. This was carried out by the nurses who staff a kidney dialysis unit which was established, initially, as a result of fund-raising by the TV programme, *Blue Peter* and the British Kidney Patient Association. In Gus's case, the nurses wheeled their equipment along the corridor to him; it was a familiar journey for the dialysis team since kidney failure is one of the most common problems in any intensive care ward. Plasma-pharesis involves the exchange of plasma which may be flawed – containing a harmful antibody, for instance – for new plasma. It is done via a cell-separator machine. Blood is taken from one vein, then spun in a centrifruge until the red cells are separated from the plasma. The red cells are returned to the body by a line into a second vein simultaneously with fresh plasma being pumped into the vein at precisely the rate of the plasma being removed. It is a delicate business, especially if the child is very young, but at any age the loss of fluid can cause nausea or weakness if it is carried out too quickly. The nurse must therefore monitor the patient's condition continually and adjust the speed of extraction to counter any signs of distress. For Gus, the process usually took about one hour twenty minutes. It didn't trouble him unduly. But it didn't work.

Eight weeks after Gus was admitted Dr Wilson and Dr Dinwiddie were obliged to exclude Guillain-Barre Syndrome as a possible cause of Gus's condition. The diagnosis was confirmed as transverse myelitis: a paralysis caused by damage to the spinal cord. This in turn was almost certainly caused by the result of a neuro-allergic reaction to an infection, probably mycoplasma pneumonia. It meant the paralysis was almost certainly irreversible. Gus would probably never regain the use of anything below the neck and so would remain dependent upon a ventilator for the rest of his life. 'The diagnosis emerged by excluding other things and by his failure to respond to treatment,' says Dr Dinwiddie. One July evening he and Dr Wilson saw the parents to break the news that they had feared and later that evening Bob Dinwiddie told Gus. 'In a sense it seemed a relief to him that he was being told the truth,' says Dr Dinwiddie. 'We could now try and recreate a life for him in his new condition.'

The 5A staff were unaccustomed to coping with the developmental needs of long-stay patients, particularly adolescent ones, but they reacted swiftly to the challenge. The next day they took Gus out of the ward for the first time; he was in a wheel-chair with nurses ventilating him by hand. With the help of such 'hand-bagging' Gus became increasingly mobile during the summer, venturing beyond the local park and shops to the British Museum, Scotland Yard and Covent Garden. Once he had a Chinese meal in Soho. By now Gus had become a firm favourite with the nursing staff. He was sometimes depressed, not surprisingly, but generally he responded well and positively to their attempts to establish a more structured day. Although Gus was physically dependent upon the nurses or his mother for mundane tasks such as eating or washing, he was mentally unimpaired; the staff therefore treated him like the teenager he was and allowed him to make decisions for himself about, say, where he went out or what he had to eat.

Filippina and Rocco Grieco had found it hard to come to terms with the apparent inevitability of their son's condition, clinging to a hope that one day, somehow, he might be able to move again. Filippina was also unhappy when, after two months or so, she and her sister were told that they could no longer occupy beds in the hospital. She continued to visit daily, usually arriving before ten o'clock in the morning and staying late. Rocco, too, visited the hospital each day, sometimes staying quietly by his son's bedside, sometimes sitting in a waiting room and sometimes wandering around the hospital from which it must have seemed there was no escape. The travelling meant a financial drain for a couple living on an old age pension, but their fierce commitment to their son never faltered. Often, though, it was a painful, tearful process. Although they found it hard to look forward rather than back, they were helped by the way Gus himself responded to a policy which one doctor described as 'firmness with warmth'. He still had his bad days, with pain or a temperature or simply depression. But more often he was quite cheerful – 'Gus has been laughing and joking this evening,' reported one nurse in the nursing notes in mid-July. He had learnt how to speak, using the air as it was released from his airway by the ventilator. He enjoyed his trips out of the hospital and nurses liked being assigned to look after him. 'It meant you got out of the hospital,' said one. On 3 September two nurses escorted Gus to his home where he celebrated his fourteenth birthday and later in the autumn he began to visit some of the nurses' homes. He even attended the wedding of Maggie Berridge, one of the staff nurses who frequently looked after him. But the biggest change to his day came with the start of regular lessons from the teachers at the hospital school.

There are twelve teachers at the school, which is funded by the Inner London Education Authority. Their transient school roll can extend from nursery-age infants to teenagers studying for GCE O Levels. Although there is a classroom and a library, most of the teaching takes place on the wards, often on a one-to-one basis. Teachers are assigned to wards which they check daily to see who might be there long enough – and be well enough – to benefit from some school work. If there is a ward which tends to be missed in the daily check, it is likely to be 5A: its children are usually too ill for even the gentlest diversion which might be offered by a teacher. In Gus's case the initiative came from the nursing staff and, in the absence of the nominated 5A teacher, it was answered by Yvonne Hill, the deputy head of the hospital school.

The high-tech ambience of 5A does not present the easiest of teaching environments and initially Gus was too depressed and lethargic to do more than listen to stories read to him by Yvonne Hill. Not surprisingly perhaps, he liked fantasy stories such as the C.S. Lewis books. He perked up even more when Fran Flynn, the music teacher, came to the ward to play her guitar and sing to him. But the introduction of a specially-adapted computer heralded the real breakthrough. Jo Douglas, the ward psychologist, had initiated a project involving another long-stay Great Ormond Street patient with similar disabilities to those of Gus. In this a computer was adapted so that it could be controlled by a wand attached to a headband. By moving the head, the wand can direct a light (or cursor) to different parts of the screen; if the screen displays symbols for the normal keyboard, for instance, the wand can activate the computer programme by directing the cursor to focus on the appropriate keys.

Jo Douglas enlisted the aid of Martina Ryan, a speech therapist who had taught the other child how to use this 'photonic' wand. At first Gus was too preoccupied with his then uncertain medical condition to display much interest; only after the doctors had told him that he was unlikely to improve did his interest quicken. He was worried that moving his head would affect his ventilation, so the physiotherapist began exercises to strengthen his head and neck. It was still quite tiring but as his fears subsided he picked up the new skills for word processing, drawing and music very quickly. Martina Ryan now began to liaise with Yvonne Hill to see how the computer – bought for him along with the special equipment such as the wand through a gift from the Friends of the Hospital – could be incorporated into his school work. The computer offered more than simply a technological advance, important though it was for Gus to express himself. 'It had been hard to get anything out of him about what his interests were,' says Yvonne Hill. 'He didn't respond much at first and if you got a shrug of the shoulders it was something of an achievement. It wasn't surprising that he was overwhelmed by his condition but with the computer he had to respond to make it work and that triggered off a lot of feedback from him.' His burgeoning self-confidence enabled him to overcome initial nerves about having his lessons with other children in one of the two schoolrooms where a portable ventilator was kept for him.

Gus began to attend school every day with proper lessons from specialist teachers in subjects such as Maths, French and English as well as Computer Studies. In the afternoons, when school is optional, he began to paint and would later joke that he seemed able to paint better with his mouth than he had ever been by hand. Whether or not that is true, his paintings formed a centre-piece of the exhibition of schoolwork put on in the school after the autumn half-term. All this time there had been little medical change. Occasional high temperatures and chest infections occurred, for which he needed daily physiotherapy, but entries in the nursing notes now took two or three lines where once there had been a page to describe a single morning or afternoon. Some days Gus would seem sad, although more often the nurses would read: 'Usual good form. Cheerful. No change in condition. Remains stable. All care continues.'

There were days when 5A's medical staff were grateful for such stability. They were concerned about Gus's future, since nobody thought he should stay on an intensive care ward for much longer, but it was sometimes a relief that one patient could be dealt with relatively briefly on the morning ward round. This round can take two or three hours if the ward is full. It involves at least one of the consultants, one registrar and the house officer plus the ward sister. Before each patient is seen there is a twelve-point checklist of topics to be discussed, beginning with respiration and ending with a review of drugs being prescribed. In between the doctors will have covered cardiology, infections, fluid balance and electrolytes, nutrition, haematology, biochemistry, liver function, general investigations and neurology plus what are loosely called social points, in other words how the parents are coping with the problem.

Jackie and Malcolm Pate had faced up to the possibility of their son's death; now they confronted the prospect that he would be crippled, losing both his hands and his legs below the knees. 'I think that was the hardest thing to take,' says Jackie, 'because you suddenly think, My God, if he's going to lose his legs and his hands, is it worth it? That was a terrible moment, when Dr Matthew explained it, but then you start to think about what, in this day and age they can do and then you think, I don't care, just let him live, let him pull through and we'll live with that when it comes. No matter what limbs are missing, he's still my son.' It wasn't easy for Jackie or Malcolm to maintain this positive approach, but they were encouraged to do so by Margaret Street, a social worker whom the 5A nursing staff had asked to talk to them. Medical social workers can often provide practical support in the form of help with travelling or other expenses, but usually equally important is emotional support. As with chaplain Derek Bacon, Margaret Street says it sometimes helps parents to talk to non-medical people. 'My role at first was to let them express their feelings – nursing staff can also do this, they don't always have the time. At first they were in a state of shock and they weren't sure whether Lewis was going to make it. He had had problems before with which they had coped but this was worse. Once it became likely that he was going to survive, their anxieties became different: if he was going to live, how disabled would he be? It was very frightening for the parents to see his blackened dead fingers. They thought they had lost the Lewis that they knew and their feelings of shock became mixed up with anger. My role was to try and channel this anger in a positive way that would be helpful to Lewis. You have to be very supportive because there is hardly ever smooth upward progress; there are setbacks which have to be coped with.'

The Pates were helped to develop a bullish attitude by some positive signs of progress, notably an improved EEG test. This measures brain activity and, if it shows no activity results, it can be an important factor in deciding whether or not to turn off the ventilator. Altered brain activity can be either the primary problem which has brought a patient to 5A or the consequence of other conditions. 'We are trying to assess recoverability,' says Dr Ann Harden of the EEG department. 'A particular problem on 5A is that even if the children are not unconscious they are given sedation which may make them appear unconscious. But with certain drugs such as barbiturates you will get no trace of brain activity and yet there will be a recovery. So we have to be very wary and you usually need two tests to establish whether any loss in activity is temporary.'

Lewis Pate was given his first EEG test on the day of his admission when, as the doctors put it, his life was on a knife-edge. A technician wheeled a portable electro-encephalogram (EEG) machine to his cubicle and connected about a dozen electrodes to his head. In simple terms, the EEG machine amplifies the electrical impulses in the brain, converts them into traces on a screen and records them on paper. By adjusting a complicated array of switches, the technician can measure differing areas or forms of brain activity. The basic test takes about an hour, longer if it includes more sophisticated techniques to measure the time taken for stimuli evoked by light, sound or small shocks to the limbs to reach the brain. Often the technician will also seek to arouse the patient, but this is not always possible if patients are sedated, as is usually the case on 5A. However, suction through a naso-tracheal tube is an alternative form of 'disturbance' which can show a reaction on the EEG traces – or, at least, the technician hopes it will. Parents do not need much medical knowledge to recognize that flat or straight lines on the EEG screen are a bad sign. Kathryn Feltham is the technician who usually handles EEG tests on 5A; she does so with tact and sympathy although there are times, she admits, when she plays dumb and passes the buck to the doctors who head the EEG department. 'It is when you are not expecting it to be flat and the parents are there, terribly hopeful and looking at it, that I start thinking "Please don't ask me",' she says.

The verdict from Lewis Pate's first EEG showed some changes in brain function, but this could have been the result of heavy sedation. Such alteration as there was, concluded Dr Harden, was 'potentially reversible'. Four days later this judgement was confirmed by a second EEG test which showed improved brain patterns. Despite his brush with death and despite his earlier brain injuries, somehow Lewis was surviving with his mental capacities potentially unimpaired. But his parents' pleasure at this news was muted by their mounting horror at the sight of his hands and feet. 'It took me a while before I could stand there and look at his hands fully,' says Jackie. 'I used to take little peeps now and then to prepare myself.'

The nurses had told them it was a form of gangrene, although Dr Matthew, worried by possible confusion with the gas gangrene of First World War trenches, preferred to use the term necrosis meaning dead tissue. Either way, it made a pretty unpleasant sight. His hands were worse than his feet which were responding better to the efforts to restore blood circulation. The poor circulation to his hands was being hindered further by swollen tissues which were compressing the blood vessels in the hands. To try and reduce this swelling first the orthopaedic specialists and then the plastic surgeons were called to examine Lewis; they sought to improve circulation (and avoid damage to the muscles) by making cuts in his hands to relieve the pressure there. When the dressings were removed the gaping wounds intensified the blotchy redness caused by the initial toxic rash. Worst of all the fingers were turning black and gnarled, twisting into a claw-like formation which Lewis found difficult to move. 'What had happened was that at an early stage in his illness, when the shock was at its worst, the blood supply to his fingers must have been so poor that the tissue died and was now shrivelling up,' says Dr Matthew.

Yet, to Jackie and Malcolm Pate, calling in the plastic surgeons seemed good news: at least it implied that the doctors were looking forward to the future where once many doubted that there would be any future at all. And apart from his hands, Lewis was beginning to look better. Four days after his admission, the slight blackening of his gums was fading and some warmth returning to his arms and legs. As the circulation improved, the initial pessimism about the demarcation line for amputation began to be revised. It now seemed likely he would lose 'only' his fingers and perhaps his toes.

This progress was matched by other signs of improvement. Kidney problems often develop as a consequence of the poor circulation induced by toxic shock and there were early indications that this was happening with Lewis; but a diuretic drug increased urine flow and as the circulation improved, so did the kidneys. The heart-rate, once over 200, was down to between 110 and 150 five days after admission. Excess fluid was aspirated from his stomach, reducing the swelling and easing the breathing so that six days after admission he was able to come off the ventilator. He breathed through an oxygen mask for a while, but had no difficulty adjusting to the change and gradually the proportion of oxygen was reduced. Lewis remained on intravenous drugs to improve the circulation to the extremities, but by the end of his first week on 5A Dr Matthew felt 'he was becoming less an intensive care worry and more a question of long-term rehabilitation'.

There was considerable satisfaction over Lewis, just as there always is when a patient recovers against the odds. Such success is a welcome fillip to morale, especially for a team braced to cope with death and especially as the work is physically as well as emotionally demanding. Dr Helen Price, a registrar on a year's exchange at Great Ormond Street from the Children's Hospital of Philadelphia, was struck by the lower number of doctors attached to 5A compared to an equivalent unit back home in the United States. Also, she says, the larger catchment area of Great Ormond Street meant that conditions here tended to be more serious with a higher incidence of mortality. Although the consultants regularly work long hours late into the night, the short-term nature of 5A's case-load means that the immediate responsibility frequently falls upon the duty registrar assisted by the houseman and the sister.

To Duncan Matthew an adequate level of middle-grade medical staffing is therefore fundamental to the work of an intensive care unit. Yet the staffing levels which struck Helen Price as low would be even worse if what is known as 'soft money' – charitable grants – was not used to supplement the two registrars whose salaries are paid by the National Health Service. Doctors hired primarily to conduct research in the hospital's respiratory unit are required to help out on the ward so that each registrar (and researcher) works one night and one weekend in five. Dr Matthew says: 'You cannot expect people to work these long days without breaks and so, from a medical point of view, we are utterly dependent upon soft money to make it work. Trying to run the unit with two registrars would be hopeless. When the registrar is on for the night he or she is often up for the whole night and is also on for the preceding day and the following day.'

The clinical work itself is taxing enough, as the check-list of twelve points to be considered in the ward round indicates. Often the registrars will have to make decisions quickly if lives are to be saved, yet few of them will have worked in a general paediatric intensive care unit before; that is why they are here – to broaden their experience – and in the British tradition they will learn largely through experience. Then there is the emotional strain of dealing with parents whose children may be dying. Here they sometimes turn to psychologist Jo Douglas for advice but generally, she says, they cope perfectly adequately. She says: 'They may be seeking reassurance that they have handled something properly or they may simply need someone with whom they can discuss their own feelings.' The consultants are well aware of the strains to which their junior staff are subjected. 'They have to work for many hours at a stretch and keep calm under stress and constant pressure,' says consultant Bob Dinwiddie. 'That's why we work as a team so we can share the burden.'

Among the 5A doctors this means that there is no division between one consultant's patients and the other's. (Nor is team spirit harmed by the practice of the consultants directing any fees for private patients into ward funds.) But it is the complexity of so many 5A cases – two out of five cases involve at least four different medical teams – which also makes teamwork essential, even if it renders diplomacy almost as valuable as physical robustness in prospective registrars. Anaesthetists are probably the specialists most closely and frequently involved, although they do not see themselves as outsiders. In the past the anaesthetists have played a greater role in the hospital's other intensive care wards than on 5A, but they have increased their commitment to ward duty so that their expertise can be provided in terms of general patient management and not simply in the technicalities of ventilation. At least one consultant anaesthetist is now on ward duty every weekday and conducts a daily ward round of all patients on ventilators.

The nursing staff, too, believe that close teamwork enables them to cope with the pressures of work. They have changed to a twelve-hour shift pattern which provides greater continuity of care, sometimes with two sisters on duty per shift, and more time off. But teamwork is not confined to camaraderie among doctors or nurses. The spirit of mutual support within the unit is almost tangible and goes deeper than the use of first names for everyone including the consultants, though this perhaps has certain symbolic value; more fundamentally, there is a recognition that skills are inter-dependent within an intensive care unit and that teamwork must embrace all these diverse skills. Duncan Matthew says: 'The first lecture which senior house

officers get is that although they are experienced paediatricians, they are not experienced in intensive care and that
they will learn as much from the nursing staff on the unit as
they do from us. We used to make them do a nursing shift so
that doctors would recognize what it involved to do such a
nursing duty.'

The short-term crisis of Lewis Pate may have passed, for
instance, but not for a week or so would he be well enough to
be transferred to the plastic surgery ward. By most normal
standards Lewis still needed intensive nursing. There were
lines into veins or arteries for intravenous drugs, feeding and
blood transfusions; he still had a catheter collecting his urine
and a naso-gastric tube through which secretions were sucked
from his stomach. Although the ventilator had gone, monitors
still recorded his heart-beat, blood pressure and temperature.
After his two minor operations to relieve the swelling in his
hands, Lewis was in considerable pain and had to be given
morphine and other pain-killers. Observations continued to be
made every half-hour and he had to be moved every two or
four hours to avoid pressure sores. Three times a day the
physio would gingerly move his hands and feet, usually giving
Lewis aspirin to ease the discomfort. Pressure bandages on his
hands had to be reapplied each nursing shift. Even for 5A it
was undemanding only in the sense that his survival was no
longer in doubt.

Jackie and Malcolm Pate were amazed by the attention to
detail displayed by the nurses. 'They were talking to the
children all the time, even though they are out for the count.
When they turn them over, it's "OK Lewis, I'm going to turn
you over" or "I'm just going to wash your mouth". At first I
wondered what the hell are they doing that for, but then they
explained that the children can hear you even when sedated,'
says Jackie. She found this somewhat unnerving and was frustrated by her inability to hold her child because of the various
lines and wires. But from the very beginning she and Malcolm
had been encouraged to help in Lewis's daily care.

'You try to offer parents something positive from the awful
experience,' says Dr Charlotte Daman-Willems, one of 5A's
registrars. 'You let them be involved in their child's care –

changing nappies, washing them and so on – so that they don't feel they have let their child down.' Parents are encouraged to become part of the team caring for their child and once the initial shock of being on 5A at all is overcome they can also be very effective in supporting more recent arrivals to the ward. Jackie and Malcolm Pate were both helped by other parents – Malcolm was moved (and surprised) when an Indian lady, whose son had just died, said she would pray for Lewis – and in the weeks ahead they would console and support others.

After a week Lewis was well enough for Malcolm to return to his job as a driver, leaving Jackie staying on in the hospital. By then she had been given a room in which to sleep but, although it was more comfortable than the camp bed in the waiting room, it was some time before she felt able to relax. 'In intensive care you are so strung up, you're on edge all the time for fear that something was going to happen at that particular second,' says Jackie. 'It's impossible to put into words your gut feelings as you sit waiting all the time for bad news.' Even when the news began to improve, she found that progress was not always achieved without some anguish; for as the sedation was reduced, Lewis became conscious for the first time. 'I was sitting with him one day, talking to him, when his eyes flickered and then he opened them. I looked at him and said "Mummy's here" and this tear started rolling down the side of his face. To see that tear was the breaking-down time. It was a feeling of relief and I just wanted to scoop him up. But you can't, so I just leant forward and kissed him, stroked him and said "Mummy's here".'

Lewis stayed on 5A for sixteen days. It was a fortnight of waiting – waiting to see if he would live at all, waiting to see whether his hands or legs could be saved from amputation, waiting to see if he could breathe without the ventilator, waiting to see if he could begin to eat after a week or more of intravenous feeding, waiting for the various tubes or lines to be removed. There were days (and nights) when he was restless and in considerable pain. His hands and feet were elevated which, although it combatted the swelling, did little for his overall comfort. Nor did the half-hourly observations, two-hourly mouth care and four-hourly turning which persisted for most of his stay on 5A. Frequent doses of morphine staunched the tears, if not his mother's anxiety. Yet, clinically, he was stable and slowly the tubes and monitors began to disappear from Lewis's cubicle.

Fifteen days after he had arrived he was well enough to be moved from the cubicle to an open section of the ward. Of the many lines or tubes which had been connected to his body, just two remained: one intravenous line to infuse the drug which improves blood pressure and circulation, one naso-gastric tube to supplement oral feeds until he could eat normally. The monitors had gone entirely and Jackie Pate was able, at last, to cuddle her son on her lap. 'Lewis seems much happier and more settled,' wrote a nurse in the daily notes. Jackie knew that the move to the open ward was a good sign, but she retained a nagging worry. 'The moment they come out of the cubicle, you know that they're not one-to-one with a nurse. That's a little bit frightening because you think, what if something happens when a nurse isn't actually watching him. But he did OK and then they decided to transfer him to 3D, the plastic surgery ward – and that's another frightening time.' At first, it appeared that Jackie's fears about the transfer to 3D were well-justified. Within hours of his arrival, he developed a temperature and Dr Charlotte Daman-Willems was summoned to see the patient she had only just transferred. There also appeared to be a minor infection affecting the abdomen where the ill-fated hydrocele repair had been made. After some difficulty finding a vein, Dr Daman-Willems put in an intravenous line through which antibiotics were infused to fight the infection. 'Most of our children are quite well, so to have someone as sick as Lewis was something of a jolt,' says Julie Simester, 3D's sister. 'It reminds you what is going on in the rest of the hospital.'

Lewis continued to pose problems for the staff of 3D for some time, but at least he had made it out of 5A. Augusto Grieco was still there. When Lewis departed for 3D, Gus had been on 5A for nearly six months. The autumn was mostly a happy time with several outings and growing self-confidence at school. But nobody was happy that he had stayed for so long on an intensive care ward. The pitfalls of such an existence were illustrated vividly a month later when, after staying up late one Saturday to watch a horror movie on television, Gus was still awake when another child had a cardiac arrest from which he subsequently died. One of the nurses noted later: 'Gus was fairly upset but realistic when we explained that this was one of the problems of living in intensive care. Tried to be positive and point out that Gus has a lot to live for as he can still use his brain and has no pain or misery; and said some children who die have such a miserable time that they are far better off when no longer in this world. A few tears shed, but then settled quickly to sleep at 02.30 hours.' The next day Gus was back to his customary form. The entries in the nursing notes provide eloquent testimony to his remarkable courage – 'cheerful', 'good form', 'great morning', 'very happy', – but the Saturday night cardiac arrest heightened the staff's concern about the unsuitability of 5A as a long-term 'home'.

In fact, the problem had been exercising the consultants ever since they broke the news to Gus and his parents that he was unlikely to recover from his paralysis. At that time Gus was among sixteen children in the country destined to be dependent upon a ventilator for the rest of their lives. One of them was a five-year-old boy in another ward at Great Ormond Street. In the New Year he would be leaving for a special boarding school in Sussex which provides medical and educational facilities for long-stay children. This school was willing in principle to take Gus, once it had seen how much work the other Great Ormond Street child had required in terms of physiotherapy and technical support. But Sussex was a long way from his parents' home in Watford, so it seemed a poor option for Gus. It was not inconceivable, in theory, for Gus to be nursed at home but his other medical problems and his parents' age made this improbable. So where should Gus live? Great Ormond Street has no facilities for long-stay, chronically sick children and, in any case, travelling to and from Watford was exhausting and expensive for his parents. Could he go back closer to his family and friends in Watford?

Dr Ganesh Supramanian, the consultant paediatrician at Watford General Hospital, was anxious to help but accommodating Gus meant finding more than a bed; he would need sufficient nurses to provide round-the-clock attention. In other words, money was required. Gus's plight had attracted some attention locally, prompting the local Rotary Club to provide transport so Gus could spend occasional days at home – accompanied, of course, by a nurse. He went home on Christmas Day, for instance, and 'had a super day'. A month later Dr Supramanian won a commitment from his hospital's authorities that extra nursing staff would be employed to enable them to look after Gus. When this would be possible, he couldn't say but the responsibility for his long-term care had been accepted; it was just a question of time.

Neither Gus nor his parents were immediately overjoyed by the news. They had grown used to 5A, for all its unsuitability, and trusted the expertise of its staff. Watford would certainly be handier and, they hoped, would enable Gus to renew friendships which had lapsed while he had been in Great Ormond Street. But any change is slightly unnerving when you are so utterly dependent upon machines and nurses to live. Even when Gus moved next door to ward 5B, it caused considerable anxiety at first.

Gus was now doing six subjects at either GCE O Level or CSE: Computer Studies, Maths, French, English, Environmental Studies and Art. He also took lessons in music and science as well as project work with other children. At school he is much more out-going than on the ward, joking and laughing with the teachers and fellow students; here, at least, he can forget his problems for a while and be responsible for his own achievements. Gus feels a particular empathy for others with problems. Once, when a child from the psychiatric unit was being teased gently by other pupils, he said: 'Leave him alone, he's all right.' Gus did particularly well with French and Computer Studies and if a predilection for musical accompaniments to his computer programmes sometimes proved distracting in the classroom, nobody complained. It was good to see him doing so well. 'Our aim is to give Gus goals and to make school life as normal as possible,' says teacher Yvonne Hill. 'We are pushing the computer work because there is some future in it – he could be given work to do and earn a living from it.' Another goal was to complete thirty paintings at which point Yvonne Hill has promised to organize an exhibition of his work; after one and a half terms, he had a dozen which he thought were good enough.

What will happen to his school work when he transfers to Watford, nobody knows. Yet school has symbolized the efforts to create a new life for Gus so somehow the activities must continue; it is another problem for Dr Supramanian to resolve and another obstacle for Gus to overcome. For his parents, the nightmare seemed unending. For them, there wasn't even the satisfaction which Gus could draw from his achievements at school or the pleasure he gains from outings as a VIP guest, say, of Tottenham Hotspur for a soccer match. There are days when his problems get him down and he feels morose or lethargic; there are still days, too, when he feels some pain. He was disappointed – and many of the staff furious – when, after months of waiting, an electric chair finally arrived only to discover that it had not been designed to carry a ventilator! Despite precise specifications being given for the chair six months previously, it was also too heavy for Gus to control by head movements as had been planned. Despite such blows Gus generally displays a fortitude which defies what fate has dealt out to him during his short life and with which, no doubt, he will face the uncertainties that lie ahead.

Lewis Pate, too, faces years of uncertainty. He stayed in hospital just over a month after his transfer from ward 5A, going home for Christmas and then returning for the next stages of his plastic surgery. Both stays were longer than anticipated because surgery was delayed by minor, but persistent, infections. For the first few weeks he was troubled by seepage from the abdominal wound where the hydrocele repair had been undertaken. Given the devastating effect that an infection here had already caused, the last thing Jackie Pate wanted at this stage – at any stage – was another infection; but this is what she, or rather Lewis, got. Jackie's anxiety was not eased by a number of occasions when Lewis unaccountably began to scream, waving his arms and legs in the air, virtually inconsolable for as long as forty-five minutes at a time. The doctors could find no physical cause for these episodes, but the most likely explanation was that Lewis was simply fed up with the discomfort, particularly when the pain was increased by physiotherapy. Certainly, the temper tantrums did not recur after he began to be given pain-killers prior to each session with the physio.

The objective of the frequent and intensive physiotherapy was to keep joints supple and tendons moving. It was part of a general programme of what might loosely be called 'damage limitation'. Barry Jones, one of the hospital's two consultant plastic surgeons, and Oliver Fenton, his senior registrar, had been involved in Lewis's care since the day they were called to his cubicle on 5A five days after his admission. Two days later, after a continuing deterioration in the condition of his hands, they conducted an emergency operation to release the tension or swelling which, they wrote in the medical notes, would otherwise cause the 'disastrous' loss of his hands. Later they added splints to keep his hands in a favourable position, but more ambitious surgery had to wait the resolution of his abdominal wound infection. By the time this had subsided it was almost Christmas and so Lewis was allowed home, returning on 2 January for what the surgeons called 'debridement' and what Malcolm Pate called 'amputation'.

By then Malcolm and Jackie Pate knew that Lewis would lose most of his fingers – one finger-tip had actually dropped off while he was at home over Christmas – but they also knew it could have been much worse. 'The blackness had begun to spread to the tips of his ears so they caught it just in time. If they hadn't worked as hard as they had, he could have been a whole lot worse,' says Jackie. Even when they were first told that his chances of pulling through were better than fifty-fifty, this news had been offset by gloomy speculation about possibly losing his hands and his legs from below the knee. Compared to that, losing only his fingers made them feel almost lucky. And they had already seen how determined Lewis was to overcome his disabilities. When he first moved to 3D, for instance, the staff had great difficulty in getting him to drink. Then, one night, a nurse left him the bottle so he could try and drink himself. Squeezing it between his forearm and chest, he tilted the bottle up and moved his head down. It looked awkward, but it worked; he could drink without assistance and from then on did so. 'I couldn't believe how well he managed,' says Julie Simester.

Kim Cecil, a physiotherapist, encouraged this independent streak and before long Lewis was using his hands to hold cups or pencils. He began to wash his face with a sponge and, by using his thumb web as a wedge, acquired sufficent control to paint and draw. And if he couldn't manage with his hands, he'd find another way, as social worker Margaret Street recalls. 'He is very determined and would pull a toy train around the ward with his teeth,' she says. 'In spite of all that has happened to him, he is a very outward-going child so that people respond positively to him. This was a great help.'

Thus, the grizzly two-year-old hooked up to a drip stand who had arrived on 3D gave way to a lively, outgoing toddler. When he returned after Christmas ward playleader Karen Bell noticed a big change. 'Before he had been very groggy with splints on his hands so he couldn't do much. His feet and legs were very raw. But after Christmas, when he was up and about, he was very active. He loved 'pushing' toys and spent a lot of time in the Wendy house making cups of tea. He was so lively that it is hard to remember Lewis as he had been when he first came to the ward. He was much more sociable and, in fact, he was a lovely boy to have around,' she says. This liveliness is characteristic of the ward as well as Lewis; its children are in hospital for reconstructive surgery, not because they are ill.

The Pate family and the staff of 3D* got to know each other better than they might have expected because, upon returning to hospital after Christmas, Lewis was found to have yet another bacterial infection. It was twenty-five days before surgeon Barry Jones thought he was well enough for the operation. Jackie and Malcolm were not worried about what the surgeons proposed to do; surgically 'debridement' is a simple process which removes dead tissue. But Jackie was worried by the memory of what had happened after another simple opera-

---

*The ward was reorganized after Christmas to include 3C as well as 3D and ear, nose and throat patients as well as plastic surgery.

tion three months earlier, especially as he'd since had so many other infections. Perhaps he would get toxic shock again? The worry had haunted her at Christmas, overshadowing her relief that he was alive at all. She need not have worried. For the first time in his stormy medical history, Lewis Pate had an operation which took less time than had been anticipated. He was soon laughing and smiling, seemingly oblivious to the loss of most of his fingers. A week later he was home. The hands had been saved but they were red and inflamed; it would be at least a year before Barry Jones expected Lewis to be well enough to begin the positive reconstruction of plastic surgery. He would then become one of the first patients, perhaps the first patient, at Great Ormond Street to undergo a 'toe-to-hand transfer'. Toes would be removed together with their blood vessels, nerves and tendons and then joined to these tissues in the hands so that on each hand Lewis had at least one 'finger' and 'thumb'. It is a technically demanding operation and Mr Jones makes no claims about the aesthetic attractions of its results. 'A toe transfer always looks like a toe, but what we are interested in is restoring some strength and function to his hands,' he says. This operation will still not complete Lewis's reconstruction since there remains the problem of his skull injury. Barry Jones, who became a consultant at Great Ormond Street at roughly the same time as Lewis Pate became a patient, believes this operation should wait until Lewis is eight by when the two levels of the cranium can be split and used to complete the repair. Until then, he said, Lewis would have to wear his cycling-style crash helmet and his parents would have to keep their fingers crossed that their accident-prone son avoids any further disasters. This might be easier said than done: just six weeks after he had been discharged, he was back in Great Ormond Street. He was admitted for two days with a suspected blocked shunt (the tube draining excess fluid from his brain). It turned out to be a false alarm, but the incident did nothing for his parents' nerves.

'I can't really believe all this has happened to us,' says Jackie. 'It's the sort of thing you read about or see in a TV documentary. I look at him now, I look at his fingers, and I don't believe this could have all happened to Lewis. And as I sit here looking at him, I think – "God, what next? What is he going to spring on us next?" I'm going to panic now if he cuts himself. What if he starts growing the bug again that caused the toxic shock? I didn't realize something like this could come out of something so simple. It really is frightening and I think I might get paranoid about it if I'm not careful. I'm scared I am going to get paranoid. But at least we've got him. A lot of children didn't make it and I felt for their parents because I know how close we came to losing Lewis. We shall be grateful to those doctors and nurses for the rest of our lives. People don't realize what's involved – the hours, the strain, especially in intensive care – until you see it for yourself.'

The staff of 5A are realistic enough to know that for some parents, the memory will be irrevocably tragic, however diligent or sensitive the unit's care. The staff certainly try hard to support families through a child's death. If necessary, the moment when machines are turned off will be delayed to help parents come to terms with its inevitability. Everything possible is done to give parents some privacy. Machines are moved out of the room, children can be dressed in their own clothes, cuddled by their parents and surrounded by favourite toys. Religious wishes will be respected so that, for instance, a Muslim child will be turned to face Mecca. But the staff worry about the adequacy of their support. It is particularly hard to help families whose children die too soon after their arrival for anyone to know them. They also worry about what happens after families have made their sad, lonely journeys home.

Parents are often offered an appointment six weeks later when they can discuss any points with the consultants. They may want to know more about why their child died and the results of the post-mortem, if performed. Or there could be a question of genetic counselling before they have another child. It is impossible for a unit as busy as 5A which draws children from a large area of southern England to attempt close after-care of its patients – or their bereaved parents. Even less busy wards fear that sometimes families slip through the welfare net with a local hospital and Great Ormond Street each assuming the other is taking responsibility. But Dr Matthew and Dr Dinwiddie have prepared a research project which will tell them how parents feel about their stay on the ward and what more could be done – inside and outside the hospital.

Death will always sadden, and often shock if it is un-expected, but there is more to 5A than bereavement. Most patients live. This record underpins the commitment of the staff and will be strengthened in the future by greater possi-bilities of organ transplantation. Yet whatever new techniques and new technology may bring, the motivation will remain very much that which first inspired Duncan Matthew when he was a registrar in Edinburgh. 'I could see then that there were critically ill children who were not being managed optimally and that to give them every chance, we needed to provide paediatric intensive care facilities in the same way as there were adult intensive care facilities,' he says. Ten years later he would like to know more about how well 5A is doing, not just in coping with the bereaved but in helping the living. 'We should be following up our children in more detail to get a better idea of how treatment has worked and, what is terribly important, what happens to the children afterwards. There is more to life than just surviving. Has it all been worthwhile?' There is no doubt how the parents of Augusto Grieco or Lewis Pate would answer: neither child emerged unscathed from their stay in intensive care, but without 5A they would never have emerged at all.

Postscript: one year later

Gus: his much talked-about move to Watford General Hospital finally happened in August 1986. This made it much easier for his parents to visit him and he was also closer to his old school friends. Gus settled into his new 'home' very well, working hard at his art, computer studies and other subjects with exams looming in 1988. He now has a battery-operated ventilator which makes him more mobile.

Lewis: he has had a good year, very lively and very determined. He faces some minor plastic surgery, but the doctors decided not to attempt the 'toe transfer' which they had once con-sidered. In the long term he faces treatment for his head injury, but for now he is leading a normal life and looking forward to his first family holiday.

2.30 p.m. *David Newton, group treasurer, convenes a meeting of the economy working party. He says the hospital has always been good at saving money 'because we have always wanted to do more than we had money for'. But the need for economies has never been greater and the working party acts as a catalyst for cost-cutting measures throughout the hospital. David Newton reckons they have already saved an average of £200,000 over the last five years and have a target of £500,000 for the next year. 'We have saved an enormous amount of money through greater energy conservation,' he says. In the past such savings have enabled the hospital to bridge the gap between its income and the cost of the services it provides. Yet it is relatively small change set against an annual outlay of around £30 million in the mid-1980s. Nursing costs alone are over £8 million a year. David Newton's financial empire must juggle with figures such as these and engage in delicate and usually protracted negotiations with the Department of Health and Social Security. At the same time it must pay the salaries of more than 2000 people – 'We're like a village or small town,' says Mr Newton – and oversee the budgets of each department and around 250 special funds associated with the hospital. David Newton also prepares the accounts of the Special Trustees, the charitable fund-raising arm of the hospital. Their funds brought in more than £1 million a year in the mid-1980s with contributions ranging from around £200,000 from the royalties to Peter Pan (the copyright was bequeathed to the hospital by J.M. Barrie) to 50p postal orders sent in by old age pensioners.*

2.35 p.m. *Alix bounces into the plastic surgery clinic to see consultant Ivor Broomhead. She is almost five years old and if she's bothered by her haemangioma, a swelling on the right side of her neck, she doesn't show it. The haemangioma is much smaller than when she was born, when it must have been a tremendous shock for her elegant mother. The swelling, which originates from blood vessels, was injected with concentrated saline when she was a baby to reduce the blood supply; this has caused it to shrink gradually over the years. Mr Broomhead shows Alix's mother how he will eventually move the skin upwards and backwards. 'It's in a perfect position for the facelift to disguise the disturbance to the* *skin,' he says. If Alix becomes bothered by the disfiguring swelling when she goes to school, he will contemplate surgery then; otherwise, he says, you get the best results when the haemangioma has shrunk to its maximum possible extent. 'The longer it can be left the better,' says Mr Broomhead. Alix is very outgoing and full of self-confidence. 'I might invite you to my birthday party,' she says brightly to the surgeon before departing.*

Other children who must wait for surgery are some with cleft lips and palates. About 650 children a year are born with this condition and of these roughly a hundred are treated at Great Ormond Street. They will have plastic surgery (and other) treatment at various stages, but the final adjustments may have to wait until growth is complete. It's a busy clinic with two consultants and a senior registrar seeing patients simultaneously. A speech therapist is also on hand to help cleft lip and palate children. So, too, is a cosmetic specialist who teaches parents and children how to disguise birthmarks, skin grafts or other scars. 'So much depends upon the parents as to how children cope,' says Mr Broomhead. One mother tells her child: 'You're jolly lucky. Not everybody can choose the shape of nose they have.'

3.00 p.m. *Chief pharmacist Heather Elliston confers with colleague Anne Pickett about the day's production of Total Parenteral Nutrition (TPN): is production on target to meet the expected demand? TPN is a pharmaceutical form of feeding which is given to children intravenously, with the ingredients as well as the volumes varied to reflect different children's needs. The feeds are made up in a special suite just off one of the hospital's main corridors. Through a small window passers-by can see the pharmacists dressed up a little like spacemen in all-enveloping synthetic suits, masks and gloves preparing the feeds in totally sterile conditions. In addition to working in this pharmaceutical goldfish-bowl, pharmacists provide in-patients and out-patients with drugs including radio-pharmaceuticals. Rare illnesses often require rare drugs and volumes must always be controlled with great care. 'You have to check your doses the whole time because every one is a fractional dose. The actual dose required for one child may be very different to that required for another, unlike adults for whom there are more standard preparations,' says Heather Elliston. The* *annual drug bill for the Hospitals for Sick Children group in the mid-1980s topped £1.6 million.*

3.05 p.m. *Cystic fibrosis is the most common serious genetic disorder in Britain, affecting one in 2000 live births. CF can now be diagnosed with great certainty by measuring the amount of sodium chloride (or salt) in sweat. There is as yet no cure, so once identified, treatment is lifelong to ward off CF's potentially fatal respiratory and dietary effects for as long as possible. Many sufferers now live into their twenties and thirties, but in the afternoon CF clinic the teenagers were visibly more affected by the condition than the younger patients. Sean, at fifteen, was pale and becoming increasingly breathless whereas four-year-old Kieran was full of vigour, reorganizing the furniture so he could drive a toy car around the room at some speed. Jill, aged six, was shortly off to Disneyworld – 'take salt tablets because of the hot weather and eat salty hamburgers, but enjoy yourself,' said Dr Bob Dinwiddie, one of the two respiratory consultants. He examined each patient, looking in their ears, nose and mouth and listening to their chests through a stethoscope. The children also saw physiotherapist Ammani Prasad, since regular physio three times a day to remove secretions from the lungs is part of the recommended treatment. Samples of sputum are taken for laboratory analysis and many patients go off for chest X-rays and lung function (or 'blow') tests. Otherwise Dr Dinwiddie works through a long list of questions about possible symptoms, diet and drugs. CF patients tend to have complicated and extensive drug regimes with antibiotics, pancreatic enzymes, vitamins, nebulizers and sometimes steroids among the daily armoury in their battle against the disease. It's sometimes hard for teenagers to maintain their determination once they know the prognosis is not so good. Yet most – like eighteen-year-old Tariq studying hard for his A Levels – react positively and strive to lead as normal a life as possible. But it is by no means easy. After a TV documentary about CF, one twelve-year-old girl was asked by 'friends' at school: 'When are you going to die?'*

3.15 p.m. *Alf Marshall, the head porter, goes to sort out congestion in the hospital driveway. It also acts as a car park for senior staff and is frequently jammed with cars. Ambulances sometimes* have difficulty squeezing through to reach the entrance for emergency admissions. Once an incubator had to be pushed up the driveway because the ambulance couldn't get beyond the entrance barrier. Ideally, Alf Marshall would like a porter controlling the entrance barrier during the day, but there is not enough staff to spare a man for the job. There are forty-two porters overall sharing duties such as sorting the post, taking children to operating theatres, taking specimens around the sprawling nine-acre site, moving beds and equipment as well as manning the reception desks in the front hall and out-patient department. The friendly service offered by these porters on the reception desks is regarded by the hospital authorities as one of their minor success stories. Minor, yet still important since the porters provide the first impression of the hospital for many visitors.

3.30 p.m. *Hilary suffers from eczema. Millions of people do and for most it's no more than a minor irritation. But for some the itching can be unbearable and produce a disfiguring rash. It is most common among young children; probably one in eight children are affected to some degree. Hilary is fourteen and as she sits talking to Dr David Atherton, the dermatology consultant, she is composed and does not scratch herself once. But when she rolls up her sleeves she reveals large and vicious scratch marks. According to her mother, she scratches herself during her sleep. Dr Atherton suggests a mild sedative to help her sleep more soundly and tries to reassure Hilary that, in time, it will get better. She is depressed because for most people of her age it has already begun to improve and adolescence is a period when individuals become more self-conscious about their appearance. 'Most people are better by now,' Dr Atherton agrees. 'But it does not mean that you are stuck with it. I am sure that it will not go on for ever.' He suggests various ointments and emulsifiers which should help control the condition until it gradually (if belatedly) diminishes of its own accord.*

Several of the patients during the afternoon clinic are eczema sufferers. Often they also have asthma, suffer from allergies or they may be growing more slowly than is normal. John, aged eleven, was in the middle of regular treatment under sun-lamps. He has a somewhat exaggerated tan, which doesn't stop him from scratching during most of his time in the clinic. Despite this, Dr Atherton is pleased by his progress and later recommends it to the parents of Sarah, a twelve-year-old girl who has already appeared on stage as a dancer. 'Light treatment has not been going for long enough to know for certain that there are no snags,' he says, 'but all I can say to you is that if Sarah was my own daughter, I would go for it.'

3.55 p.m. *Laura, a four-year-old West Indian girl, is sent from the plastic surgery clinic to have her photograph taken. Her scalp had been badly burned and the doctors wanted a photographic record of the current state of repair. She goes with her mother to the medical illustration department in the old hospital building. Each year the department takes photographs of some 3000 patients with dermatology, plastics, dental, ophthalmology and orthopaedic departments being the heaviest users of their services. Usually the photographs show only part of the body – an inflamed hand or deformed jaw, for instance – but they have to be taken with great precision so that comparisons can be made of progress over a period of time. Film or video records are also made to show how a child is moving. Medical photography is highly specialized and may use ultra-violet, infra-red or fluorescent techniques. The department also produces booklets for parents explaining forms of treatment plus graphic illustrations and slides for use in textbooks or lectures at the Institute of Child Health.*

Casualty

It was not a good start to the day. Shortly after nine o'clock Joel, a feverish two-month-old boy with bronchiolitis, vomited while being examined by Dr David Goldblatt, the duty casualty officer. Joel was his first patient of the day and quick reflexes avoided too much damage to his clothes. Fourteen hours and twenty-five patients later Dr Goldblatt would leave the casualty department, although not for long: he would remain on call throughout the night and return the next day until around five p.m. – thirty-two hours after Joel had provided such an inauspicious start to his shift.

There is nothing particularly unusual in such shifts for junior hospital doctors, or 'house officers' as they are called; at weekends the hours are even longer and it is possible to find consultants who believe junior doctors are mollycoddled in comparison to their days. Nor is a child's vomit an unusual hazard of life in a casualty department. In the first of Dr Goldblatt's two days of duty he and his colleagues would encounter most things from convulsions to coughs, cuts to burns, asthma to diarrhoea. Eighty-six children would be seen of whom eight would be admitted to the wards. Both figures are slightly below the daily average for the casualty department of the *other* Hospital for Sick Children in the Great Ormond Street group – Queen Elizabeth Hospital for Children in the East End of London.

Queen Elizabeth's is only three miles away from Great Ormond Street but it might as well be in another world. Great Ormond Street is far from opulent; it is overlooked by fourteen-storey blocks of council flats and hemmed in on three sides by traffic-clogged streets. But Queen's, as it is known, lies on the borders of Hackney, which according to government statistics is the most deprived borough in Britain, and Tower Hamlets, which is not that much better off. Unemployment is high, housing poor, the ethnic mix complex. These factors intensify the contrast between the two children's hospitals. One offers specialized, high-tech treatment for the most serious and rarest of illnesses; its patients come from all over the country, some from all over the world. The other hospital also possesses great expertise in certain areas, such as gastro-enteritis, but mostly it now serves the local community. Nowhere is this seen more clearly than in the casualty department – or, indeed, in the existence of such a department at Queen's and its absence at Great Ormond Street.

Queen's is sited on a main road and there are times when its casualty department seems just as busy a thoroughfare. The hospital's main ground-floor corridor runs right through the middle of the department. On one side are three examination cubicles and a cramped office, on the other the waiting area and larger treatment rooms. During the day people seeking out-patients, X-rays or the pharmacy constantly wander up and down the corridor. The reception desk for casualty is itself further down the corridor so first-time visitors frequently lose their way before arriving in the waiting room. This can seat about two dozen people and, with parents accompanying children, it soon fills up. So it did this Monday: a day in the life of casualty.

No day in casualty is ever truly typical, but it usually begins quietly. There had been only three patients overnight before Joel arrived at eight o'clock. The nursing staff changed at seven-thirty. For Mary Brackett, the senior of casualty's two sisters, and the other three nurses on duty, the day begins unexcitingly with cleaning and stock-taking. Because it was Monday, it would be busy; some children seen over the weekend would return for further checks at a time when the hospital was fully staffed. It was also winter, which meant more colds than in summer. Colds and coughs are not necessarily mild. Two months earlier, a routine chest X-ray of a child with a cough revealed leukaemia. 'Colds' can also be bronchiolitis or pneumonia, especially in an area such as Hackney; poor living conditions render children more vulnerable to disease. Yet at least the weather was kind. There would be no broken bones caused by icy pavements or playgrounds. And Queen's does not cater for road accidents. It was the walking wounded who made their way or were carried to casualty.

For the first hour after the doctors arrived at nine, their customers were mostly babies. Eugene, a five-year-old Irish boy, was the oldest. He had cut his palm when trying to smash open a glass money box, succeeding only too well. The cut was cleaned and examined; it did not need stitches. Otherwise the first hour brought one case of earache, one nosebleed, one vomiting, one diarrhoea, one bronchiolitis, one to have stitches removed, one to have a weekend thumb injury checked and two children for the 'gastro' clinic – four mornings a week a registrar sees children who have suffered from gastro-enteritis to check their progress. The work is often as much education as medicine.

Daniel's West Indian parents, for instance, were worried by his diarrhoea. He was only two months old, but in order to tackle what they regarded as a problem, Daniel's parents were cutting back his milk. Dr Chris Ingall, the registrar, asked them a number of questions about his general health: any fever or colds? any vomiting? any problems with urine? how frequent was the diarrhoea? what was his diet? Daniel, like all children visiting casualty, was weighed and his temperature and pulse were recorded by the nurses. Dr Ingall also examined him, checking his ears for any viral infections and listening to his chest. Daniel, said Dr Ingall, seemed basically healthy. 'I think,' he told the parents, 'that you should concentrate on the child, not the stools. "Starving" a child to get rid of diarrhoea is a common reaction but it isn't really a good idea. Give him more milk, slowly increasing the strength and I think you'll find it clears itself up.'

'Education to correct misinformation and reassurance that a child's problems are not abnormal are a large part of paediatrics,' says Dr Ingall. Occasionally parents resent this. 'If I'd have sent them home with a drug or given the child an injection, I'd have been a real superstar,' said another doctor later in the day, after declining to offer one family anything but advice. Reassurance is not always possible. Clair, a sixteen-month-old baby, was brought to casualty with a painful right leg. She was examined by Dr Rob Ross-Russell who, like Dr Goldblatt, was a houseman rotating between duty in casualty and the wards. He took a detailed medical history, paying particular attention to the ages at which she smiled, crawled and sat. He flexed Clair's legs, causing her to wince. To her mother's surprise, and dismay, Dr Ross-Russell decided she should be admitted to Bailey ward.

He explained that Clair had what is called an 'irritable hip': inflammation was causing tenderness and limiting her movements. This was not uncommon and usually settled down of its own accord within a few days. 'Just occasionally there are problems which don't go away so we always take it seriously. It's a question of being safe,' he told Clair's parents soothingly. She would be given some traction and blood tests, just to make sure more serious problems did not develop. Clair was the second admission of the day. She had been referred to the hospital by her GP, but her parents had never anticipated that she would stay. Other parents would be similarly shocked during the course of the day. And the doctors never forget that amid apparently routine complaints lurk potentially serious problems.

The generally low use of GPs in the area is one reason why the casualty department checks the general health of its patients and why the doctors take extensive medical histories; otherwise problems may remain undetected. Most patients are seen in one of the three examination cubicles. Children requiring dressings are taken to a separate room where wounds can be swabbed or stitched and foreign bodies removed. Seven-year-old Dean, for instance, had managed to wedge a piece of popcorn down his right ear. This was a job for a doctor, but dressings can be changed and stitches removed by a staff nurse. Nurses also exercise an initial judgement about which patients need to be seen first – and where.

At noon Jason, a thirteen-year-old asthmatic, became the first patient to use the emergency room on this particular Monday. He was seen by a doctor within five minutes. The room contains two beds and all the equipment which might be needed in an emergency — intravenous fluids, 'drip' stands and electronic monitoring equipment, oxygen and ventilating tubes, heart stimulators, resuscitation drugs, suction catheters and the like. Jason's breathing difficulties were not acute enough to warrant any of these aids. What he needed was a nebulizer. This is a mask through which a patient breathes a drug that has been transformed into droplets, inhaled with oxygen from a cylinder. Jason, whose ambition is to play football for West Ham, was something of a veteran in casualty and could give his own medical history. 'I'm so used to talking to parents, I've almost forgotten what it's like to talk directly to a patient,' Dr Goldblatt told him. Jason had been treated at Queen's many times before, but it was his first asthma attack for almost a year and relatively mild. After a chest X-ray was added to his bulging file, he went home.

Jason came to Queen's because his mother knew that the casualty department was equipped with nebulizers. In this way, the expertise of Queen's reinforces a traditional East End reliance upon hospitals for problems which elsewhere would be dealt with by general practitioners. The historical reason for this was a shortage of GPs: patient lists were large and surgeries often conducted from lock-up shops with minimal after-hours cover. A few health clinics have been opened recently by groups of doctors, committed to the challenge of inner city health care. But so far another factor has outweighed their impact – immigration.

By the mid-1980s forty per cent of Hackney's population were classified as 'ethnic minorities' and they are among the casualty department's biggest users. Overall numbers visiting the department have risen from around 16,000 a year at the end of the 1970s to 25,000 in the mid-1980s. Dr John Black is a consultant paediatrician who was appointed to recommend ways in which the casualty department might adjust to the challenge, such as the appointment of bilingual community health workers. He says there are two broad reasons why the local Bengali community, in particular, prefers the hospital: 'The first is, again, tradition. They don't have many GPs in India or Bangladesh so, if they go anywhere when they are ill, it is to hospital. The other factor is that many mothers don't speak English and so they wait until their husbands come home from work so they can be escorted. This is why so many people turn up in the evenings when GPs are not available, although the threat of racial harassment is another element in the women's reluctance to come here alone.'

On this particular Monday all but six of the patients came from North or East London postal districts. The majority were white East Enders, but among casualty's international clientèle were families originally from Ghana, the West Indies, Bangladesh, Pakistan, India, Cyprus and Ireland. Language is generally less of a problem for the medical staff than different feeding traditions. This is why Queen's plans to send bilingual health workers into the local communities to educate families about diets. In the short term, though, there is no prospect of Queen's shedding its role as a source of basic health care, however odd this may seem to Whitehall administrators bent on economies. Yet Queen's is also far more than just a local hospital.

Queen's dates back to 1868 with Charles Dickens among the earliest visitors. He described the hospital as 'a haven to the children who came from the length and breadth of East London'. Originally there were two separate hospitals, one on the present site in Hackney Road and the other in dockland at Shadwell. These amalgamated under the present title in 1942. The next administrative changes came in the 1960s with the closure of the Shadwell branch of the hospital and the amalgamation of the Hackney hospital with that at Great Ormond Street under one board of governors as the Hospitals for Sick Children.

Queen's is a rather bleak, four-storey Victorian building on a busy main road. Many of the nearby shops are protected by metal grilles, although valiant efforts are being made to improve the environment through the creation of a new park next door to the hospital. Inside the front door, however, Queen's has a more intimate atmosphere than that of Great Ormond Street. This is partly a function of size – 133 beds compared to 331 and not all those fully occupied – and partly because relatively fewer children are so acutely ill. The staff are also less isolated than their more specialist counterparts at Great Ormond Street so that everyone seems to know each other. But their affection for the hospital is often tinged with defensiveness or vulnerability. Many feel they are the poor relations in the group; few of the pop stars, sportsmen and other celebrities who visit Great Ormond Street ever make the trip to Hackney. A more widespread worry is that as medical technology becomes ever costlier and funds apparently ever shorter, any decision by the government to concentrate specialist skills and equipment at Great Ormond Street could undermine the ability of Queen's to maintain its own areas of excellence.

Queen's pioneered significant treatment for cystic fibrosis, spina bifida, gastro-enterology and surgery for new-born babies. It performed a bone marrow transplant before Great Ormond Street. The combination of specialized medicine and large numbers of patients has made Queen's a place where hundreds of medical students receive their paediatric training each year. The medical schools of the London and St Bartholomew's hospitals have established an academic unit of child health here which not only conducts research but is responsible for a third of the medical work in the hospital's seven wards. Queen's also provides an essential training ground for, among others, the Charles West School of nursing based at Great Ormond Street. The wards of Great Ormond Street itself have become so specialized that they can no longer offer the all-round experience required by student nurses. Concern about the future of Queen's is therefore not confined solely to the East End of London.

Yet, overall, Queen's gains by association with Great Ormond Street. Administratively, its status within a health authority directly responsible to the government offers greater protection than would exist if Queen's were part of a regional board. Medically, several consultants work at both hospitals and the Great Ormond Street laboratories provide a twenty-four hour service which is invaluable for a department such as casualty. For casualty never closes. Even Christmas day tends to be busy with sixty or more patients most years.

No day, though, is ever predictable and it is this which appeals to the department's two sisters, Mary Brackett and Karen Cleaver. 'You have to be a bit more outgoing to work in casualty,' says Karen Cleaver. 'You have the opportunity to work more on your own initiative which means you enjoy your work more, but you have to have the confidence to do so. In the wards people are generally grateful for what you do, but in casualty you get a lot of aggression. People have to wait and often they think we are not doing anything and this is often the cause of the aggression.'

The need for confident characters who can cope with, let alone enjoy, casualty work is one reason why the department has two sisters and a low proportion of student nurses. Another is something which has become known simply by its initials – NAI. This stands for non-accidental injury and is something for which all casualty staff must be on their guard. Mary Brackett says that although social workers often alert them to a possible case of NAI, student nurses are taught to be aware of the possibilities on all occasions. How did a child break his arm? Could a fracture occur accidentally if a baby was not yet mobile? Are the burns accidental? Is it likely that a child could fall not once but twice against a radiator causing burns on *both* sides of the body? Is a child's malnutrition the result of poverty, ignorance or deliberate neglect? 'You can become very cynical, but if you do make a mistake and miss something it can have tragic consequences,' says Karen Cleaver. 'After my lecture students spend the rest of the afternoon suspecting everyone of inflicting injury.'

No cases of NAI were suspected by the staff on this particular Monday. There was one minor burn caused by hot tea and a couple of head injuries caused by falls. Alannah, for instance, arrived at two o'clock with a gash in the crown of her head. She was a pale English girl of six who had fallen at school. The wound was not too serious, but it did appear to require stitches. Sister Cleaver, though, recalled a ploy she had seen when working at Guy's Hospital near London Bridge. If the hair was long enough, she could bind the wound by tying the hair tightly together; this also avoids shaving the head. 'All you have got to do is to keep infection or germs out. It doesn't have to be too neat in terms of a scar because for a girl it will be under the hair,' she said. And so Alannah left Queen's unstitched and unshaven.

Not all the customers were quite so satisfied. Michael, a puffy faced four-year-old Cypriot boy, arrived with a recurrence of a long-term kidney problem for which he had frequently received treatment at Queen's. It was not too serious, Dr Rob Ross-Russell told his parents. A course of steroids should solve the problem: come back in a week's time. 'We can't,' said his father. 'We're off to Tenerife tomorrow.'

Dr Ross-Russell said he would have to consult Profesor Chris Wood, the head of the academic unit who was in overall charge of Michael's case. The casualty officer's own view was clear. 'The effect of steroids is to stop the kidneys leaking protein. We can then gradually reduce the steroids and the problem is usually resolved. But if it doesn't respond, it becomes more worrying. Michael is well enough to go home, but I would want to see him for checks. I am unhappy about him being away for such a long time.' So, too, was Professor Wood. Nobody, though, was unhappier than Michael's parents. They saw their holiday and hundreds of pounds disappearing. Dr Ross-Russell sympathized and said that the hospital could provide letters which should help get their money back. At first Michael's father contemplated ignoring the medical advice and going ahead with the holiday. But you do not lightly risk the health of your child and eventually they bowed to the inevitable; one week later Michael would be back in Hackney, not Tenerife.

Michael had arrived shortly after five o'clock in the afternoon. He was patient number sixty-five. Sister Brackett and the early shift of nurses departed at four-thirty, along with Dr Alex Furtado, a part-time casualty doctor who saw fifteen patients during her six hours on duty. Now Sister Cleaver and the three nurses on the late shift were bracing themselves for the early evening rush. Already the day had been busier than most, although there had been no real emergencies – so far. 'Children do die in casualty from time to time,' says Mary Brackett. 'Not often, because we don't take road accidents. The more common emergencies are children who arrive unconscious, with breathing problems or suffering from fits or burns. The thing about casualty is that you can never tell what's going to happen next.'

The oldest child seen this Monday was Peter, a fourteen-year-old with a painful leg. The youngest were a couple of one-month-old babies who seemed to their mothers to be wheezy.

Some complaints are so common that the casualty staff log them simply by initials: 'Ds and Vs' are diarrhoea and vomiting, 'FB' a foreign body. Today's FB count was light: one in the ear, one in the nose. Otherwise there were cuts to fingers, toes, lips, heads, palms and noses but just one broken bone – a shoulder. There were coughs, earache, sore throats and runny eyes. Some coughs, though, are taken more seriously than others. Dale, a one-year-old girl, arrived at teatime and was seen quickly. Why? Because she had leukaemia. But tests showed that she could wait until her next out-patients appointment in two days' time. Only two children were admitted up to six p.m., lower than average. But six more children would be transferred to the wards before the evening was over.

Usually there is a two-hour wait during the evenings, partly because there are fewer doctors on duty. It is then that tempers begin to fray. Queen's has done its best to make the waiting room bright and cheerful. There are paintings on the walls (as well as exhortations to immunize children against various infectious diseases), a table at which children can draw or play, a rocking horse, a fish tank and cuddly toys as well as books and magazines. During the day a playleader spends some of her time playing with the younger children, but there is less she can offer to entertain either babies or older children. The waiting room is inevitably at its worst when it is busiest. Less room to play and longer to wait causes frayed tempers; older children will get bored and babies will begin to cry, particularly if they are in pain. 'What parents don't understand,' says Karen Cleaver, 'is that we don't necessarily see people in the order that they come in. The most urgent cases are seen first and then there are other factors such as how quickly we can find their medical records. If it's busy and a child comes in with a non-urgent problem, we tell them – yes, we'll see you but you may have to wait a long time.'

Some children, of course, are seen immediately. Sarah arrived at six twenty-five p.m. with croup, a hacking, racking type of cough which is uncomfortable to hear, let alone experience. She was sixteen months old and accompanied by her father, an orthodox Jew. She had been referred to the hospital by her GP after the cough had failed to respond to steam inhalations at home for several days. She was examined in the emergency room by Dr David Goldblatt who listened to Sarah's breathing through a stethoscope; he was in no doubt that the GP had done the right thing. But Sarah's age did not make it any easier for the doctors to help her.

First, the doctor attempted to put a nebulizer face mask on Sarah but she wriggled and coughed so much she probably lost much of the benefit. Then Dr Goldblatt tried to insert a glucose 'drip' into a vein. But the veins of babies and very young children are often difficult to tap and it was only at the fourth attempt that Dr Goldblatt succeeded with Sarah. Next came a chest X-ray. This showed traces of pneumonia in the mid-zone of the right lung. Dr Goldblatt conferred with Dr Deirdre Kelly, the duty registrar. Sarah would have to be admitted, but the doctors were unsure about the cause of her difficulties. Was it a bacterial infection of the larynx or could she have inhaled a foreign body? A sample of blood was taken and sent to the haematology laboratory at Great Ormond Street where the ear, nose and throat specialists were also alerted. Sarah, meanwhile, was admitted, still coughing, to Connaught ward.

In this case Sarah's father was almost relieved that she was admitted to hospital. He had arrived with an obviously sick child and needed no persuasion that hospital was the best place to treat her. Other parents were shocked by their child's admission. Terry, a twenty-one-month-old boy, was brought to casualty at twenty past seven with a cough and a high temperature. Nothing too serious, his mother thought, but best to check. Certainly, he looked well enough in himself and the nurses saw nothing to warrant any queue-jumping. Yet when the routine chest X-rays returned to the casualty office the doctors said: 'Good God!' It showed pneumonia in the middle lobe of the right lung and in the lower lobe of the left. Terry would have to be admitted. Where Sarah's father had experienced relief, Terry's parents – both local East Enders – now felt concern because the admission had not been expected.

The evening rush failed to materialize. Apart from the time the doctors went to supper, waits averaged about thirty minutes, much as they had all day. At twenty minutes past eight, for the first time since a lunchtime lull, the waiting room was even empty. Yet fourteen patients had still to arrive. There would be more 'Ds and Vs', more coughs and more cuts. And three more children were admitted, again producing contrasting responses from their parents. Louis, a three-year-old, was suffering from convulsions which were clearly best dealt with in hospital. Forty-five minutes later another three-year-old arrived: Samuel. He was wheezy and accompanied by his parents and grandfather, a North London GP. His parents hoped that a nebulizer would be sufficient, as it had been for Jason, the twelve-year-old asthmatic, earlier in the day. It was not to be: to his mother's surprise and natural disappointment, the doctors wanted Samuel to stay overnight.

Samuel left casualty for Barclay ward just before eleven o'clock. There were still some children and parents in the waiting room and others in the treatment cubicles. From five o'clock the casualty staff had taken over from the pharmacy, dispensing drugs from their own emergency supplies; from ten o'clock the two night nurses have to find the medical records themselves. These could be bulky – doctors would groan at the sight of bulging files for fear of the complications that might await them – and elusive. It took fifteen minutes to find the records of Jonathan, a five-year-old with a croupy cough and wheezy breathing. 'I feel like giving people a kiss when they say they've not been here before,' says staff nurse Christine Johnson. 'Otherwise there are about five different places the records could be.'

Jonathan became the seventh patient to be admitted to the wards on this particular Monday. He was followed, shortly before midnight, by Ojo, a ten-week-old boy with suspected meningitis. Eight admissions, yet the day had been neither dramatic nor exceptionally busy. The night nursing staff came on duty at nine-thirty p.m.: they would go home at seven-thirty the next morning. The doctors would be summoned from their rooms on the top floor of the hospital as often as patients arrived. The only certainty about the night ahead, as with the day that was just ending, was its unpredictability. It would be wrong, for instance, to imagine that night-time patients are necessarily seriously ill. At eleven o'clock Karen was brought in by her parents. She'd had diarrhoea for two weeks and it could well have waited till morning. And at a quarter to midnight three-month-old Mustafa became the day's final visitor to casualty – patient number eighty-six. What was the problem? Well, he seemed hot and hadn't been feeding well. Anything else? 'Yes, he's crying.'

Stacey

Stacey Tyrrill was a Christmas baby. Labour was accompanied by the sound of *Silent Night* sung by the Salvation Army and ended as church bells pealed at five minutes before midnight on 24 December 1978. But it was to be five years before Stacey spent Christmas Day at home and another twelve months before she had her own bed there. In those six years Stacey spent just two nights out of a hospital bed. These were years when Stacey's story involved four hospitals and twenty-three operations, years when her problems pushed her parents' marriage to breaking point, but years too when a sickly, premature baby survived against the odds to become an attractive, charismatic young girl.

Not that her problems were by any means over. At the age of six she still breathed through a tube inserted directly into her windpipe at her throat. She was still fed largely through another tube, this time into her stomach. In the coming year she would face five operations at Great Ormond Street and she would sleep overnight at Queen Mary's Hospital in Carshalton, Surrey, for a further nine months. And while doctors would strive, with some success, to tackle her breathing and feeding difficulties, one problem remained beyond them. Stacey was almost totally deaf. Of all her problems, deafness was the only one which does not appear to have been with her from birth.

Nothing in Stacey's life has ever gone easily. She was born seven weeks premature after Pauline her mother, had endured a difficult pregnancy. She had suffered severe headaches and stomach pains. And as she swelled – her normal waistline of twenty-two inches became forty-eight inches – Pauline became convinced that something was wrong with her baby. She hadn't felt like this with her two sons from her first marriage. Tests appeared to confirm her anxiety: there was too much fluid in the womb. More seriously, other tests showed that the baby was not getting enough oxygen. Labour would be induced at noon on Christmas Eve.

Pauline had been warned that the baby's lungs would be weak because birth was going to be early. Yet, at first, Pauline's fears appeared unfounded. Stacey weighed in at 2 kg (4½ lb), not bad at all for so premature a baby. 'She looked perfect and I'd longed so much for a girl. They gave her to me to cuddle and she seemed to be OK,' recalls Pauline. Her relief was short-lived. After barely a minute, Stacey started to turn blue and the doctors, worried about her breathing, gave her oxygen. She was placed in an incubator and hurried to the intensive care unit. It would be almost two days before Pauline saw her baby again and by then Stacey would be dependent upon machines to keep her alive. What should have been the happiest of Christmases had become a nightmare. Pauline was surrounded by joyful mums, proudly showing off their perfect babies to visitors, while she could not even see her child.

Stacey had been born at St Helier hospital, half a mile from Pauline's home in Morden, South London. Here, on the third day of her life, the first of Stacey's problems was diagnosed. She was born without a normal oesophagus or gullet. This is the tube which takes food and fluids from the mouth to the stomach. When there is a gap in the tube it is known as oesophageal atresia. It also seemed likely that there was a link between the oesophagus and her windpipe which caused food to spill over into the windpipe, known technically as the trachea. This is called a tracheo-oesophageal fistula or TOF, for short. Within a few days these unheard-of, almost unpronounceable terms would become as commonplace to Stacey's parents as chickenpox or measles. In fact, neither of these abnormalities is particularly rare: oesophageal atresia affects one in 3000 live births and of these approximately three-quarters also have problems with the windpipe. But the treatment required more specialized surgical skills than those available at a district general hospital. Stacey was therefore transferred just over two miles across South London to Queen Mary's Hospital for Children at Carshalton. Pauline watched the ambulance leave, never dreaming that Queen Mary's was to be Stacey's home for nearly seven years.

At just four days old Stacey Ann Tyrrill experienced the first of what would be many visits to operating theatres. Her weight was down to just over three pounds. Back in St Helier hospital Pauline could not imagine how anyone could operate on so tiny a baby. Nobody sought to minimize the difficulties – or the dangers. One doctor told Pauline that Stacey's lungs were so weak she had only a forty per cent chance of surviving for long after the operation. Statistically, the odds were even worse.

Herbert Eckstein, the consultant surgeon, found that there was, indeed, a link or fistula between the gullet and windpipe. He closed this link but decided that the gap in the gullet or oesophagus was too large simply to be stitched together. Stacey, however, was too weak to withstand more ambitious surgery. Mr Eckstein therefore had to devise a way for Stacey to be fed without food spilling into the windpipe and lungs. He did this by inserting what is known as a gastrostomy tube into her stomach through which liquidized food could be pumped. He also cut into the side of her neck to insert what was effect-ively a 'drain' into the upper part of her gullet. The idea behind this was simple. Although Stacey would actually be fed via the gastrostomy tube, it was important that she learned how to suck and swallow. The drain in the neck – an oesophagostomy – would remove fluids from the throat before they could spill over into the windpipe. It also allowed 'sham feeding' until such time as a permanent repair of Stacey's insides could be tackled. Or so the doctors hoped.*

Stacey had come through the operation, but the first time Pauline visited her baby at Carshalton all she could see of her was a chin. She was a mass of wires with a ventilator breathing tube up her nose and a drip feed connected to her gastrostomy tube in the stomach. Worse still, other tests showed some signs of brain damage. For Stacey's parents, this marked the lowest point in her life. What would they say if asked whether the life-saving machines should be turned off?

Pauline and Phil Tyrrill had known each other for little

---

*See Robert's story for more about operations to tackle oesophageal atresia and tracheo-oesophageal fistula.

more than a year. They had each been married before and were awaiting divorces so they could marry. Stacey's problems were to put her parents' eventual marriage under great strain, but in those early months and years Pauline and Phil were close and happy. Stacey had not been planned – Pauline had been taking the Pill at the time – but there was never any thought of an abortion. 'I loved Phil and his child meant a lot to me. I never thought about other people's reactions,' says Pauline. Phil moved into Pauline's house on a spruce council estate between Morden and Sutton. They were both South Londoners, then in their mid-twenties. Their personalities, though, were very different.

Pauline, as Phil recognizes, is the stronger character of the two and it was she who, in the years to come, would chase and chivvy the innumerable doctors, nurses and officials who figured in Stacey's life. She is an attractive, slender woman, happier in jeans than skirts, with dark hair and eyes which hint at an inner toughness that belies her slight build, trim appearance and infectious chuckle. For her own sake, as well as Stacey's, she has needed to be strong. Her own family was large – she was one of nine children – but not especially close. She worked as a secretary for a bank in the City of London after leaving school until, at the age of twenty-two, she became a mother herself. She has two sons from an unhappy first marriage: Karl, who was five when Stacey was born, and Tommy, who was three.

Stacey was Phil's first child. 'I never knew that the birth of a child could change your life so much,' he says. He was working as a minicab driver when Stacey was born – 'it helped not being tied down to set hours and the firm helped by pumping good jobs my way' – and found some escape from Stacey's problems by tinkering with cars. 'I must have got through twenty in that first year, but at least I didn't lose any money on them. It took my mind off things.' However, the worry affected Phil differently to the way it affected Pauline. He was always the more easygoing character of the two and, as Pauline became more stubborn and determined, he grew more withdrawn and fatalistic. Increasingly, he would look at Karl and Tommy, who were fine, and blame himself for Stacey's problems. 'You ask yourself, is there any justice? What have you done to deserve this?'

Stacey's first brain test was their first crisis. Until then, Pauline and Phil had felt helpless, knowing there was nothing they could do. Now they could face a life-or-death decision. Pauline says: 'We decided that if she was going to be a vegetable, rather than make her suffer endless operations, we would rather she went in peace. It may seem strange but once we had made that decision, Stacey seemed to decide otherwise. She began to fight back. She progressed a little. They did another test and this suggested that her brain was not damaged as much as they thought. The first one had been done before a normal baby would even have been born. She still had blue spells but, if she's going to fight, you've got to give all you can to help her. Every ounce she put on was a victory for us.'

In April, when Stacey was four months old, she returned to the operating theatre at Carshalton. Now Mr Eckstein, the surgeon, was to attempt a permanent repair of Stacey's misformed oesophagus. He took a piece of the colon and transplanted it into the gap in the oesophagus. And that should have been that. Food and fluids should have gone down the oesophagus via the colon transplant into the stomach. The gastrostomy tube could then be removed. Although Stacey did well immediately after the operation, she began to be sick and to lose weight. Another operation removed a blockage in her bowels, yet still Stacey suffered from vomiting, blue spells and chest infections. There must, her doctors concluded, be another problem.

On 11 June 1979 Stacey arrived for the first time at the Hospital for Sick Children in Great Ormond Street, one of the few British hospitals with paediatric consultants for ear, nose and throat (ENT) problems. She was just under six months old. Stacey had been referred here by Mr Eckstein, who worked as a consultant paediatric surgeon at Great Ormond Street as well as at Queen Mary's in Carshalton. He suspected that Stacey had a problem with her windpipe which was still causing food to spill over into her lungs. Stacey's arrival at Great Ormond Street epitomizes its role as a place to which most patients are referred by other hospitals rather than their

GPs. In official jargon, this makes it a tertiary referral hospital.

The undoubted world reknown of Great Ormond Street hospital is not immediately apparent. Indeed, it would be hard to imagine a greater contrast between two hospitals than that encountered by Pauline and Phil Tyrrill. Carshalton is on the southern fringes of London where leafy suburbs give way to open countryside; Queen Mary's comprises a series of single-storey buildings separated by spacious lawns. It is so spread out that doctors sometimes do ward rounds by car. Great Ormond Street is squeezed between three roads in central London. When Stacey first arrived, as indeed for most of the next seven years, a new cardiac wing was being built noisily next door. As first impressions go, the outside face of Great Ormond Street wins few prizes.

Stacey was admitted to ward 2C on the second floor, overlooking the driveway to the hospital's main entrance. 2C had just been designated as a specialist ward to look after children with tracheostomies – tubes placed directly into the windpipe or trachea through which a patient breathes. Tracheostomy was yet another strange word with which the Tyrrills would become all too familiar.

Gill Tym is the ward sister on 2C, a tall and athletic Yorkshirewoman who was then just twenty-three. Along with Pat Carter on the oncology ward (see Anna's story), Gill Tym was the harbinger of a new breed of youthful ward sisters at Great Ormond Street. Simultaneously, and perhaps not coincidentally, the wards have become more specialist so that sisters have acquired great expertise. So rare are many of the conditions treated at Great Ormond Street that a senior ward sister will frequently be more familiar with the problems than a junior doctor on a three or six-month stint as a house officer. In the coming years Gill Tym would write articles about tracheostomy care for medical journals and win a travelling scholarship to America in order to study US nursing practices. Such specialization deprives nurses of the variety found in general hospitals, but Gill Tym believes it is better for the patients. 'Children with tracheostomies can develop problems in no time at all. We must have nurses who know what to look out for and know what to do instantly.'

Stacey Tyrrill would need all 2C's specialist skills. On 12 June 1979 she went to Great Ormond Street's seventh-floor operating theatre for the first time. Stacey had been starved for four hours before the operation was due. Forty-five minutes before going to theatre she received a pre-medication drug to dry the body's secretions. Then, her identity band checked, Stacey was taken to the anaesthetic room next door to the theatre. At that stage John Evans, one of the hospital's two ENT consultants, did not know exactly what he would be doing. It would depend upon what he found by looking down Stacey's windpipe. For the upper airways the process is known as a micro-laryngoscopy, for the lower trachea and passages leading to the lung it is a bronchoscopy. Both procedures involve inserting a tube down the patient's throat; a light is then directed through the tube which acts, in effect, as a microscope. What John Evans saw, magnified approximately forty times, was a large cleft or gap in the larynx.

The larynx is often known as the 'voice box'. This is because within its complex collection of cartilages, ligaments, muscles and membranes are the vocal cords. When speaking, air passing over the cords from the lungs causes them to vibrate, rather as a musician blows over the reed in an oboe. The tension and length of the vocal cords can vary, producing different notes which become the sounds required for speech. This alone makes the larynx crucial, but it has other functions too. Its muscles enable us to cough and remove mucus or phlegm from the chest. The larynx also forms a barrier between windpipe and gullet every time we swallow. In Stacey's case, however, there was a gap in the larynx. This cleft, as it is called, allowed food to spill into the windpipe and mucus to stay in the chest, causing infections.

A cleft larynx is extremely rare. John Evans has seen just twelve in ten years, yet even this is probably more than any other surgeon in the world. He was appointed an ENT consultant at Great Ormond Street in 1972 at the age of thirty-seven. He is well over six feet tall and his height conveys an impression of aloofness to some parents. Surgeons are inevitably less visible figures than doctors on non-surgical wards, if only because they spend so much time in operating theatres. In

John Evans' case, this apparent remoteness was reinforced by the part-time nature of his consultancy at Great Ormond Street; he is also a consultant at St Thomas's Hospital, across the Thames from the Houses of Parliament. However, the long-term nature of tracheostomy care is gradually forging a closer relationship between surgeons and patients; it has also changed the traditional balance between hospitals and homes and introduced other specialists into a child's care.

There are many reasons for a tracheostomy or a trachy*, to use the usual abbreviation. It can be a short-lived emergency procedure for a patient in intensive care. It can be an interim measure while doctors seek to repair some congenital malformation, such as Stacey's cleft larynx. There is a third reason which has caused the numbers of children having tracheostomies to double over the last decade. Ironically, this stems from the increasing ability of hospital neonatal units to keep alive premature babies who once would have died. Breathing tubes inserted down tiny windpipes can damage the tissues and cause scarring or a narrowing of the airways known as sub-glottic stenosis. Tracheostomies enable such children to breathe until either natural growth or surgical intervention widens the airways sufficiently for normal breathing.

Stacey Tyrrill required a trachy because it would enable her to breathe more easily and the dangerous mucus secretions could be sucked out via the tracheostomy tube. The cleft larynx itself would be repaired later. For the initial examination during that first visit to the Great Ormond Street operating theatre she had lain on the operating table fully visible. For the trachy to be inserted, green surgical sheets covered all but her neck. This was swabbed with iodine and then wiped clean. A sandbag was placed under her shoulders so that her neck would be fully extended for surgery. But before the surgeon picked up a scalpel, he felt and prodded Stacey's neck with his hands.

In a child the larynx is higher than in adults and the softness of the surrounding tissue can make it difficult to identify the key cartilages. The surgeon has to make his incision below the

---

Sometimes spelled trache, but always pronounced 'track-ee'.

larynx, finding the right spot by feeling. He is aiming for a position between the third and fourth 'ring' in the trachea or windpipe which, at Stacey's age, would have been barely two inches long. Having found what he believed to be the right place, John Evans made his first incision – a horizontal cut just under two centimetres long. Nurses sucked away the trickle of blood which seeped from the wound; junior surgeons held back the skin with tiny clamps as Evans cut deeper. Each layer of skin or fat was cut so that it remained flush with the edge of the wound. When he reached the trachea, the surgeon placed his finger in the hole; it was as deep as his finger-nail. He wanted to be certain to cut into the trachea at its centre.

The smallness of the windpipe was highlighted by the size of the plastic tracheostomy tube which was inserted: it was just three and a half millimetres in diameter. The hope was that after the larynx was repaired, the tracheostomy could soon be removed. It would be there for a maximum of six months, Pauline Tyrrill was told. It turned out to be there for six years.

The increasing numbers of children requiring trachies and the long-term nature of their treatment lay behind Great Ormond Street's decision to devote the best part of a ward to caring for such children. Yet outside one or two centres – Liverpool's Alder Hey Hospital is another – childhood tracheostomies remain rare. Even Great Ormond Street cared for only 242 children with trachies in the first six years of 2C's existence. This, though, is probably as many as any hospital in the world.

Stacey's six years with a trachy is longer than most, but even the two-year average makes it impossible for all the children to remain in hospital until the trachies can be removed. It is not just impossible but undesirable, given the known harmful social and educational effects of prolonged hospitalization. Parents have thus been embraced as partners in the care of their trachy children. A map hangs on a wall of ward 2C, dotted with pins representing families with a trachy child at home – from Cumbria to Cornwall, Glamorgan to Tyneside.

In each case these parents have learned to become nurses, able to suck mucus from the windpipe and lungs via the tracheostomy and to change the trachy tube itself. Initially, most people shy away from the prospect. The first time Pauline Tyrrill did it, she was nearly sick. But for her, as with most parents, it soon became routine. Essentially, it involves inserting a tube called a catheter into the tracheostomy so that the lower end rests in the windpipe. The catheter is then connected to a pump which sucks out any secretions in the windpipe as the catheter is withdrawn. It doesn't take long in itself, but there are related tasks, such as using a syringe to instil saline into the trachy and the need to sterilize equipment each time it is used. The trachy tube itself needs to be changed at least weekly.

Most parents master the mechanical skills within a fortnight. The problems then become ones of responsibility and exhaustion. Will they recognize the warning sounds of laboured breathing? Supposing they don't wake up if their child gets into difficulty at night? Some children – Stacey Tyrrill was one for a time – need suction every few minutes. Many need suction every hour. How can parents cope with this night after night? For this reason Gill Tym, the ward sister, tries to teach both parents the necessary skills, although the prime burden usually falls on the mother. Even when the parents do share the responsibilities, they often feel isolated. It is quite likely that neither their GP nor their local health visitor has any knowledge of trachies. Gill Tym and her staff nurses on 2C therefore receive a regular flow of calls from parents seeking advice – day and night.

Stacey Tyrrill, though, did not return home with her trachy; she returned to the hospital in Carshalton. This was not because Pauline or Phil were unable to cope with the trachy, but because of Stacey's other problems. She still had frequent attacks of breathlessness, turning blue with alarming speed. She was still being fed through the gastrostomy tube into her stomach. Yet for Pauline there was something more upsetting than any of the tubes which were attached to her daughter's body. Because Stacey now breathed through her tracheostomy, no air was passing through her larynx. She had therefore lost her voice. She could not even cry. There seemed nothing more pitifully heart-rending than silent tears.

Luckily a personality which outshone all Stacey's problems

had begun to emerge. She smiled a lot, laughed often and hardly ever complained. Her parents had visited her every day since she was born, but only now was the bond becoming close. Initially, Pauline resisted becoming too attached because she feared Stacey would die. 'I had never experienced before anyone being so ill. It's the sort of thing you never think can happen to you. But she was fighting so hard, we had to be positive. She did not cry or complain very much and she had this terrific smile. There were days after operations when all you could see were her eyes or her mouth, but she never looked miserable. Her eyes always looked bubbly and happy, despite the pain she must have been in. To give up on her now would be impossible.'

In August Stacey returned to Great Ormond Street for her cleft larynx to be repaired. She was patient number two on the surgical list, arriving in the anaesthetic room next to the operating theatre at just before nine-fifteen in the morning. Anaesthetizing any young child is difficult and delicate. The veins can be hard to find and the oxygen required per kilogram of body weight is greater than for adults. Some operations involving the windpipe can pose additional difficulties when both surgeon and anaesthetist share the same airway, but on this occasion the tracheostomy helped by providing a secure airway below the larynx.

The cleft in Stacey's larynx was large, extending almost the entire depth of the cricoid cartilage. John Evans, the consultant, decided to approach the larynx from the right-hand side of the neck. This would be less likely to damage the vocal cords than a frontal approach. Although Stacey was light for her age, she had long, spindly legs. Yet here, on an operating table large enough for gangling adolescents, she seemed minute. She was surrounded by a dozen people – surgeons, anaesthetists and nurses. The object of all this attention was a larynx barely half an inch long. Smallness causes myriad problems for paediatric surgeons; tiny bodies require tiny instruments and gossamer-thin thread. 'The longer you can delay any operation, the technically easier it will be,' says John Evans. Another hazard for any paediatric surgeon is that he or she is repairing a body which must be able to grow – in the case of Stacey's larynx,

from around one centimetre to adulthood's five centimetres –
with all its functions unimpaired.

The operation took most of the morning. The lateral
approach meant that after the surgeon had reached the larynx,
he had to rotate it by fifteen to twenty degrees in order to make
the repair. He had to cut through several muscles and avoid
damage either to these or the cartilages of the larynx. Closing
the cleft required work of great precision, as John Evans
explains:

'If you tied it up too tightly, the cords would not open sufficiently. If it was too loose, you would still get overspill into the
lungs. But Stacey's case was complicated immensely by the
fact that in addition to a cleft larynx, she had had an oesophageal atresia [the gap or hole in the gullet]. The operation which
had repaired this caused scarring of the tissue which made it
that much more difficult to repair the larynx and had also left
her with an oesophagus that couldn't work too well until her
larynx was repaired.'

This, though, was spoken with hindsight. The scale of
Stacey's problems would only become apparent after succes-
sive failures to repair the cleft larynx. But the omens were
scarcely encouraging. Almost as soon as Stacey returned to
ward 2C from theatre, she was in difficulty. She developed
chest infections and saliva seeped from the neck wound made
by the surgeons. She was feverish and frequently turned blue.
Thick, mucus secretions oozed from her tracheostomy. For
forty-eight hours a drain collected fluid which seeped from her
neck wound.

Stacey was not, in short, an easy patient to nurse – for all
2C's expertise. The nursing requirements were spelled out in
the Cardex file kept for each patient. Reading it, you wonder
how Stacey ever got a moment's rest. For forty-five minutes
every hour liquidized food was pumped down the tube into her
stomach. Every half hour dextrose-saline solution was added
via another tube. The trachy was sucked as necessary, which
generally meant every few minutes. Her pulse and breathing
were checked every hour, sometimes every fifteen minutes.
Every two hours her temperature was taken and Stacey was
turned over to avoid sores developing; the inside of her mouth

was swabbed two-hourly to fight infection. Six times a day she underwent physiotherapy treatment. And once a day, at least, the dressings on her neck and stomach wounds were changed.

Stacey was nursed in a cubicle, propped in an upright position. At night she slept in a plastic tent, breathing humidified air. One problem for any child with a trachy is that air entering the windpipe via the tube is cold and dry, whereas the normal route via the nose makes it warm and moist. If the air is too dry, secretions can become encrusted and block the tube. Beside Stacey's cot, among a vast array of specialized equipment, was an oxygen breathing circuit in case she still had any difficulties breathing. She did.

Two days after her operation, doctors from the hospital's respiratory unit were called in. As a result, yet another tube was inserted into Stacey's body – this time into a vein on the top of her head. Through this, antibiotics were given to fight the chest infections which had developed. Other drugs were prescribed either to keep Stacey continent or to loosen the mucus secretions in the lungs. The physiotherapy was also intended to assist the removal of these secretions; if they stayed in the lungs, they might cause serious chest infections. The physiotherapist therefore sought to shift the secretions from the lower airways to a point where they could be sucked out via the trachy tube. The physiotherapist does this by, first, instilling saline solution into the trachy tube to loosen any secretions and then by gently pummelling each side of the chest with cupped hands. The technique is known as percussion. After the percussion comes vibration – a gentle, but firm, shaking of the chest until the patient coughs or can be given suction. The treatment can take ten or fifteen minutes and in Stacey's case it was given up to six times a day.

The combined effects of intensive physiotherapy and the antibiotics gradually began to work, but progress was anything but smooth. As late as three weeks after the operation, the respiratory specialists were back in her cubicle in the early hours of the morning attending to a breathless and distinctly blue Stacey. A chest X-ray was taken and oxygen given. She was propped up because that seemed to help her breathing. More antibiotics were administered. And to cap it all, in the middle of the night her feeding tube somehow came out.

Despite these misadventures Stacey was eventually discharged from ward 2C to Carshalton. Not for long, though: two months later she was back at Great Ormond Street, this time for a microscopic examination of her larynx in the operating theatre. The repair attempted in August had broken down. They would try again on 20 November 1979. It turned out to be as dramatic – and perilous – as any day in Stacey's life. She was then just under eleven months old.

She went to theatre just before nine-thirty in the morning. Once again John Evans, the surgeon, attempted the delicate task of repairing the larynx. This time, though, he inserted a silastic roll into the upper windpipe at the level of the larynx. This is a piece of plastic material, cut and rolled up like a Swiss roll. It keeps the airway open and, by exerting pressure on the walls of the windpipe, helps the tissue to regenerate without infection. If all went well, it would be removed in roughly six weeks' time. In fact, it lasted barely four hours. Stacey coughed out the silastic roll at two-thirty in the afternoon. She would have to return to theatre.

Pauline had grown to hate waiting for operations; if something went wrong, she would rather hear the news at home. But when she had phoned at lunchtime, she had learned that Stacey was fine. Now Pauline arrived with Phil to find their daughter being prepared for her second general anaesthetic of the day. Pauline says: 'Stacey went to theatre at about nine o'clock and we went to a waiting room down the corridor. We just didn't speak. What made the waiting worse was the fact that, just a few hours earlier, we'd been told she was fine. We had felt like walking on air because, once again, she had come safely through the operation.'

Four floors above them, there was rather more activity. At first, all went smoothly. The neck wound was reopened and a silastic roll was reinserted. But towards the end of the operation, things began to go wrong. Stacey was having great difficulty breathing and her pulse rate was dropping. In particular her right lung was not inflating properly. Pauline Tyrrill says that one doctor told her that Stacey had actually stopped breathing at one point. Although this is not recorded in the official notes of the operation, Stacey was certainly in severe difficulties. It was a question now of keeping her alive so she was given one hundred per cent oxygen. Her trachy tube was changed. This had no apparent effect but when saline was flushed into the tube, it released – according to the operation notes – a 'thick, tenacious plug of sputum'. Her breathing began to ease. She was pulling through.

Stacey returned to the ward shortly before midnight. Her condition was described as 'shocked'. Her pulse rate was 210, her temperature 39.5 – figures of 110 and 36.9 would be normal. She was nursed sitting up in an oxygen tent. Once again she was launched upon a round of antibiotics and physiotherapy to fight off infections. That first night, the duty physiotherapist came every two hours. Her blood was checked, a chest X-ray taken. Because her pulse rate had been low in the theatre – known as bradycardia – the heart specialists examined her. Her breathing was rattly and frequent — sixty times a minute upon return from the theatre. The site of her stomach tube was oozing stale blood. Not surprisingly, she was restless and agitated, finding it difficult to sleep. She was not the only one.

Pauline and Phil Tyrrill had finally gone home at one o'clock in the morning. Neither slept much. Phil suffers from asthma which always seemed to be worse every time Stacey had an operation. That night was no exception. The next day Pauline was back on ward 2C. She sat by the cot all day. So, too, did a nurse since Stacey's condition was critical enough to warrant her being 'specialled'. She was still in her oxygen tent and the round of X-rays, physio, antibiotics and frequent observations continued. 'She did not move or open her eyes all day,' says Pauline, 'but at least she was breathing a little easier. By the time Phil came to pick me up at nine o'clock that evening I was mentally exhausted.'

Stacey was not well enough to be discharged to Carshalton for more than two weeks; it would have been even longer if she was to return to her home rather than another hospital. So, again, the 2C staff only saw Stacey when she was really ill. 'In those days we almost used to dread her coming in,' says ward sister Gill Tym. 'She was the little girl who was always going blue. It was only later that we really got to know Stacey and Mrs Tyrrill.'

Stacey spent her first birthday and her second Christmas in ward B4 at Carshalton. In one sense Christmas was like any other day for Pauline and Phil, travelling to and from a hospital. But at least Stacey had got this far. Pauline could also spend this Christmas with her two boys. Stacey had occupied so much of her time – and thoughts – that she had begun to worry about neglecting Karl and Tommy. But still, a New Year was coming when, surely, Stacey would soon be coming home? And 1980 would see Pauline and Phil free to marry at last.

The New Year began well enough. Early in January Stacey returned to Great Ormond Street to have the troublesome silastic roll removed. The surgeons also wanted to look down her windpipe and oesophagus. The larynx appeared watertight, but the oesophagus was harder to examine. X-rays later suggested that it was still partially blocked at the point where the colon transplant had been made. But this narrowing could be because the cleft larynx had meant Stacey had never used her oesophagus. She had taken all her food and drink through the gastrostomy tube into her stomach. If the larynx was now watertight, this might correct itself. When Stacey returned to Great Ormond Street, it would therefore be with the aim of removing the tracheostomy. One worry clouded this apparently improving picture. Stacey now appeared to be deaf.

Pauline says she had begun to notice a change in Stacey after that traumatic day of two operations the previous November. 'She didn't seem to hear anything any more,' says Pauline. The Carshalton surgeons asked the ENT specialists at Great Ormond Street to investigate Stacey's hearing and these confirmed her deafness. 'I had known I was right **for** quite some time, but having it confirmed that she was stone deaf made me feel very bitter,' says Pauline. 'All I could think was, why *her*! What had she done to deserve all this? How could my baby, who had fought so hard for life against all the odds, be deaf for the rest of her life? If there is a God up there, He must be very mixed up.'

Nobody knows for certain what caused the deafness. Was it the result of one of the antibiotics given to fight the chest infections? Deafness is a known side-effect of one particular drug, but the levels were monitored carefully to try and prevent this disastrous outcome. Or was it the result of Stacey's difficulties in the operating theatre on 20 November? Too little oxygen can destroy hearing. Pauline Tyrrill attributes no blame, accepting that the deafness is probably the inadvertent consequence of other measures which kept Stacey alive. Nevertheless, it was a devastating blow, particularly when attempts to use hearing aids failed. Stacey showed no response whatsoever. 'I still get very uptight over her deafness,' says Pauline, 'because I know they cannot operate to try and put it right the way they have with everything else.'

Compared to the news about Stacey's deafness, the failure to remove the trachy seemed a minor disappointment. The delay, Pauline and Phil were told, was temporary. Upon examination – Stacey's tenth visit to an operating theatre – the larynx remained watertight, but some scarred tissue was found at the site of her tracheostomy. Removing the trachy would have to be postponed. Pauline wanted to believe the doctors that all was well, yet she had her doubts: 'Great Ormond Street said Stacey could now swallow safely – she had simply lost the instinct to do so. But neither I nor the nurses at Carshalton could make her swallow and when food was put in her mouth, she didn't like the taste. She was losing weight she could ill afford to lose, so we had to go back to the gastrostomy tube in her stomach.'

The return to gastrostomy feeding and an operation to repair a hernia had swift results. Indeed, Stacey had never been better. Her parents had double cause for celebration. At the age of seventeen months Stacey was well enough to be taken home – only for an hour, but a milestone nonetheless. Then, on 20 June 1980 at Morden Register Office, Pauline and Phil were finally married. Among the guests – and rivalling the bride and groom in winning attention – was Stacey. Several nurses from Carshalton also attended. 'They had been like extra mothers to Stacey,' says Pauline. 'She was special to them, too, and they spoilt her a lot.'

The optimism did not last. By the end of July Stacey's larynx was discovered to need a further repair. This disappointed but did not surprise Pauline since in the previous few weeks Stacey had suffered repeated chest infections and attacks of breathlessness. It was a low point for Pauline and Phil. There were money worries and frequent rows. 'Everything seemed to be going wrong,' says Pauline, 'I was just about at the end of my tether. People around us had all been kind, but deep down they did not seem to realize how hard it was getting for us to be a normal family. We'd visited one hospital or the other every day for the past eighteen months.'

Even when Stacey was well enough to come home for longer periods during the day, she still dominated family life. By now Pauline was thoroughly skilled in the techniques of tracheostomy care. And as parents can recognize their own child's cry, Pauline got to know from how Stacey cried whether she needed suction. But Stacey was particularly prone to excessive secretions and frequently required suction every few minutes. The living room was full of medical gear – assorted tubes, creams, catheters, syringes, tapes, pumps and medicines. Portable suction gear and oxygen had to accompany Stacey everywhere she went and family outings were further restricted by the gastrostomy feeds. Each took forty-five minutes, at first hourly and eventually three hourly. 'I never had to look at the clock – I knew the time by the gaps between the feeds,' says Pauline.

'I tended not to go out with her that much. If I'm honest, it was too much effort carting around all the gumph and sucking out her trachy every fifteen minutes or so in the street. Even at home I always seemed to be either feeding her or sucking her out, so there wasn't much time to play. I used to give her toys to play with but she was never very interested. She followed me around the house in her baby walker and slept quite a lot. I used to get tired and depressed, but there was never a feeling of "Oh, God, I've got to do it all over again" because she was always good company. She makes you laugh.'

What with feeding, bathing and transporting Stacey to and from hospital, Pauline also had little time for the boys. 'Karl and Tommy used to go with Stacey to the hospital in the evening because they were then too young to be left. And they were dragged off there in their holidays, but they never once complained about this. They've never taken it out on Stacey, or said they resented her, although they did sometimes take it out on me,' says Pauline.

Her only break from the unrelenting pressure came on Saturdays when she did the family shopping – and at night. Years later Pauline would feel guilty about her 'failure' to keep Stacey at home overnight. 'I would take this bouncing, energetic kid back to hospital each night and feel awful about it,' she says. Few people, if any, agree. Coping with a tracheostomy tube is demanding enough, let alone a gastrostomy tube. Sue Fisher, a speech therapist at Carshalton, speaks for many: 'Pauline runs herself down, but we have all been amazed at how well she and Phil have coped. It's hard to imagine how they have managed to cope so well, let alone imagining that they could have done more.'

When you have been told that your two-day-old child has only a forty per cent chance of surviving, every birthday seems extra special. So it was with Stacey's second birthday. She was becoming a very pretty as well as a cheerful, somewhat artful little girl. Her mischievousness had almost been her undoing shortly before her birthday: she pulled the trachy out of her neck. She passed out but, luckily, she was in hospital and not at home. A tube was reinserted and she survived. Christmas, too, was not uneventful. It was to have been Stacey's first Christmas Day at home. She came home for her birthday – and celebrated it by walking unaided for the first time – but became feverish and had to return to hospital. Despite this, it was a good Christmas. Pauline and Phil were happier but, always at the back of their minds, hovered the next operation, yet another attempt to repair the cleft larynx. Would it be the last chance to get it right?

Early in the New Year, back at Great Ormond Street, Pauline and Phil watched Stacey return from the operating theatre, still partly sedated but restless. They then waited all day to see the consultant. When they did, they were in for a surprise. To John Evans, at least, it was not the last chance. If Stacey could fight so hard, who was he to give up on her? He also confessed that he did not know whether or not the repair would work. Oddly, perhaps, this declaration of fallibility by

282

the country's leading paediatric ENT surgeon struck a chord with the Tyrrills. 'We seemed to get on much better from that day,' says Pauline. 'We'd had years of promises. Maybe this would work, maybe that. Each time it didn't work it just meant more pain.'

Yet again they had been given hope. Yet again they would have to wait and see if the larynx repair had worked. Yet again they would be first encouraged and then disappointed. During the course of 1981 Stacey made three further visits to Great Ormond Street – once for a check-up which revealed no cleft, twice for check-ups which did reveal a cleft. The cleft seemed to be getting smaller so that repairs could now be attempted internally via the throat without cutting open the skin. Not that this made her post-operative care any easier. She could still change dramatically in a matter of minutes, one moment charging around the ward in a baby walker, the next gasping for breath and going blue. At Carshalton she came through a major stomach operation at Easter 1981 to stop reflux and regurgitation of stomach contents into her colon transplant, although not without the aid of a ventilator machine to assist her breathing. Again, the doctors said it was going to be a slow business. She moved to a new ward – B3 – for older children, something which heralded a new beginning and time to take stock.

Pauline and Phil were planning a week's holiday in Cornwall, their first in four years. Hospitals, and waiting for the next operation, had become a way of life – and the strain was beginning to tell. Because it seemed so unending, and so unreal, Pauline wrote an account of Stacey's life at about that time: 'I wanted to be able to remember, whatever happened.' In it she described family life:

'It affects the boys differently. Karl [the eldest] does not do well at school when Stacey is ill. He takes it all inwardly and when on the rare occasions she is well enough to come home he devotes all his time to her. Tommy gets very aggressive and bad tempered, not being really old enough to understand fully. Phil was working nights and wasn't getting much sleep. The nights I spent on my own became very depressing. I began to think we were all drifting apart and I was in the middle of it all.

I had to be the hard, strong one – the boys came to me, Phil needed more of my time. I began to wonder how much more I could take.'

It would not have provided much consolation – or help – for Pauline to have known that her problems were not untypical of families with trachy children. May Bywater is a social worker at Great Ormond Street with responsibilities for, among others, tracheostomy children. She says: 'The responsibility of looking after a trachy child can push a family to breaking point. The main burden usually falls on the mother because the father has to work. She is often up all night and is living with constant uncertainty. The trachy child needs so much attention that other children get less and the husband sometimes gets less so their relationship can suffer.' Jenny Jenkins, a psychologist at Great Ormond Street, agrees. 'We have to encourage parents to have a good, strong relationship with their sick child without allowing the child to take over to such an extent that everything else goes into abeyance.'

Pauline and Phil got their holiday in Cornwall. The weather was good and, for once, they could relax. Yet, to Pauline, the boys' enjoyment only served to underline the problems at home. 'They were so good and so different from the way they were at home that I had to admit Stacey was a bigger problem than we had realized. I could now see that the boys were beginning to resent the attention she received.' It scarcely helped when, on returning to London, Stacey showed resentment, too. 'She totally ignored us, as much as to say – why did you leave me? I've missed you! At that moment I'd have given anything to have been able to tell Stacey just why we'd left her for so long. But you can only *show* love to a deaf child. It's so hard to explain.'

These problems of communication were also causing the Carshalton hospital staff to take stock of Stacey Tyrrill. She had survived against the odds. She was going home regularly during the days. But there was no prospect of her going home for good: the hospital was therefore responsible for her development as well as her health. Stacey was consequently referred for speech therapy. This tends to conjure up an image of elocution lessons or, maybe, help for stammerers. More

accurately, it means communication therapy and its importance for trachy children has only recently been appreciated.
Debbie Sell, a speech therapist at Great Ormond Street, has
thus become an integral member of the 2C ward team along
with Jenny Jenkins, the psychologist, who helps with broader
problems of development and family relationships. Debbie Sell
says: 'Many children with tracheostomies face potentially
severe delays in their ability to communicate which can affect
other aspects of their development.'

Speech is only possible if air is expelled from the lungs
through the vocal cords in the larynx through to the mouth. A
child with a tracheostomy breathes out through the trachy tube
and so will not normally be able to speak. This condition is
called aphonia. A few children can manage to talk if the trachy
tube becomes narrower than the diameter of their growing
windpipe. This allows air to leak past the tube and reach the
vocal cords. There are also types of tracheostomies which
incorporate an inner tube with a hole allowing some air to
reach the larynx. This is called a 'speaking tube' but it is
usually made of metal, which children under four often find
difficult to tolerate. At first it did not work for Stacey Tyrrill.

In fact, Stacey presented a considerable problem for any
speech therapist. She was not merely aphonic, but deaf. She
could not, or would not, swallow. She was already two and a
half years old, an age by which she should have begun to
construct simple phrases or sentences. She had spent her entire
life in hospital and thus missed much of the social benefits of
play with other children. But she did have something going for
her, as Sue Fisher, her speech therapist at Carshalton, recalls:
'Stacey appeared to be bright, alert, without speech but very
communicative.' It was Sue Fisher's job to develop this natural
instinct to communicate in ways other than speech.

'I saw her three times a week to develop some sign language.
There was also one session a week to teach ward staff and also
to teach parents. Everyone was terribly enthusiastic. The ward
staff took it seriously and Pauline stood no nonsense, telling
her family that they had all got to do it. A whole lot of them
attended evening classes in sign language. Stacey was so little
and cute, so winning, that this made people determined to do

their best to help. She wasn't at all resistant to sign language. In fact, she had begun to develop her own gestures. She loved it because she could go and be rude – or cheeky rather – to people. The ward sister sometimes caught her standing behind a doctor doing the sign for pig! We also half-regretted teaching her the sign for stupid because she'd run all over the ward doing it. But it made us realize how bright she was.'

Where Sue Fisher was less successful, however, was in trying to help Stacey eat food orally. Speech therapists are involved in feeding problems because these involve tongue movements and the mechanics of swallowing. In Stacey's case, Sue Fisher tried to develop a sense of taste by giving her lollies to suck or by smearing jam on bricks when she was at the sucking stage of play. It never worked and the constant battles over feeding began to stir some resentment at Carshalton. What was happening over the larynx problem? Would it ever be resolved?

In two years Stacey only went to Great Ormond Street twice. Each time the larynx repair broke down. John Evans thought that time and natural growth might make a permanent repair easier. But as the months, years, dragged by Stacey's parents became exasperated by the delay. Pauline thought it was time for a second opinion and, after much perseverance, she took Stacey to the Brompton Hospital in West London. It was the fourth hospital in Stacey's life and she was a month short of her fourth birthday. 'Phil would take things as they came but I wasn't prepared to wait for doctors to call her in when it suited them. They might want to wait a year but I wasn't to know that next year would ever come for Stacey. I had to do all I could in the time we had, just in case the worst happened,' says Pauline.

Pauline had pushed hard for the Brompton because another child from Carshalton, with apparently similar breathing problems to those of Stacey, had improved dramatically after treatment there. This did not happen for Stacey and Brompton confirmed that Great Ormond Street was the only place likely to succeed in healing the cleft larynx. However, Brompton did achieve one significant success. Dr John Warner, one of its consultants, fitted Stacey with a 'speaking tube' type of tracheostomy. It would not help her speak, because of the damaged larynx, but Dr Warner thought it might enable her to cough up mucus. Such a tube had been fitted at Great Ormond Street without success. This time, perhaps because she was older and bigger, Stacey was able to tolerate it. Within a few days, her chest infections began to diminish.

For two years or so something approaching stability reigned in Stacey's life as the Great Ormond Street team waited to see if growth would help to solve her problems. They were not, however, easy years for her parents. Two miscarriages intensified the stresses, especially for Phil who blamed himself for the problems. As Stacey got better, the rows at home became worse. Only over Stacey was the family united. Hospital staff continued to confess their admiration for Stacey and her parents. Dr Warner at the Brompton, for instance, wrote that Pauline and Phil had 'coped magnificently with Stacey ... who is obviously an intelligent child'. Sue Fisher, the speech therapist at Carshalton, says: 'We couldn't have done what we have done without the support of the family. There were so many different people involved — different hospitals and later different education authorities — that Pauline used to chivvy us to make sure things got done. Quite rightly, she wouldn't let us treat her as "just the Mum". She knew more about Stacey's problems than most of us.'

An educational assessment shortly before her fourth birthday rated Stacey not far behind other children and her language was good compared to other deaf children. But her concentration was poor; she was too easily distracted. She also lacked experience of playing with other children. For a time her favourite playthings were hospital tubes, syringes and other equipment – it was all she had really known. She joined sessions at the hospital with mentally handicapped children, largely to learn how to play. Nobody was very happy about this as a long-term prospect. 'Stacey was out-stripping all of us in sign language,' says Sue Fisher.

The problem was resolved by one of the few instances of unmitigated good fortune to occur in Stacey's life: the opening of a special unit for children with hearing difficulties at Green Wrythe Lane primary school, less than half a mile from her parent's home. She was luckier still to find in Ann Pascoe a teacher willing to take on a child who was not only deaf but dependent upon a tracheostomy. Many playgroups and schools are reluctant to take trachy children.

At first Pauline stayed with Stacey all day, not just in case there were problems with the trachy but also to feed her. Feeding Stacey was invariably traumatic. Doctors wanted Pauline to persist with oral feeding in the belief that only by using the repaired foodpipe would it stretch to normal size. So each day she would sit for an hour or more coaxing her daughter to swallow mashed-up food. Stacey used all her developing wiles to avoid eating. She would cry, grimace, cough, even appear to choke and wave her hands to plead that this apparent torture should end. Yet seconds later, distracted by something in the classroom, she would be laughing and happy. 'It makes you feel so cruel,' says Ann Pascoe who eventually took over the lunchtime feeds from Pauline. It could also be extremely messy. 'I used to go home looking like someone's dinner,' says Pauline.

Mealtimes were a daily battle and, ultimately, unsuccessful. Stacey did not eat enough to manage without three night-time 'feeds' via the gastrostomy tube – and this, on top of the frequent suction, was why she continued to sleep overnight at the hospital in Carshalton. 'I feel I copped out badly,' says Pauline, 'but there was no way I could look after her twenty-four hours a day as well as the boys. I felt guilty, partly because at the back of my mind was still the fear of getting up in the morning and finding she wasn't alive. If it happened in hospital, it wouldn't be your fault. The first time Stacey did sleep at home – on the night of her fifth birthday – it was so nerve-racking I stayed awake all night. She slept on a sofa downstairs. She didn't have her own bedroom. It was as though Stacey didn't exist.'

Stacey only began to sleep at home regularly when she was six years and nine months old. She did so then in preparation for an attempt to remove her trachy – more than six years after it had been inserted rather than the six months which had first been mentioned. The previous twelve months had seen a marked increase in the number of visits paid by Stacey to Great Ormond Street. Between May 1982 and September

1984 she had been there only twice; in the following twelve months she had been admitted on no fewer than eight occasions. These were mostly for checks on the state of her larynx. The cleft definitely appeared to be smaller, small enough to be tackled within the windpipe without cutting through the skin. Not that this spared Stacey a visit to the operating theatre. Each endoscopic repair, as it is called, and each internal microscopic examination requires a full anaesthetic. Stacey also developed tonsillitis during this period so the tonsils were later removed. But, at long long last, the cleft appeared healed.

Initially neither Stacey nor Pauline had felt at home at Great Ormond Street, compared to the more familiar surroundings of Carshalton. However, the frequent visits not only transformed their feelings but had made Stacey a firm favourite among the nursing staff on 2C. Gone was the sickly infant who was 'always going blue'. Now an effervescent six-year-old scampered around the ward playing with the other children. 'You often forgot Stacey was deaf,' says ward play-leader Joey Fox. 'Other children didn't seem to know or care because she was so good at communicating through gestures.'

The nurses particularly admired Pauline Tyrrill's combination of patience and firmness. 'A lot of trachy mums would let their children get away with everything, but not Mrs Tyrrill,' says nurse Carol Mason. Pauline can sound quite tough with Stacey, particularly as she cajoles her into eating an unappealing mishmash of mince, peas and potatoes. She says: 'Stacey gets a lot of attention in hospital. She's quite an actress and turns on the charm, but I don't want her growing into a precocious little brat. So, if she's naughty, I tell her off like you would a normal child because, to me, she is a normal child.'

Teachers at the hospital school also noted changes in Stacey. Angela Bell was one who would visit the ward with her 'school in a basket' — a collection of educational games and materials for drawing and writing. She says: 'Stacey wanted to learn and, although she was still easily distracted, her application to school work was better.' Music teacher Fran Flynn organized sessions with other children who would clap, stamp, march and generally make a vaguely tuneful noise. Although deaf, Stacey learned how to keep in time with the rest of the group, partly by watching others and partly through a natural sense of vibration. 'She seemed more able to enjoy the sessions, more able to succeed, more aware of what was required and more able to laugh at herself and the activity,' says Fran Flynn.

The countdown to removing the trachy began at home, long before she arrived at Great Ormond Street. The tracheostomy tube was blocked to see if she could manage to breathe normally through her throat – at first by day and then also overnight at Carshalton. Breathing through the larynx is three times more difficult, in terms of airway resistance, but Stacey was able to cope. After almost seven years at Carshalton, Pauline therefore decided it was time for Stacey to come home – for good she hoped.

Trachies are normally removed without a visit to the operating theatre. And so, shortly after the doctors' regular ward round at eight-thirty one September morning, Stacey's trachy was simply pulled out by ward sister Gill Tym. A dressing was put over the hole and the job was done. Stacey ran off to the ward playroom. Here Pauline saw her moulding some play dough when she arrived a few minutes later. 'It was as though she had completely forgotten about it. She said it had hurt a bit, then carried on playing. I had wanted to be there for that moment when they did it. I really wanted to shout and say "For Christ's sake, we have really got there," but there was no one to share it with.'

It is always an emotional moment for any parent, however long the wait. The longed-for achievement therefore constitutes a high point in ward life. Other parents at earlier stages of living with a trachy will draw encouragement from each success. 'It's the best part of my job,' says Gill Tym. Frequently it is a time for tears and Sister Tym could see that Pauline Tyrrill was close to weeping. Pauline agrees: 'It had been so long coming that when it was taken out it was like winning the pools. I felt like crying, but that wouldn't be tough little me. Not many people have seen me cry.'

The veneer of toughness also spelled caution. There had been so many setbacks in Stacey's life that Pauline was reluctant to believe the trachy had gone for good. She would wait and hope. Stacey coped well without the trachy and did not

need humidification at night. But, twice, bad nights with difficult breathing and a temperature delayed her discharge home.
Her swallowing problems were now emerging as the greatest
obstacle to full health. Until Stacey could eat normally, she
would be dependent upon the gastrostomy tube for at least the
night-time feeding.

It had always been hard for medical staff to establish how
genuine were the swallowing problems. So much seemed to
depend upon Stacey's moods. One way of checking was to
arrange a 'barium swallow'. This is a process used by the X-ray
department to record the movement of a liquid through the
body. The drink looks (and tastes) rather like a strawberry
milk shake but contains barium, a radio-opaque substance
visible on X-rays. In Stacey's case it showed no problems with
the larynx but suggested a slight narrowing or kink in the
oesophagus at the point where the colon transplant had been
made six years earlier. If this did not correct itself with use, it
might have to be dilated or stretched, which would mean
another operation with a full anaesthetic – and the anaesthetist
might have to put a ventilating tube down a windpipe still
scarred by the recent presence of a tracheostomy tube. As this
could conceivably damage the windpipe, the dilation would
have to wait. Try it too soon and the trachy might have to go
back in.

For the first time, Stacey left Great Ormond Street for
home rather than another hospital. For the first time 'home'
became her way of life rather than a place to visit or to stay at
occasionally. The electric suction pump and other tracheostomy gear were pushed to the side, but the neat house still had
corners which looked like a chemist's shop. A drawer under
Stacey's bed was filled with creams and tubes for her gastrostomy tube; a shelf in the living room near an aquarium held
the daytime supplies. Each night Pauline had to feed Stacey
through the gastrostomy tube, relying on a three a.m. call from
a relative's minicab business to wake her. ('What the guy
thinks about this strange woman who likes to be woken at
three in the morning, I've no idea.')

Stacey returned to school after half-term, proudly showing
off the small scar on her neck where the trachy had been. She

was well enough now to play in the playground with the rest of the pupils disappearing in the throng like any other active child. She also started school dinners, but eating remained a battle. For her parents, once again, the hope prospect of further surgery threatened – this time to dilate the foodpipe. Pauline and Phil knew this had to be done, but they wanted life to settle down at home. John Evans, the ENT surgeon at Great Ormond Street, was less willing to wait.

When he saw Stacey as an out-patient he asked her to breathe deeply which – after Pauline had translated this into sign language – she did with Chaplinesque flourishes. Having asked how the feeding was going, the surgeon said it was time to attempt the dilation. Her breathing appeared to be fine: she should be able to cope with the anaesthetic. As the surgeon and her parents talked, Stacey appeared to be playing but she knew exactly what was at stake. When the adults stopped talking, she turned to her mother and pointed to the gastrostomy tube. You didn't need sign language to know that she was asking if it could come out. 'Not yet,' replied Mr Evans with a smile, 'not yet – but soon if we can sort out the swallowing.' 'Not until you start eating properly,' was Pauline's somewhat liberal, if characteristically firm, translation.

Shortly before Christmas Stacey returned to Great Ormond Street. More than two months had passed since the trachy was removed, but it still seemed worryingly quick to her parents. Stacey sensed the anxiety. When Pauline told her that tomorrow she'd be going to the operating theatre, Stacey immediately became agitated. She pointed to the scar on her neck where the trachy had been and shook her head vigorously. 'No, no,' replied Pauline. 'The doctor wants to see why you're not swallowing. He's not going to put the trachy back.' The surgeons planned to probe the oesophagus or foodpipe to establish the extent of any blockage. The process is called an oesophagoscopy and, if a blockage or narrowing was found, the oesophagus would then be dilated or stretched. And that, fingers firmly crossed, would be all.

It turned out to be a morning of surprises. To a non-medical person, the surprise was the discovery that a rigid twelve inch metal tube could disappear down anybody's throat, let alone that of a child's. Never again would the performances of circus sword-swallowers seem quite so astonishing. To the surgeons, the surprise was that there appeared to be no blockage of the oesophagus at all. First the rigid endoscopic tube was eased thirty centimetres (twelve inches) down Stacey's oesophagus and then a flexible, fibre-optic tube went thirty-five centimetres deep. Looking down the tubes the surgeons found some food deposits and lots of mucus lining the oesophagus; but they had reached the stomach without any blockage. The suspect junction where the colon transplant had been made was anatomically sound.

At lunchtime, after completing his morning's operations, consultant John Evans toured the ward to tell parents what had happened. 'The good news,' he told Pauline and Phil Tyrrill, 'is that there is no physical obstruction so we didn't have to dilate the foodpipe.' Pauline's relief that Stacey would not need the dilation was tinged with mild regret however: if there had been an obstruction, it would have explained the feeding difficulties and its removal would offer the hope of a quick improvement. Mr Evans offered no such prospect. He said: 'Stacey obviously has some difficulty in the mechanics of swallowing, but this should sort itself out naturally with practice and in time.'

In other words, there appeared to be nothing more that he could do. Stacey (and her parents) would simply have to persevere in the hope that feeding would eventually become easier. Pauline was sceptical: 'I'll believe it when it happens. Stacey has been eating orally for a year and, if anything, it's got worse since the trachy came out.' Still, she emphasized the doctor's verdict to Stacey: 'The doctor says you can eat normally.' And, despite the somewhat quizzical look she received from her daughter, Pauline decided to cut back the gastrostomy feeds, beginning – to no one's surprise – with the one at three a.m. 'I'll just hope that by giving her less by night she'll get hungry enough to eat more by day,' she says.

There is no doubt that Stacey would love to be rid of her gastrostomy tube. Often sore, it curbs her ability to play games or sports. She loves running and horse-riding, but gymnastics and swimming pose some risks until all her tubes have gone.

But at least Stacey could prepare for her birthday and Christmas without the shadow of further operations. She would have to return to 2C for the trachy hole to be closed surgically, but by her standards this is minor indeed. Otherwise she will simply be an out-patient.

Her seventh birthday and her eighth Christmas were the most normal she had ever known. As soon as she saw the decorations go up, she asked (in sign language): is it my birthday today? Her presents included a Cabbage Patch doll which goes everywhere with her and for which Stacey insisted on buying nappies. 'Each night she takes the doll to bed and says – "Ooh, it smells", so we have to change its nappy,' says Pauline. It was also the most normal Christmas which Pauline had known since Stacey was born. Previously, when Stacey had been well enough to come home, Pauline stayed awake with her all night to ensure she didn't have any difficulty breathing. This time she got a night's sleep, more or less. There was still the midnight gastrostomy feed and Stacey's general excitement kept her perky long after everyone else flagged. And yet a cloud hung over the celebrations. Pauline and Phil were drifting apart. Phil had got promotion – he is now a foreman in a building firm – and was increasingly preoccupied by work. As Stacey got better, the rows at home got worse – never over Stacey, but often over Pauline's children from her first marriage. The family were together for Stacey's birthday and for Christmas, but the strains rarely disappeared far from the surface.

It has been a long, hard road for the Tyrrills. They have got further than they often dared to hope. And they have a daughter who, without saying a word, is invariably the centre of attraction. She oozes charm – if she wants to. She is cute – without being coy or winsome. She is bright – although Pauline worries that she is falling seriously behind at school. Although her larynx has been repaired, Stacey still cannot speak; the delicate vocal cords have sustained too much damage over too long a period. Stacey's future, unlikely to be easy, will probably involve a boarding school for deaf children which would separate mother and child more than hospitals ever did. Even this may depend upon successfully ending all the gastrostomy feeds. And although Stacey was eating more – and more quickly – her weight began to fall after Christmas. It was another worry which Pauline Tyrrill faced effectively alone, spurning tranquillizers, somewhat resenting Phil's freedom yet retaining the spirited determination that served Stace, as she calls her, so well.

'Doctors have said you look sad or depressed, would you like some Valium? But tablets are not going to make problems any easier or take them away. I find time hangs heavily on my hands now. I haven't got to go to a hospital. I haven't got to go to the school. I haven't got so many feeds or any suction to do. If I go out on my own I feel like I have lost something. You put so much into her she becomes your life. Looking back, I don't know how I managed to do so much and I do not seem to be coping as well now as I did when she was really ill. I've had to be stubborn and tough for Stacey's sake but being hard doesn't make you much fun to be with. I get angry with myself for shouting at the boys if things go wrong. Basically, I suppose I'm just fed up with things going wrong. I don't understand why it was less of a strain on our marriage when things were really bad than it is now.

'I do not know how I would cope if I lost Stace. I suppose it is more frightening to think of her dying now or dying unexpectedly. Perhaps subconsciously I am still listening to hear her breathing, but as she gets better you don't tend to worry so much. You ease off. You don't expect trouble. Life starts to be normal, although it is at the back of your mind that something might go wrong. I have worried myself sick about her losing weight, for instance, and the possibility that there may be something else wrong.'

According to the doctors who have successfully healed one of the rarest of abnormalities – her cleft larynx – time will resolve Stacey's feeding problems. Maybe time and relative normality will also heal the strains within the Tyrrill family which were wrought by seven years of unrelenting pressure. At least Stacey's irrepressible spirit appears unaffected by the difficulties of the family around her. Pauline says: 'There were times when we wondered whether Stacey would ever come home. Well, she's made it. And if something did happen to her now, I could say that she has made people laugh a lot. I think she will probably go through life like that – for all her problems.'

Postscript: one year later
She has had a reasonable year. She still doesn't eat well or easily, but she is eating without any tubes and has put on weight. She still has regular check-ups at various out-patient clinics, but her education is becoming the major worry; if extra help cannot be provided by her local school, she may have to go to a boarding school for deaf children. The highlight of her year was presenting a bouquet to the Queen.

4.00 p.m. *Deadline time in the milk kitchen. With so many of the patients under one year old the dietitians and their staff are responsible for preparing about 500 milk feeds for an average of around a hundred children a day. This is more complicated than it may sound; there are about thirty-five different ingredients used at any time. The evening and night-time feeds must be ready by four o'clock for distribution to the wards. The dietitians must also devise special meals for around thirty children a day. These are produced by their own staff in the diet kitchen. This kitchen also produces so-called 'sterile' meals – ordinary food prepared separately in clean conditions for children at risk from infection. Many of the conditions treated at Great Ormond Street require complicated (and often expensive) diets so the dietitians have to produce attractive meals which contain sufficient protein, calories, minerals and vitamins for the child to grow without, say, the ingredients to which children may be allergic. Diets need to be tailored to an individual's age, height and weight and often involve a range of ingredients calculated and measured to decimal point accuracy. When a child goes home such precision is often impractical so the dietitians suggest diets which meet the medical needs in such a way that the child can be managed at home and if possible eat with the rest of the family. This is particularly important for conditions like PKU which will involve many years' adherence to a strict diet and Dorothy Francis, the chief dietitian and one of the world's acknowledged authorities on paediatric dietary problems, will spend many hours teaching families how to cope with their child's complex dietary regime.*

4.10 p.m. *Philip Ransley, the urology consultant surgeon, sees his twelfth patient of the afternoon clinic: one-year-old Joseph has hypospadias, a malformation in which the urethra (which carries urine from the bladder) opens on the underside of the penis. The baby is very well otherwise and the repair will be straightforward. Joseph's mother asks what caused the condition and whether she can do anything to avoid it happening again if she has another child. Mr Ransley tells her that no one really has the answer to her questions. The latest theory is that while the baby is still in the womb he puts his foot in the wrong place while the penis is developing. There is a waiting list for the operation, but he* *promises to try and tackle Joseph's repair before too long. If at all possible, he avoids operating when a child is between eighteen months and three years because this is such a difficult age to win a child's co-operation.*

In all Mr Ransley sees fifteen children, some with urological problems or renal failure which require surgical investigations, one or two with abnormal genitalia, one a little girl born with two closed bladders. He operated on the girl when she was new-born and she is making such good progress that her parents are beginning potty training. This kind of reconstructive surgery is one of the most exciting parts of the work, but other cases are less dramatic and may involve long-term follow-up. To two sets of parents Mr Ransley suggests they try a diet which eliminates tartrazine – a red and yellow colouring found in many foods – from the child's diet to improve general behaviour, irritability and possibly bedwetting.

4.30 p.m. *Anne Carlisle, the accommodation officer, is rung by a ward sister to see if there is a bed for a mother whose child has been admitted as an emergency from an out-patient clinic. There is no bed available this late in the day but, luckily, somebody agrees to leave a day early. Otherwise Mrs Carlisle would have to ring round her list of local hotels, but this is unsuitable if a child is really ill and the ward may have to contact the mother during the night. Since she was appointed, Anne Carlisle has increased the number of beds available by substituting bunks for single beds, even though this does make the rooms more crowded. Rarely does she have empty beds and there are usually several parents sleeping on camp beds in waiting rooms or playrooms. The standard of the accommodation varies: some is cheerful and nicely decorated – thanks to private donations – but other rooms can be cold in winter. Most parents are grateful to be put up inside the hospital near the child and don't complain; most are also considerate and supportive to each other, although inevitably there is the odd one who creates a disturbance. Priority goes to mothers who are pregnant, breast-feeding or where the child is under five, but the main factor is the seriousness of the child's condition.*

4.45 p.m. *Mrs Caroline Bond convenes the monthly meeting of the board of governors for the two Hospitals for Sick Children –*

Great Ormond Street and the Queen Elizabeth Hospital in the East End of London. Together the hospitals form what is known as a special health authority which means that they do not come under a regional health authority but are directly answerable to (and funded by) the Department of Health and Social Security. This status recognizes the role of Great Ormond Street as a specialist centre serving a far wider catchment area than any one region of the country. It also reflects the research role of the Institute of Child Health to which the hospital is closely linked. There are twenty members of the board and they sit around a large conference table with about a dozen senior hospital employees, doctors and nursing officers as well as administrators. The board, too, is composed of lay and medical members with the former chairing sub-committees which appoint consultants and which hear staff appeals against dismissals.

Mrs Bond became chairman of the board in 1982, succeeding Mrs Audrey Callaghan, the wife of the former Labour Prime Minister. A former ward sister (although not at Great Ormond Street) Mrs Bond spends on average three days a fortnight at Great Ormond Street, usually queuing up in the canteen at lunchtime with the rest of the staff. She conducts the board meeting with grace yet firmness. The first half of the meeting is open to the public and press, although few outsiders usually attend. In this open session board members hear of administrative overspending (largely due to the need to hire agency telephonists because basic pay is too low, explains the treasurer); a new complaints procedure; the temporary acquisition of a neighbouring building to provide office accommodation during future rebuilding; the implications of the departures of the two hospital administrators; the report of an organ transplant working party (kidney transplants yes, heart transplants maybe – in the future); and the need for a second paediatric dermatology consultant.

Afterwards, Mrs Bond said it was a pretty dull meeting, no real fireworks or arguments. The only real passion flared over the discovery that building works at Queen Elizabeth had caused the closure of twenty beds at its busiest time of the year – winter. To make matters worse, sick children could not be transferred to Great Ormond Street because beds were closed here owing to insufficient money to pay enough nurses. The explanation that the building *work had to take place before the end of the financial year was accepted somewhat reluctantly. 'To have to close beds for financial matters is just terribly wrong, especially as we all know that the pressure on the beds at Queen Elizabeth is in the winter months,'* says Mrs Bond. Nobody disagrees.

5.00 p.m. *The evening shift of cleaners arrive. There are around 160 domestic staff, but if there are vacancies they are likely to be on the evening shift. The low wages make it hard to get regular workers for evening work. It is also hard to clean old buildings, especially with so much equipment overflowing into corridors. Special extra-powerful vacuum cleaners are used for all patient areas including intensive care wards, operating theatres and the TPN suite. Each ward has its own cleaner (or domestic assistant as they're officially called) and on many wards the cleaner is very much part of the ward team and gets to know the parents as well as the children.*

5.30 p.m. *Phyl Howard and Della Boyd load a three-tier trolley with sweets, crisps, toiletries, stationery and books. Both are volunteers and Phyl has been taking the trolley round the wards one day a week for seven years. She likes the feeling of going right through the hospital and knows that for many parents, as well as children, the evening trolley round offers a welcome diversion. Occasionally a parent will buy an armload of sweets. Phyl and Della are among a hundred people who work regularly at the hospital as volunteers. They help playleaders, escort children from admission to wards, serve in the hospital shop, act as interpreters and run the hospital radio station which was due to go on the air shortly. Many are people whose children were once patients and want to show some gratitude in a practical way. Most are women, but few accord with the image of do-gooders. There are also young men looking to broaden their experience before starting careers in childcare or community services.*

6.00 p.m. *Derek Bacon, the hospital chaplain, begins the service of compline in the chapel. It is described as 'short, simple prayer for the day's end, valued by those who are wearied by the changes of this fleeting world'. Reverend Bacon is one of three chaplains, but the only one who is resident in the hospital. For six days a week –*

Saturday is the day off – he is on call. A softly spoken man, he will frequently be called by wards to talk to parents whose child is critically ill or possibly dying. He also attends many ward meetings and provides a lay view on the hospital's ethical committee. This is one of the more important hospital committees, especially for an institution at the frontiers of medical research. It vets proposed changes in treatment to try and ensure that the interests of the children are not subordinated to those of research; it is a difficult and delicate balance to achieve but this committee ensures that the hospital never forgets its motto – 'The child, first and always'.

Kristie

Even before she was born Kristie McWilliam was destined to become a Great Ormond Street baby. She is the victim of a rare and eventually fatal condition for which the only treatment is a bone marrow transplant. She was to be the youngest-ever patient to receive a transplant at the hospital, from the healthy bone marrow of one of her parents. For months she would live in the protective isolation of a plastic bubble while doctors treated her with techniques which were at the very frontiers of medical research.

Her parents held the key to Kristie's illness. Although at first unknown to them, Steve McWilliam and Debbie Morgan are both carriers of a rare recessive gene – called recessive because it only transmits its characteristics if both parents share the same gene. The chances of two such people meeting and having children are fantastically against the odds. But in Steve and Debbie's case, any child born to them would have a one in four chance of being stricken by Severe Combined Immune Deficiency (SCID) – a fatal congenital illness in which the baby lacks the immunological mechanisms for producing the white blood cells vital to fighting off infection. Steve and Debbie had already lost one child and the events which were to bring them and their daughter to Great Ormond Street began during the previous year with the birth and short life of Kristie's brother, Daniel.

To say that Steve and Debbie are young, unemployed and unmarried – which was the first, somewhat unpromising, description which the medical and social worker team at Great Ormond Street had of them – does not do justice to them. They are quick-witted and outgoing, generous and sensitive to other people. Steve, slight and fair, was only twenty-one when Kristie was born, and Debbie, dark and pretty, was three years younger. Their relationship, though it was to be tested by the boredom, anxiety and confinement of months spent living at

Great Ormond Street, was stable. Both had enthusiastically taken to parenthood when Daniel McWilliam was born in Liverpool on 4 July 1984.

Typically – for a SCID baby — Danny seemed normal at birth; he was born at full term weighing 3.9 kg ($8^1/_2$ lb). He was a hauntingly attractive baby with large eyes and fine features. There was no reason to suppose that there was anything wrong with him and both parents welcomed him with open arms. In the absence of a job, Steve threw all his energies into fatherhood and Debbie, a warm-hearted and very feminine girl, had always wanted babies. Although they had decided that 'marriage was just a bit of paper', the couple had known each other for four years. They had set up home in a renovated Housing Association property in Wallasey in the same street as Debbie's family; Debbie is close to her family and she has aunties and grannies who are uninhibited Liverpool characters. Steve's mother was also a frequent visitor. Capable and likeable, Steve has worked at several casual trades – in a garage, in a second-hand shop, on building sites and fitting kitchens. But living on Merseyside has produced in him a fatalistic acceptance of the lack of permanent jobs. Debbie has an O Level in Biology but, also a product of the depressed climate in which she grew up, did not consider any career except raising a family.

Debbie loved being pregnant and Daniel's arrival went well. But soon she became convinced that there was something wrong. From birth Daniel had problems feeding and although the midwife said not to worry, he was constantly being sick, sometimes with projectile (or forcible) vomiting. During the two weeks that Debbie and Steve had him home they were constantly to-ing and fro-ing to their GP. He could not perceive any specific problems, though Debbie's instincts insisted that all was not as it should be. Daniel continued to lose weight. He was admitted to the isolation ward of the local maternity hospital where he had been born and then transferred to Alder Hey Hospital, a regional paediatric centre in Liverpool, a couple of bus rides (or a bus ride and a ferry) from where Steve and Debbie live.

Here Daniel was put on to naso-gastric feeding and tests

were started. At this tense time his weight had dropped from his birth weight to 3.4 kg (7lb 7oz). It seemed to his parents that the doctors did not know what was wrong with Daniel nor how to treat him, and that not enough was being done. Debbie's Mum came with them and she insisted on answers from the hospital. Daniel had thrush – a fungal infection – and a lung infection. After a while he gained weight, though he kept picking up infection after infection. 'They told us,' remembers Steve, 'that they were going to send his blood off to London. It was for something extremely rare. Of course it came back positive. Then we finally knew what was wrong.'

Although his parents came to the hospital every day, willing and praying for him to make it, and although he was in the hands of a specialist unit, the baby himself lacked the most basic defences against illness. He had been diagnosed as immuno-deficient: his body could not make the white blood cells necessary to fight infection. These cells are produced by the bone marrow where they begin life as primitive, multi-potential 'stem' cells. Some mature to function as cells known as macrophages which will absorb or eat up bacteria while others are able to recognize and kill cells infected by viruses. Yet another group of white blood cells produce proteins, known as antibodies, after contact with an infection, which a normal person keeps in their blood to provide long-term immunity. All these defences were missing in Danny.

It was hard for Steve and Debbie to begin to understand this complex illness. Immunology is a fairly new science which even non-specialist doctors find difficult; SCID itself was only recognized in the late 1960s. Debbie sat in Wallasey Public Library attempting to read up on genetics. But just at this point, when the diagnosis had been made and the Alder Hey doctors had begun to consider transferring Danny to London, his chest infection got worse. Debbie spent the day with him; part of the time he seemed fine and smiled at her, so she went home. But by the time Steve arrived to spend the night there, Danny had been rushed into intensive care. 'I could tell by what they said it was bad, and I thought, how much worse is it going to get? They told us his chances were fifty-fifty.' Steve hurriedly summoned Debbie and her parents by phone. 'We were just waiting and waiting; Danny was on all these machines.'

Daniel McWilliam died on 2 October. He had lived just ninety days. His short life had been, in fact, typical of a SCID baby. Family history is important in diagnosing SCID for often there are early and unexplained deaths of infants in the family, perhaps put down as cot deaths. The babies look normal at birth and at first have some immunity from their mothers; but gradually they succumb to a variety of infections. They may develop diarrhoea and be treated for gastro-enteritis or simply thought to be 'failing to thrive'; however, without the root cause being suspected, they become progressively weaker and more vulnerable to infection. The only cure for the condition is a successful bone marrow transplant which will provide the baby with the crucial stem cells which develop into white blood cells. Today, as the condition becomes better known, a diagnosis of SCID is more likely to be suggested earlier. It can be confirmed by a simple blood test and also when the baby is still in the womb through amniocentesis. Because of this Daniel's death was to give Kristie her great advantage, for the early, pre-natal diagnosis would identify the baby for treatment before repeated infections had taken their toll.

After Daniel's death, an Alder Hey paediatrician explained to Steve and Debbie for the first time the nature of the illness, how they both carried the gene which caused the condition, and how there was a one in four chance that any future children they might have would be affected. He suggested that they visit Guy's Hospital in London, for further tests and in January 1985 Steve and Debbie had an interview there. It was explained how tests could be done in a future pregnancy by analysing foetal cells obtained at amniocentesis to determine if the child was affected.

As it turned out, Debbie was rapidly pregnant again and in May she returned to London – this time to King's College Hospital – for an amniocentesis test in which a sample of the amniotic fluid which surrounds the baby in the womb is taken and tested. The test was done when Debbie was about sixteen weeks pregnant but the results, which did not come through until four weeks later, were not a hundred per cent clear.

Debbie recalls being told that the fluid had become blood-stained from an earlier threatened miscarriage, which allowed a small element of doubt to creep in about whether this baby was a SCID baby, too. She remembers that there was a ten per cent chance that the baby was all right, but the Great Ormond Street doctors say the chance was much smaller. The result of the test had been telephoned to her by the maternity hospital where Daniel had been born and Debbie says she was asked: 'When are you going to have an abortion?'

Termination is never a comfortable option and, at this late stage of twenty weeks, can be an appalling experience to go through emotionally and physically. The intensely maternal Debbie found herself unable to accept the prospect. It was an emotional decision but Debbie decided that, given the slight doubt about the certainty of the test, she would carry the baby through to the end of the pregnancy 'to give it the extra chance'. Her decision was at odds with the position of the doctors. They would not influence the choice of the parents, but they would not have performed an amniocentesis, which carries a slight risk of miscarriage, without an understanding that should the results be positive, the pregnancy would be terminated. It is pointless, otherwise, to have the test and expose what could be a normal baby to that risk. (Pre-natal diagnosis of SCID has now been developed by the Institute of Child Health as a service for most of Europe; they are close to perfecting a test which can be done in the first three months of pregnancy.)

Kristie was born on 24 October 1985 in the same maternity hospital as her brother fifteen months earlier. On that foggy night they could hardly see the bonnet of Debbie's mother's car as they rushed to get to hospital in time. To Steve the baby seemed blue at first and it was a long time before she cried. She was a good weight, 3.9 kg ($8\frac{1}{2}$ lb) like Daniel, but also rather like her brother she didn't seem to like being picked up and handled. The day after she was born the last element of doubt was removed: Kristie was tested for SCID and found to be positive. Debbie, perhaps unrealistically, had been clinging to that small chance of a normal result but now 'that little bit of hope was gone'. As Steve took in the news he felt: 'Here we go, here comes the battle.' They knew that Kristie was on her way to Great Ormond Street for a bone marrow transplant; they also knew that one of them would be the donor of the healthy marrow she needed to survive.

Most of the SCID children born in Britain are referred to Professor Roland Levinsky of the Institute of Child Health, which is closely linked to Great Ormond Street. A tall and imposing figure, he came to London from South Africa at sixteen to go to medical school, became a paediatrician and via an interest in kidney disease became involved in the problems of immunity; he now heads the Department of Immunology at the Institute and is also a consultant at the hospital. For the previous four years before Kristie's arrival at Great Ormond Street, his team had been perfecting the techniques of treating SCID children with bone marrow from 'mismatched' donors and this would be the type of transplant which Kristie would have.

The first condition for ensuring a successful transplant is to choose the donor carefully. From the very first bone marrow transplants which were carried out in the 1960s, it was clear how vital was the closeness of the match between donor and recipient. The first successful transplants were carried out between identical twins. For the transplant to 'take' – or not to be rejected — donor and recipient must be as compatible as possible, within the same genetically determined tissue type groups. Each person's tissue type is inherited from their father and mother and there is a one in four chance that two siblings will be an almost identical match. Transplants carried out for SCID in these circumstances are almost invariably successful.

But the small families in Western society and the plight of children with no normal brothers or sisters mean that the parents are the next best choice of donor. The chances of finding a match outside the immediate family are logistically difficult; hence the research programme to enhance the prospects of these 'mismatched' transplants, which use a new technique to treat the marrow so that it will be accepted. The results have been very encouraging, but not all aspects are yet fully understood; for instance one group of transplants did not take and the doctors do not know the reason why. 'The parents have to accept that what we do is not foolproof. We offer them the chance of a cure, but at the same time we point out that our results are not a hundred per cent, though they are improving all the time. They go into the transplant understanding all that,' says Roland Levinsky. The risks are high because these children are already seriously ill and because the transplant itself carries risks.

At first, until the transplant has taken, the child has no immunity from infection at all. So he or she must go into protective isolation inside a cubicle until tests have shown that the bone marrow has 'engrafted' and begun to produce sufficient white blood cells in the recipient. The isolation period may last weeks or months so that all the stress of confinement is added to anxieties about the illness. The problems are severe: both for the parents, who will have to endure a long, tense hospitalization and for the doctors, who still have major conceptual advances to make and who find it distressing and discouraging when they fail to save these children. Yet the risks and setbacks, and even the tragedies for individual families, have to be seen within the context of these fatal illnesses: SCID children have no future at all without a transplant and they do not often have a matched sibling donor. Until the success of the mismatched transplants, which have only come about since 1982, a child like Kristie would have been sent home to die. The other groups of illnesses in which bone marrow transplants have given promising results are also life-threatening.

Great Ormond Street transplanted more than a hundred children in the first half of the 1980s. The largest group were leukaemia patients under the care of haematology consultant Dr Judith Chessells, and here the results have been very encouraging, particularly in those types of leukaemia where chemotherapy is less likely to cure the patient, such as acute myeloid leukaemia. There is also more than one kind of bone marrow transplant: in an autograft or autologous transplant some of a patient's own bone marrow is removed and then 'cleaned up' and returned to the patient via an intravenous line. The cleaning process involves the removal of any leukaemic or cancer cells in the bone marrow (this is described in

308

detail in Anna's story). The application of this technique to children with cancer means that they can receive high doses of chemotherapy or radiotherapy (or both) which otherwise would irreversibly damage their own bone marrow; treatment can be more intensive if some of their bone marrow can be removed and returned unaffected by the drugs afterwards.

Roland Levinsky was pleased to have Kristie admitted so soon after birth, before repeated infections had weakened her and lessened her chances of coming through the transplant. But the bad news was that Kristie's form of SCID – ADA deficiency – is the most intractable to cure; she lacks a vital enzyme involved in the natural breakdown of substances which form the building blocks of our basic genetic make-up. Because of this missing component, there is an accumulation of other metabolic products which are very toxic to the white blood cells which control the immune system, and consequently she has very few of them. Only once before has the Great Ormond Street team successfully transplanted a child with this most difficult form of SCID with a mismatched donor: can Kristie be the second?

Kristie's greatest hazard will be infection. Just before and after the transplant, the tiny bit of immunity she has of her own and which she may have received from her mother, will be depleted by a pre-conditioning programme of immuno-suppressant drugs. These will make her more likely to accept the transplant. But the same mechanisms are at work in fighting off foreign tissue – now suppressed by these drugs – as in fighting off germs. So at the same time she will be at her most vulnerable to infection until the new marrow starts growing and producing a functional immune system. As arrangements proceeded – before Kristie was even born – for her to come to Great Ormond Street, the hospital therefore prepared every possible precaution. Professor Levinsky arranged for a bubble tent to be placed inside an isolation cubicle on Cohen ward which would reinforce further the child's separation from the impurities of the outside world. Sister Annabelle Dale came into the hospital on her day off, twenty-four hours before the baby's transfer from Liverpool on 12 November, to watch its installation and check that everything was all right.

The 'bubble' is a transparent plastic tent, about ten feet by eight feet, with its own air filtering system. Strict precautions control entry into the bubble. Steve and Debbie will have to put on mask, gown and plastic overshoes before going into the cubicle, then wash their hands before unzipping the door into the bubble which holds just the baby's cot and one nursing chair. Inside Kristie will be cuddled, breastfed and loved as a normal baby would be but she will only know her parents' faces half-hidden by hospital masks. Later, doctors were to say to Debbie that it wasn't necessary for the parents to wear masks constantly, bearing in mind the psychological need for the baby to bond to her parents' faces and, eventually, to begin to vocalize. But Debbie replied that she would rather take every possible precaution and the masks stayed on.

The bubble was paid for, not by the National Health Service and the hospital budget, but by the Great Ormond Street Bone Marrow Research Fund, a charity largely established by parents of earlier transplant patients at the hospital. It was ordered by Professor Levinsky because of the danger from airborne infection caused by aspergillus fungi, whose spores live in building dust. At the time of Kristie's arrival, work was just beginning three floors above Cohen ward to install two Laminar Flow isolation cubicles on Ward 3A. These cubicles, with their moulded plastic furniture, plastic walls and their own filtered air, have a space-age appearance strangely different from the clutter of the rest of the ward. They will be used to isolate and protect transplant patients and are vital at Great Ormond Street where there has been building work associated with the ill-fated Cardiac block* alongside the main hospital for virtually a decade with the prospect of further redevelopment to come in the years ahead.

The Laminar Flow cubicles (also paid for by the Bone Marrow Research Fund) took two years of fund-raising and planning. The dimensions of the existing cubicles were so small that fitting complicated systems within them caused the hospi-

---

*The Cardiac block was finished in 1980 but then found to have such fundamental structural faults that it required an extensive and costly rebuilding programme, due for completion in 1987.

tal works department prolonged headaches. In fact, the two new cubicles occupy the space of three old ones so the gain in quality of nursing care has been achieved at the expense of the quantity of beds in one of the hospital's busiest wards. Kristie could not wait for the cubicles to be completed (which turned out to be in January 1986) and so the bubble was erected to provide a similar, air-filtered environment. Yet useful as it proved, the most important ingredient of Kristie's protection would be the meticulous and experienced care of the nurses.

Cohen ward is used to taking meticulous care over infection. It is formed of two wings on the ground floor of the hospital; one ten-bedded wing looks after neurology and dermatology patients, the other with eight beds has SCID patients and children with infectious diseases. Some of the latter are children with cancer who have to be isolated because they have developed infectious illnesses. Even chickenpox can be fatal to these children whose immunity has been suppressed by chemotherapy drug treatment, so these illnesses have to be isolated quickly.

As many a hospital administrator or consultant will remark, it is the ward sisters who run the hospital and Sister Annabelle Dale, who has been in charge of Cohen since 1980, is the sort of sister whom anxious parents get to know with relief. She was in her mid-twenties when appointed a ward sister and exudes the blend of warmth and authority typical of a Great Ormond Street sister. She will need both on this busy ward, which often cares for seriously ill children and where there are many times of anxiety and tension. Annabelle Dale is responsible for training her team of nurses in infectious precautions and making sure that standards are maintained at all times; it isn't possible for anyone to have an off day when children such as Kristie are so vulnerable. Detailed routines thus have to be observed at all times, such as the rules governing entry to the bubble, its daily cleaning, the restriction of visitors and the twice-daily change of bedlinen — with fresh sheets always taken from the middle of the pile in the cupboard because those on the top will have been in contact with the air. The baby herself must be watched carefully for any small sign of infection, such as a rash or rise in temperature.

All this calls for painstaking nursing on an already emotion-ally demanding ward. Because many patients are long-stay, the staff get to know them and their families very well. 'They care very much about the whole family, not just the condition,' said another Cohen ward mother. It can be very hard for the staff to struggle for a child for a year or more and then lose them. In the last year or so an additional strain has been added to the ward's duties, although the nursing staff does not make a fuss about it: nursing a small number of AIDS patients, mainly babies who have contracted AIDS through blood transfusions. The nursing care for these patients involves strict infectious precautions and, as at present there is no cure, nurses must reluctantly accept that there is little they can do for these chil-dren.

Destined for this highly specialized ward, Steve, Debbie and Kristie arrived by ambulance from Liverpool at three p.m. on Tuesday 12 November. The previous week they had been allowed to take their baby home for a few days so that they would have experienced having Kristie at home, whatever might happen in the future. Family photographs show the two grannies, faces masked, holding the new baby. They were given a great send-off from the street; neighbours had not been allowed into the house to view Kristie, but had come and peered at her through the windows and promised a party to welcome her home when she returned.

Ward staff expected the young couple to be slightly bemused by their arrival. Except for the two brief visits to doctors, neither of them had been to London before. But the nurses were favourably impressed by the couple's attitude and the sensible questions they asked about Kristie's treatment. Steve and Debbie went through the familiar double-take, common to most Great Ormond Street parents on their first visit: they could not believe that this nondescript building was really the world-famous hospital. To Debbie, Cohen ward seemed very big: 'It was just like your first day at a new school,' she says. Jean Simons, the medical team's social worker, was on hand to advise about financial problems and to give the couple an initial payment, later paid back, until their social security book was processed through from Liverpool. She may have expected to act rather more as Steve and Debbie's 'minder' in the first few weeks than proved to be necessary; for such parents, unemployment provides one of its few advantages.

A prolonged hospital stay for a child can cause major problems for a family, as eventually it would for Steve and Debbie. A husband may be at home many miles away caring for other children who are disturbed by the family crisis while his wife, in hospital with the sick child, becomes more and more institutionalized and obsessed by the hospital world, the couple communicating only by telephone calls. A bone marrow transplant, which is life-threatening and in the SCID patients may take months to accomplish, is particularly fraught; the psychological stresses are currently being studied by Carien Pott-Mees, a psychologist based at Westminster Children's Hospital. At least Steve and Debbie had each other's company. At first they were sustained by the drama of the situation, including the euphoria of having a new baby, even though she was so seriously ill. They were enjoying getting to know the hospital and talking to other parents about their children's illness and treatment.

Anne Carlisle, the hospital's accommodation officer, showed them to a small but adequate bedroom, up several flights of stairs in the oldest wing of the hospital. The new parents' sitting room on the fifth floor of the main hospital was an altogether more cheerful prospect and here Steve and Debbie were to spend much of their time in the weeks ahead. The sitting room and kitchen had recently been upgraded and redecorated, along with an adjacent wing of mothers' bedrooms, by Marks and Spencer. After decorating The Sick Children's Trust house for parents nearby, the company asked Anne Carlisle if there was anything else on her 'shopping list'. She took them to see the existing sitting room, a cheerless and badly furnished place, where a television set blared incessantly. Marks and Spencer took on this challenge and the result was a newly-carpeted and curtained room in warm reds and browns, with well-planned new seating which seemed to invite conversational groups to form. They had come up with all kinds of extras, too: plants, soft lighting, books and linen. By refurnishing the bedrooms with bunk beds, they had also gained space for five more mothers. 'They did everything I asked and more,' says a gratified Anne Carlisle. The room now offers physical comfort to the many parents who sit there while their children undergo surgery or intensive care. Instead of television, conversation could develop over a cup of tea or coffee with other parents linked by the common bond of shared experiences. Soon Steve and Debbie would be the veterans of the parents' sitting room who would encourage others to relax and chat. Three weeks later Steve was to sit all night with another parent who was on her own in hospital as her son approached death on ward 5A.

Anne Carlisle, a former nurse who still retains a strong Northern Irish accent, is deeply sympathetic to parents but she has an unenviable job. Yet it is an important one. In the 1950s the pioneering work of James Robertson showed the serious adverse effects on children in hospital deprived of their mothers: they became withdrawn, angry and developmentally delayed. This was followed by the campaigning of the National Association for the Welfare of Children in Hospital (NAWCH) to establish the principle that children in hospital ought to have their mothers with them as much as possible. Therefore basic overnight accommodation has to be available — yet it is always limited. In a tertiary referral hospital such as Great Ormond Street, where patients have mostly been referred from their local hospitals, many parents will have travelled sufficient distances to make getting home overnight impossible. In Great Ormond Street, too, there are a high proportion of seriously ill children whose parents will want to be readily available overnight and who are passing through a crisis in their lives when the family ought to be together. But the hospital was built in a very different age – the 1930s. Wards display signs saying 'Parents welcome at all times' but when they are full they are not large enough to contain easily even the daytime presence of parents and friends.

In principle, the hospital now gives access to all parents without being able to offer accommodation to everyone who wants it at all times. A typical ward, when busy, might have a mother sleeping in a cubicle built onto a balcony adjoining the ward, a couple of mothers sleeping on fold-up beds in the ward waiting room or playroom, and others sleeping in hospital accommodation which, in the main hospital, is mostly small rooms with bunks to give maximum use. (The beds in cubicles are popular but limited; the building programme had to be halted when it was found that the balconies could not support the extra weight.) Anne Carlisle will also arrange hotel accommodation in nearby Bloomsbury and with families who put up parents on a bed and breakfast basis for a small charge. And the Sick Children's Trust has acquired a second house which it plans to renovate for parents (and families) to stay.

Steve and Debbie's small room became their base for what everyone knew would be a long stay of weeks, possibly months. On the Monday following their arrival they met Dr Hilary Blacklock, the haematology consultant in charge of the bone marrow transplant programme. She repeated the explanation about how blood tests would enable the doctors to find out which of them would be the more compatible donor for the transplant. If these tissue-typing tests showed that both were equally compatible, other factors, such as the absence of viruses, which could be transmitted to Kristie, would decide the issue. If it were Steve, he would be urged to give up smoking and either way, the donor would have a chest X-ray, heart and blood tests to check that they were in good general health. 'We are very careful about our donors and do more tests on them than a patient normally undergoes to be absolutely certain that they are fit to have an anaesthetic – because although the harvest is vital to their sick child, it is not necessary for their own health,' says Dr Blacklock. It would be a few days before Steve and Debbie would know which one it would be; each was fully prepared to be the donor, though Debbie felt that, as Mum, she had a particular right.

Hilary Blacklock also went through the details of how the marrow would be 'harvested', as the process of removing the marrow is known. Great Ormond Street is not suitable for adult patients so an arrangement has been made with a neurology consultant to 'borrow' one of his beds at the National Hospital for Nervous Diseases in Queen's Square, just round the corner from Great Ormond Street. The donor would be admitted to the National Hospital the night before the harvest was due; there would be nothing to eat from midnight and the donor would be visited by an anaesthetist to check that there were no lung or other complications. In the morning the donor would be prepared for theatre where the harvest would be performed by Dr Blacklock, assisted by a registrar. The marrow would be taken mainly from the hip bones in the pelvis and, if necessary, from the sternum or breastbone. It would be extracted by penetrating the bone with a needle and drawing up the liquid marrow through a syringe. Afterwards the donor would feel bruised, but should be back to normal in a day or so. Only about one per cent of the donor's own marrow is taken, and this quickly grows again so that no deficiency is caused in the donor.

While they waited for the tests to identify the most compatible donor, Steve and Debbie got to know Cohen ward and settled into a routine. This included giving almost all of the baby's feeds and doing most of her care. Debbie continued to breast-feed and began to express breast milk which could be given by bottle. The night-time feeds were usually given by Steve who took considerable pride in being able to get 100 or even 150 millilitres into the baby. After a week or so Sister Dale commented that the bubble had not given her as many nursing problems as she had anticipated – or none that they had not been able to overcome, such as taking an X-ray through the walls of the bubble. Space was very tight since the cubicle was barely four metres long by little more than two metres wide; but this was not such a severe problem with a cot as it would have been with an older patient. Conditions certainly were not ideal for cosy breast-feeding and it occasionally annoyed Debbie that visitors would peer through the windows. However, she successfully kept the supply going.

Other personalities on Cohen gradually became familiar to them, among them Dr Parvis Habibi, the registrar. He had cared for a number of transplant families on the ward and he gave Steve and Debbie a practical tip: make sure you get enough time out of the hospital, play with Kristie when she is awake, but when she is asleep, get away and do something different. Another member of the close-knit and informal ward team is Helen Gascoine, the playleader. She spends her time

mainly with the older children on the ward, believing it important to offer them opportunities 'to express the aggression they
must feel at being stuck in this awful situation'. And so there is
rough and tumble play, punching clay or bashing a punch bag.
There is also 'hospital play' which involves medical procedures
such as giving Teddy injections or bandages. 'I don't like to be
seen as just the play lady, the Goody Two Shoes, who does the
nice things,' says Helen. She likes to work with the doctors, for
example holding a child when a blood test is done. After a few
days Steve, too, was helping the doctors when Kristie was
having a blood transfusion, by holding the line when it was
being clamped.

Nine days after Kristie arrived on Cohen her plastic bubble
became the location for an unusual, perhaps even unique,
event – her christening. Derek Bacon, the hospital chaplain,
performs many christenings in Great Ormond Street, sometimes when a child is very ill; if there is not enough time to
summon him (although he carries a bleep six days a week), a
ward sister will sometimes say the words of baptism over a
baby. In Kristie's case, the ritual had to circumvent – but not
undermine – the strict infectious precautions surrounding the
baby.

When the chaplain arrived to christen the baby on a late
November afternoon, Annabelle Dale had ready sterile water
and a sterile container plus a canister of antiseptic spray. Derek
Bacon brought with him candles, flowers, fresh linen and a
silver cross. Outside the cubicle, Sister Dale sprayed the cross
and two pink roses with the antiseptic before they were taken
into the bubble. Kristie wore a new frilled christening gown,
bought by her godmother – the godparents were fellow Great
Ormond Street parents. Gowned and masked, the chaplain was
allowed the rare privilege of entry into the bubble with Steve
and Debbie; here he conducted the service with a congregation
of nurses and other parents clustered together in the corridor,
listening through the intercom. It was a relaxed and happy
occasion, although the precarious situation of the baby was in
everyone's minds. Afterwards Steve and Debbie gave everyone
wine and sandwiches in the parents' sitting room upstairs.

On the day of the christening Debbie and Steve were told

that Debbie would be the donor. Kristie herself had already been to theatre to have a Hickman Catheter* inserted, for blood transfusions and for her to receive the marrow. The tissue-typing tests had also thrown up a bonus. Both Steve and Debbie had been reasonable matches for Kristie, with Debbie slightly better. And part of the genetic inheritance which Kristie had from Steve was similar to part of Debbie's genetic make-up. This meant that the match between mother and daughter was closer than could have been expected. The good news added to Steve and Debbie's optimism.

The date for the bone marrow harvest was set for Monday 2 December. By then Kristie would have been in her bubble for virtually three weeks. In the week before the harvest, Kristie began her programme of immuno-suppressant drug conditioning; this was vital in preparing her to accept bone marrow from a donor who, despite the similarities, was still a mismatch. Her programme was worked out very carefully. The chances of a graft taking are higher the more a patient is pre-conditioned; but these drugs make her even more likely to be overwhelmed by infection, so the doctors have a difficult balancing act to maintain. Too little may result in rejection, too much and the patient may die from the treatment or an infection. The drugs which kill off the cells which will reject the graft may also damage normal cells and can make the patient very ill. Even though the doctors have a range of sophisticated drugs which are targeted to select certain features and be less harmful to other cells, and even though they can also reduce the drug dosage by using 'monoclonal' antibodies which are very specific and not toxic, the treatment may still have consequences. Because Kristie was so young and because her likely resistance to the graft was known to be very low as a result of her type of SCID she was given a mild programme of pre-conditioning. And she remained well while it was being given.

On the evening of 1 December Debbie reported, as arranged, to the National Hospital, feeling a certain amount of butterflies. Early the next morning Hilary Blacklock walked along the basement passage connecting the two hospitals,

---

*See pages 93-4 for description of this procedure.

carrying a tray of surgical implements. Inside the theatre, Sarah Johnson, the haematology sister, prepared a trolley of equipment which included a filtering system for the collected marrow. The marrow was aspirated (or extracted) from many different sites in Debbie's hip bones and sternum, averaging about four to five millilitres each time. Anti-coagulant was added to the marrow to avoid it clotting and the resulting mixture – which looked like blood, although somewhat thicker – was passed through the filter to remove bits of fat and clumps of cells. The harvest went normally; indeed, Debbie proved to be an ideal subject so that a large quantity of marrow was able to be taken.

Immediately after the harvest, as Debbie slept on in the recovery room near the operating theatre, Dr Blacklock's registrar took the marrow to the Institute of Child Health and gave it to Dr Gareth Morgan, an important member of Professor Levinsky's research team. Under his supervision the bone marrow that had been collected from Debbie was first spun very fast in a centrifuge to separate the marrow (which has a different weight) from blood plasma and red blood cells. These two layers were discarded and the marrow was washed with a special solution and spun again so that everything would be eliminated but the bone marrow cells.

The next step was to kill off the T-lymphocytes, the white blood cells in Debbie's bone marrow which would recognize the baby as foreign tissue and react against her. This could cause 'Graft Versus Host Disease' in the baby, a serious hazard in transplantation; it can involve catastrophic damage to the skin, intestine and liver. This T-cell depletion, as it is known, uses monoclonal antibodies – synthetic antibodies which are targeted specifically against T-cells. The monoclonal antibodies, mixed in a solution with the bone marrow, coat the T-cells and a reaction is set off which destroys the T-cells. Only the bone marrow cells, carrying the stem cells which will develop into white blood cells, are left.

The technique of T-cell depletion, and the experience doctors now have in using it, are what have made the successful mismatched transplants possible. Finally, the bone marrow, now greatly reduced in volume, was washed and spun again to get rid of excess antibody and dead cells and checked to see if all the T-cells were gone; this was satisfactory and it was carried back to the hospital. That same evening, about fifty millilitres were transfused, via her Hickman line, into Kristie. It would find its own way into her bone marrow.

By about one p.m. that day Debbie had come round from the anaesthetic. 'It wasn't as bad as I expected. The National Hospital was very nice, but I missed the baby being over there. It was painful but in the evening I got up and started to walk. Jean Simons (the social worker) popped over to see us. Then about midnight Steve phoned up to see how Kristie was and found out that she had had a reaction from the transfusion. I was a bit worried, and wanted to get back to Great Ormond Street, so they wheeled me back in a wheel-chair.

'Kristie didn't look too well. She was a funny colour and she choked on her feed. There was a little blood in her urine at first. I was upset, had a bit of a cry. I went upstairs and sat in the parents' waiting room on my own. But the next morning when I got there she looked better and fed beautifully.' Gareth Morgan reassured Debbie and Steve about the blood in the urine and said the doctors were watching it, but that there was nothing to worry about.

Everyone knew that it would be weeks before any significant signs of a 'take' appeared. Kristie was watched closely but showed no symptoms of Graft Versus Host Disease. In the couple of weeks that were left before Christmas, her parents' confidence was kept high. Debbie visited Oxford Street and shopped in street markets, often buying a toy or a dress for the baby. As Christmas approached Steve put up the Christmas tree and decorations in the parents' sitting room; Anne Carlisle thanked him but Helen, Cohen's playleader, complained that her stores of green foil had been raided. They joined the audience for the hospital's Christmas show, an uninhibited affair produced by some of the sisters and junior doctors but also featuring many of the consultants who give bravura performances, forgetting dignity and status. Some were almost unidentifiable beneath their bizarre costumes, but Roland Levinsky (whom Steve and Debbie had already come to know as a friendly and helpful person despite his intimidating intellect) was unmistakable. Sister Annabelle Dale, too, had literally let her hair down for the night.

By Christmas the results of Kristie's daily blood tests looked increasingly promising. Immediately after a bone marrow transplant, the 'count' of white cells in a blood sample falls – perhaps to zero – because of the drug treatment which is wiping out the little bit of immunity the patient has. Blood contains different types of cells and the first signs of the marrow engrafting would be these blood cell lines growing in the daily counts produced by analysis of Kristie's blood in the haematology laboratory. Kristie's blood counts began to show this happening. At first the haemoglobin (or red blood cells) was low, but this was the first to increase. The next cell line to recover was that of her platelets, a type of cell which helps blood to clot. The crucial white blood cell line was slower to grow, but did show signs of recovery as the count came up to 0.5 and 0.9 and then to 1.2. Steve copied out the results of the blood tests each day to keep with his photographs of the baby; he and Debbie were thrilled that the first signs looked so good.

The doctors, though they never committed themselves totally, said that it was encouraging. Also significant, although not conclusive, was a test which showed a high proportion of T-cells in Kristie's blood; this was very suggestive, as they knew she had so few T-cells of her own. From a research point of view, they were longing to bring off what would be only their second successful mismatched transplant on a child with the same form of SCID as Kristie. Other research teams all over the world had had the same problem with this notoriously difficult form of SCID. Four weeks after the transplant, in the early part of the New Year, Kristie's blood was sent for a more elaborate, tissue-typing test to see if cells which were Debbie's could be identified; this would provide final proof that the transplant had taken.

Steve decided to go home to Liverpool over the New Year, feeling so happy that he wanted to tell everyone the good news. Though he went home with only £7 in his pocket, he bought a bottle of whisky and raffled it in his local pub, bringing back £30 for the Bone Marrow Research Fund. (Later he organized a sponsored darts marathon which raised a great deal more.)

Irresistibly, the thoughts of Steve and Debbie flew to Kristie being allowed out of the bubble, even to taking her home. By now they had accumulated such a lot of soft toys, presents and clothes for her that it was going to be a problem getting it all back to Liverpool.

The results of the blood test to see if the baby had any maternal cells were due in the first week of January. Steve and Debbie waited on edge for what they hoped would be confirmation that the transplant had really taken. Four days earlier, Steve had fallen down a staircase and bruised his foot in his haste to get to the ward to hear what was said during Professor Levinsky's ward round. At all times the doctors kept the couple fully informed of what was happening, even though it often meant long explanations. But now they entered a phase when the doctors would be imparting less encouraging news.

The tissue-typing blood test to see if Kristie had any of Debbie's cells proved negative. The doctors were disappointed, yet still felt that it was possible that a graft had taken place but was still very immature. This test was later repeated but the results were either equivocal or negative. The doctors stressed that time was important: they must wait. Then Kristie's white cell and platelet counts began to fall, then go up again; from now on, the counts would circle up and down at a low level. Periodically she had diarrhoea and did not feed well; her feeds were changed in an effort to find something she could absorb.

The transplant had been performed at the beginning of December. January and February, as the outcome began to look more uncertain, developed into a tense period for Kristie's young parents. When the white blood-count was low, they waited anxiously for it to come up. Friction developed between them and after a row Steve would go back to Liverpool for a few days. At times they were able to accept the situation, at other times the frustration and the feeling of being cut off from normal life became too much. Debbie especially did not understand the complexities of the condition. They had no experience, as the doctors and nurses had, of the length of time it usually takes to accomplish a successful mismatched transplant. Appalling ordeal as it would be for any parents, Steve and Debbie had extra problems: they were very young, they were not married or employed and they had already lost one child through this dreadful illness.

Though, essentially, they had a good relationship with the ward, the tension occasionally broke out into arguments here, too – especially when Kristie was unwell. Once Debbie threatened to discharge Kristie because she didn't understand why the doctors didn't do something when they seemed to know that the graft had not taken. 'They are very frustrated. They have patiently waited all this time and now, it seems, the graft hasn't taken,' said Dr Parvis Habibi, the ward's registrar. 'It may seem clear to the lay person, but they don't understand the details, they only see the simple black and white features.' The explosions were over quickly, however. Steve and Debbie are people who keep their feelings out in the open and the doctors understood why the couple became emotional.

By March Steve and Debbie were somewhat reconciled – both to each other and to the situation, which had not changed. It remained a waiting game. The doctors knew that these low levels could still be the prologue to an engraftment. They repeated that it was necessary to wait to establish for certain that the transplant had taken, but they began to suggest that a second transplant was on the cards. Because Kristie still had diarrhoea, which showed she was not absorbing her feeds properly, she was put on a course of Total Parenteral Nutrition, an intravenous pharmaceutical 'feed' which would ensure that she didn't lose weight. The diarrhoea was typical of a SCID child, because chronic low-grade infection slightly damages the gut. However, she remained – for a SCID baby – very healthy and if she were to undergo a second transplant she needed to be as strong as possible.

Kristie had developed from the tiny three-week-old baby whom the ambulance had brought down from Liverpool into a happy five-month-old. When she was well she enjoyed her feeds and Steve and Debbie had always spent so much time with her inside the bubble that she was very responsive. She was quick to smile and play. She would play with her activity centre and gaze at her teddies; she rarely cried. But she had never been part of life in a family home, never been taken for a walk outside. An immaculate pram waited unused in the small house in Wallasey, where her grannies and aunts had to make do with photographs. Visitors who wished Kristie well could only get an obscure view of her through the glass wall of the corridor and the plastic wall of the bubble. Kristie was underweight for her age and, as she grew older, the confinement and lack of stimulation would pose a serious problem. But there was never any doubt of her parents' commitment to her, either in the amount of loving care they gave her every day or in the intensity of their anxiety.

Debbie prayed frequently in the hospital chapel where an intercessions book is placed for parents to record their feelings. Her prayers had gone from 'Dear Lord, please help my darling baby daughter to accept her transplant. I love her so much, please let me keep her for ever' to 'Please, please, help Kristie to make her white cells, don't let the heartache start again'. As hope of the transplant faded, the prayers ranged from the desperate 'Please, Lord, I can't pray any harder' to the simple 'Lord, please look after Kristie tonight and for ever'.

At the Institute the doctors reviewed the scientific position and took the decision to re-transplant. 'I think the graft actually did take initially and then it was gradually rejected,' says Professor Levinsky. 'Because we didn't give enough drugs to wipe out her immunity, it came back before the graft had been fully established, then it took over and wiped out the graft. We had also been giving her blood transfusions to clear the toxic products which are the result of her enzyme deficiency. By doing that we also restored a little immunity. These immuno-suppressant drugs are highly toxic and we were very anxious not to give too much. It is a balancing act and this time we just didn't get it right. For the second transplant we are going to increase the pre-conditioning.'

Kristie's treatment has been very new and experimental. 'Four years ago the SCID children without a matched donor all died, but now with T-cell depletion and the mismatched transplants, we are getting fifty to sixty per cent cures overall, with Kristie's group remaining the most difficult. We never dreamt that we would be this successful. In the beginning I used to say to parents that the treatment was at a trial stage; it might work for their child, but if it didn't at least they were probably helping future children. Well, some of those children unfortunately did die and they did help the future, but others came through it and are very well.'

Groups like Professor Levinsky's team are at the forefront of research in evolving new procedures which very rapidly become routine treatment. He says: 'What we have in the back of our minds as eventual treatment is replacing the defective gene, which sounds still in the realms of science fiction, but is probably only five or ten years off. We already have the theoretical knowledge for doing it, but we need to perfect it in the laboratory. It will also require ethical approval.' (New treatments have to be approved by the hospital's ethical committee which includes lay as well as medical representatives; the committee has to be satisfied that a proposed treatment offers sufficient benefits to justify any additional risks or burdens it places upon the patient. SCID research led the way in perfecting the mismatch techniques experimentally because for SCID children there was no alternative treatment.)

Although SCID is a rare disease, it is possible that many children who die from obscure causes have various forms of immuno-deficiency. The research at Great Ormond Street also benefits leukaemia patients so that a lot of Professor Levinsky's support comes from the Leukaemia Research Fund because the Fund recognizes how the two fields are interrelated. In a world context, the number of Nobel prizes that have been won in the field of immunology in the past decade or so reflects the importance of this kind of research to humanity.

Professor Levinsky's team is heavily financed by the Bone Marrow Research Fund and this, allied to the support it receives from the Leukaemia Research Fund and the Lee Smith Research Foundation, shows how dependent this pioneering work is on private funding. Professor Levinsky estimates that he spends a third of his time soliciting money for research. He would like to see more Sick Children's Trust houses for parents as well as more research staff and technicians. 'The facilities are appalling. It's amazing that we do any decent medicine or keep sane and smiling,' he says. 'It is also emotionally destructive working in this field. One year when we lost a number of children I just wanted to quit, but another family turns up and you go on. You have to be an optimist.'

It takes a special kind of doctor to carry on this pioneering work but their determination is fuelled by the knowledge of what has already been achieved. The disease is invariably fatal without a successful transplant. 'The successes we have achieved are real numbers, not the isolated case. And from our progress it extends to different hospitals around England and the world, and so it's worth it,' says Roland Levinsky. For Steve and Debbie, it is impossible not to go on, too. Whatever it takes, they will be there. Although they have seen the worst happen to other parents – many of whom they had got to know well – during their time at Great Ormond Street, they can hardly imagine it happening to them. 'But if it takes months and months and then she is better, it will be worth it in the end,' says Steve. And if not for Kristie, it will be worth it for other children in the future, for whom Great Ormond Street is giving the chance of life.

Postscript: one year later

She had her second bone marrow transplant when she was six months old. This time it was successful and her recovery was straightforward. After one short trip home, she returned to Merseyside in time for her first birthday which she marked by appearing on breakfast television. By then she was walking, eating normally and free of infection. Despite inevitable anxiety when Kristie catches a cold, she and her young parents have had a happy year.

6.30 p.m. *Parents or relatives who have been working call in on their way home. Otherwise, as the evening draws in, the hospital begins to empty. If they are lucky, and there are no particular crises, doctors will be handing over their wards to the registrars and housemen who will remain on call through the night. These doctors on the night rota could also be lucky and have a quiet night; but they must be prepared to be up for much of the night, if necessary, and then work through the next day without sleep. Downstairs, a film show begins for children (and parents) in a basement lecture theatre. This fortnightly treat is provided free – by the father of a previous patient – and is followed two hours later by a film intended for adults, staff as well as parents. Apart from these films (and television) any entertainment has to be provided by the parents or nurses since by now the playleaders have finished for the day. Supper will have been eaten by five o'clock and many younger children are being prepared for bed. In the front entrance hall queues form for the telephones as parents wait with pocketfuls of change to send progress reports home.*

7.15 p.m. *It's 'Kids and Us' . . . one of the regular programmes put out by Radio GOSH, the hospital's own radio station, broadcasting from its eighth-floor eyrie at the top of the building. The station has been broadcasting on average eleven hours a week since 1981. It's run by the Maccabi Association London, a large youth-oriented Jewish sports and social group in Camden. 'Kids and Us' features interviews with three patients who talk about themselves and their favourite music. Sometimes the children go to the studio (a former laboratory) but if necessary one of the volunteers who run the station records the interview in the ward. In all about thirty people help Radio GOSH at the hospital. Some are professionally involved in the music business, radio or television but for many it's a rewarding hobby that offers something different from their working life. The DJ tonight, for instance, is Howard Robinson, a university student from Queen Mary's College, London, while the engineer is Serina Torz, a clerical assistant in the Foreign Office. Programmes are a mixture of record requests, story reading and magazine items which are sometimes produced in conjunction with the hospital school. Older students have just been rehearsing their own play – Charlie and the Chocolate*

Factory – for transmission on the air. The costs of Radio GOSH are met through a combination of individual donations and fund-raising stunts such as broadcasting marathons and celebrity sports matches. And not every radio station can boast Paul McCartney, Paul Daniels, Lulu and Chas and Dave among their regular contributors: all have recorded special messages of good wishes to the station which broadcasts one evening a week and all day Sunday.

8.45 p.m. *The night nursing staff arrive. Only 1A, the intensive cardiac ward, and ward 5A, the general paediatric intensive care ward, will have a sister in charge tonight. Elsewhere it will be a staff nurse. Staff shortages and sickness can cause problems finding people with the appropriate experience to run wards at night. Some of the gaps are filled by agency staff who are mustering in a waiting room at the nursing office. They are allocated to wards by the night nursing officer and two night sisters who are on duty. As they do so, wards report how many children they have, how many need special nursing and whether their staff have turned up. For the next hour the nursing officer will juggle her staff, moving nurses and auxiliaries from ward to ward to provide nursing cover where it is most needed.*

9.30 p.m. *The night cleaning staff arrive for the operating theatres. There is also a night nursing staff for the theatres to cover emergency operations. Any emergencies will be handled in either the first or sixth-floor theatres. If it's quiet, they will do some stock-taking and re-ordering, as necessary, to replenish the supplies of drugs, gowns and other equipment used in theatres. They will also clear up anything left behind from the evening and prepare the instruments for sterilization for the first operations on tomorrow's list. Meanwhile the cleaners work their way through the theatre suites, also getting them ready for the morning.*

10.00 p.m. *Gillian Bosworth, the senior night nursing officer, now knows the worst: as a result of staff sickness she is twelve nurses short for the night. There are 221 children in the hospital of whom thirty are being 'specialled' on a one-to-one basis by nurses. Two wards lack staff nurses but former Great Ormond Street nurses among the agency staff have been put in charge. Ward 1A is particularly busy and Miss Bosworth moves someone in from 1C.*

It's not simply a question of numbers; she must ensure that wards have sufficient trained staff to administer intravenous drugs. There must also be sufficient people to allow staff meal breaks during their eleven-hour shift. When the juggling has been completed, Miss Bosworth and the two night sisters tour the hospital. Each has certain wards for which they are responsible, although Gillian Bosworth tries to visit all wards at least once. Many wards are very quiet with the lights dimmed and the children asleep. On others, where the patients are older or sicker, there is more activity. Ward 6A, the neonatal surgical ward, is ablaze with light and preparing for the arrival of an emergency admission. Ward 3AB, the oncology and leukaemia ward, still has parents sitting alongside their children or chatting to each other in the kitchen and playroom. A few teenage children are watching television. But generally it is a peaceful scene with fewer people around than by day and less crying as sleep stifles the tears. Even children hooked up to intravenous lines can look tranquil when asleep. Many are wearing their own pyjamas and sleeping under colourful, hand-made blankets; for once this is not an economy measure, but intended to make the children feel more at home, more relaxed.

10.30 p.m. *The first of two emergency admissions arrives – a three-day-old baby for ward 6A suffering from a suspected intestinal blockage. She is immediately surrounded by doctors and nurses. Her condition does not appear to be too critical but a number of tests are initiated. The duty radiographer wheels her portable X-ray machine to the ward and samples of blood are taken for laboratory analysis. Two floors below, on the general surgical ward of 4AB, a much larger patient is being admitted: a fifteen-year-old boy so tall that his legs would dangle over the end of the bed if he did not curl them up. He has a suspected blocked shunt (a device to drain excess fluid from the brain) which is causing bad headaches and disorientation. He has been treated at Great Ormond Street in the past but had theoretically been transferred to the nearby National Hospital for Nervous Diseases. He's come to Great Ormond Street by mistake but ward 4AB will look after him for the night. He, too, will have various tests including an X-ray and he's destined for a more unsettled night than the baby on 6A. Two emergency admissions during the night are by no* *means unusual. A trolley plus emergency medicine box are kept by the main entrance all night, just in case. Over twenty-four hours around ten children are usually admitted as 'emergencies'. Miss Bosworth hopes there will be no more than two tonight. The signs are up on the wards saying the hospital is on 'restricted admissions'; this applies primarily for patients requiring intensive care because there are not enough nursing staff currently available during the day. The hospital doesn't have a casualty department but some children are still brought there directly by their parents. 'We always see them. We don't turn them away,' says Miss Bosworth.*

11.00 p.m. *Errol Henry, the night telephonist, starts his nine-hour shift. It can be a lonely vigil with few calls after midnight until six a.m. when parents start to phone to inquire about their children's condition and staff start to call to say that they're sick. There is a bank of alarms alongside him – burglar alarm, fire alarms and refrigerator alarms for blood banks. An important duty might be to alert medical staff if there is a cardiac arrest. One special phone only rings if any child has a cardiac arrest; if it rings the telephonist must summon the duty anaesthetist and the appropriate doctors plus the nursing officer. Sometimes you can get five arrests in a week, at other times you can go for weeks without one. Every day, though, at 9 a.m. the procedures and lines are tested, just in case. Nine o'clock is also the start of the busiest period for the antiquated switchboard. It handles 50,000 incoming and outgoing calls a week – excluding 55,000 internal calls dialled directly. A new electronic switchboard should make life easier but it will not solve the underlying problem of low pay which causes staff shortages; staff can get £20 a week more working on the switchboards of neighbouring hotels than in the hospital.*

11.15 p.m. *A mother makes her way through a dank and dingy corridor to the old hospital building. She shares one of the parent's rooms here but before climbing the stairs pauses to visit the chapel. The chapel is always open and many parents pray here last thing at night. Some also write down their thoughts and prayer in the intercessions book. Some are simple: 'Please look after (our daughter) in this difficult time.' Some are thanks: 'We thank you for (our*

330

son's) life and all the help you have given him and us over the past weeks and we ask you for your continued blessing.' Some are desperate: 'Please, please make my baby better. Don't let the heartache start all over again.' Some are almost angry: 'Please rid her body of this evil disease.' Some come after their child has died: 'Dear Lord, I come to you at this sad time and pray that you will be with all the staff that gave (our son) all the love and care they did. Thank you that you took him without any pain. I know that he's gone to be with you in a much better place and that you will be with all my family. It's such a sad time. Take care of us and take care of him. I don't feel bitter because I know he's in a better place without any pain.'

12.35 a.m. *A ten-year-old girl walks down from 3AB to have a chest X-ray accompanied by a staff nurse and her mother. She's suffering from asthma and feeling breathless. She has had a nebulizer to ease the difficulty in breathing but the doctor wants a precautionary X-ray taken. Two registrars are in overall charge as Resident Assistant Surgeon and Resident Assistant Physician, but housemen will be handling the more routine calls. On-call doctors (including an anaesthetist) are given rooms in the hospital where they can sleep, if they're lucky. They won't finish until five p.m. today – thirty-three hours after starting their shift – but it's even worse at weekends. Then the housemen are on duty or on call from eight a.m. Saturday until five p.m. Monday.*

1.30 a.m. *The canteen is running out of hot suppers for the night staff. It usually serves about forty meals during the night but after two o'clock, sometimes a little earlier, it offers only tea, coffee and snacks. The canteen closes at five o'clock.*

2.00 a.m. *In the biochemistry lab, a technician is finishing the last of her tests – or so she hopes. They are routine blood and urine tests for the baby admitted to 6A earlier in the night. Unless other tests are ordered, she will then go to sleep in a room provided in the nurses' home. The haematology lab also has a technician on call throughout the night and other labs have staff who can be called in from home if required. But in areas such as microbiology and virology the tests tend to take too long to produce quick results and therefore do not warrant overnight manning.*

2.15 a.m. *A cardiac arrest on 1A. Each ward has its emergency
kit for coping with an arrest but 1A, the cardiac ward, is naturally
one of the best equipped to handle such an emergency. It doesn't
always activate the standard procedures involved by dialling 555.
When it does so, the telephonist summons the anaesthetist, either
the surgeons or physicians (depending upon whose patient it is on
1A) and the nursing officer via a special bleep number. A minute
or two later the telephonist checks to see that they've all arrived,
just in case their bleeps aren't working. Initially the medical staff
will try to get the heart working by external massage and by ensuring the patient has a clear airway. Oxygen is almost always given
and frequently the children have to be intubated. Drugs can also
help the action of the heart, so intravenous lines must be established. This child recovers and stays on 1A; if it had happened on
less-intensive wards, he could have been moved to 1A or 5A where
the specialist equipment and nursing is concentrated. As soon as
possible, it's time to contact the parents. If they are not staying in
the hospital, the night nursing officer may have to contact the
police to deliver the news. 'You have to be very careful what the
police tell them because it's going to be a terrible shock for any
parent,' says Miss Bosworth.*

2.45 a.m. *Gillian Bosworth is called in by a nurse to perform an
intravenous drug injection for which one ward's staff lacks a
sufficiently-qualified nurse. She finds that the doctors have not
written up the prescription properly; she doesn't know how much
to give. The doctor will have to be woken up to rewrite the
prescription before the drug can be given.*

3.40 a.m. *A sixteen-year old boy sits up reading on ward 4B. He
can't sleep or get comfortable. The night sister pops in to see if he's
all right but as he is causing no problems, he's left alone. Night
staff don't like children to spend too long awake because it leaves
them tired for whatever lies in store during the day.*

4.00 a.m. *Clarissa Mossop, the duty physiotherapist, is having a
busy night. Usually they try to let children sleep from midnight
unless their condition would deteriorate without treatment and the
physio can get some sleep. But tonight she has been giving chest*

physio to a baby on 6A every two hours and there have also been calls to 1A and 4AB. Chest physio helps children to clear secretions and keeps their airway clear. She once got as far as preparing for bed, then the bleep summoned her back to duty and now she's abandoned any thought of sleep during the night.

4.30 a.m. *The fifteen-year-old emergency admission to 4AB is becoming increasingly agitated and restless. Guy Adam, the resident assistant surgeon, has been to see him and has called in doctors from the National Hospital. They are not too worried and say they will make the necessary arrangements to transfer him later today. Mr Adam has been busier during the night than his non-surgical counterpart, Dr Sally Mitton. He has also had to check the baby admitted to 6A (who was now stable) and an eleven-month-old girl on 5A who was recovering from a major stomach operation. The nurse looking after the girl on 5A had become concerned by her peripheral circulation and her poor urine output. They always take a nurse's concern seriously, but there was particular reason to do so on this occasion: the nurse was a ward sister from 4AB doing a spot of agency work during her week's 'holiday'.*

5.30 a.m. *The porters unlock the main front door ready for a new day. It's been locked since midnight, more to keep out potential dossers than errant boyfriends seeking the nurses' home. One of the three night porters has stayed at the door to let in parents or doctors called in from home. It's been a quiet night with no emergencies after midnight. Night duty is always unpredictable. Sometimes ambulances have to be summoned to take people away from the hospital; parents, for instance, can get ill or even go into labour. A nursing officer answering her bleep may find it's about anything from a leaking lavatory to a child whose condition is suddenly worsening. A child may die and the cries of the parents will echo round the stillness of the hospital. But not during this night: 223 children, including the two overnight admissions, are awakening to face the challenges of another day. For some there will be tears, for others triumph; for all of them, thanks to this most famous of children's hospitals, there will be hope.*

APPENDIX ONE: What people are paid

Salaries in hospitals are immensely complicated. They will vary according to seniority, overtime, night shifts, weekend work, standby allowances and other more specialist factors. However, the list below indicates the basic annual salary ranges of some hospital posts at Great Ormond Street (including, where applicable, London weighting) as at 31 March 1986.

Grade	Basic £	Including night duty and weekend duty £
Senior nurse, grade 8 (clinical nursing officer)	9537–11,337	10,572–12,372
Ward sister, grade 1	9537–11,337	10,363–11,972
Ward sister, grade 2	8357–10,877	8992–11,703
Staff nurse	6877– 8052	7477– 8748
State-enrolled nurse	6147– 7377	6813– 8179
Student nurse: 3rd year	5457	6177
2nd year	5152	5872
1st year	4966	5697
Nursing auxiliary	4827– 5997	5403– 6673
Consultant (plus possible distinction awards)	22,337–28,577	
Senior registrar	13,257–16,507	18,182–21,432*
Senior house officers	10,357–11,637	14,845–16,125*
Porter — Senior	5567	
Basic	5043	
Telephonist	5528–5739	
Cook	5316–5669	
Canteen assistant	4773–5316	
Cleaner	4773–5316	
Radiographer: Basic	7333–8583	8659–9909*
Superintendent	13,358–14,618	

Pharmacist: Basic	8147–9968	
Grade 5	19,243–20,983	
Physiotherapist: Basic	7333–8583	7845–9095*
Superintendent I	13,358–14,618	14,108–15,368†
Playleader	5507–5997	
Laboratory technicians:		
Junior 'A' MLSO	4436–6212	
Principal MLSO	14,576–16,588	

* *including standby or on-call assistance (not night or weekend payments)*
† *including training allowance*

APPENDIX TWO:
How to donate money to Great Ormond Street

As *Children First and Always* has revealed, the Hospital for Sick Children relies on private donations to pay for many projects, services and equipment which cannot be provided from its National Health Service budget. Money donated to the hospital is kept separate from day-to-day running and Special Trustees decide how contributions should be spent. Many people like to donate money to support particular aspects of the hospital's work and information about specific needs can be obtained from Robert Pike, the appeals co-ordinator, whose address is given below. But the Trustees are always grateful for general donations, not earmarked for particular purposes, which can be spent on unforeseen needs, research or large-scale enterprises such as a new whole-body scanner costing £400,000. Robert Pike says: 'We can assure everyone that every donation, however small, will always be spent in the best possible way for the benefit of our young patients. The treasurer will be pleased to provide details of other methods of payment such by deed of covenant or by legacy. Or if anyone would like more information about the work and needs of the hospital, they should contact me.'

Robert Pike
Appeals Co-ordinator
49 Great Ormond Street
London WC1N 3HZ
Telephone: 01-430 0784